Functional Neurosurgery: The Essentials

Jeffrey A. Brown, MD, FACS, FAANS
Neurosurgery Director
NYU-Winthrop Hospital CyberKnife® Program
Private Practice
Neurological Surgery, PC
Lake Success, New York

Julie G. Pilitsis, MD, PhD
Chair, Department of Neuroscience & Experimental Therapeutics
Professor of Neurosurgery
Department of Neurosurgery
Albany Medical College
Albany, New York

Michael Schulder, MD, FAANS
Neurosurgery Program Director, and Vice Chair and Professor
Department of Neurosurgery
Donald and Barbara Zucker School of Medicine at Hofstra/Northwell
Hempstead, New York

70 illustrations

Thieme
New York • Stuttgart • Delhi • Rio de Janeiro

Executive Editor: Timothy Y. Hiscock
Managing Editor: Nikole Y. Connors
Director, Editorial Services: Mary Jo Casey
Production Editor: Torsten Scheihagen
International Production Director: Andreas Schabert
Editorial Director: Sue Hodgson
International Marketing Director: Fiona Henderson
International Sales Director: Louisa Turrell
Director of Institutional Sales: Adam Bernacki
Senior Vice President and Chief Operating Officer: Sarah Vanderbilt
President: Brian D. Scanlan
Printer: King Printing Co., Inc.

Library of Congress Cataloging-in-Publication Data
Names: Brown, Jeffrey A., author. | Pilitsis, Julie G., author. | Schulder,
  Michael, 1957- author.
Title: Functional neurosurgery : the essentials / Jeffrey A. Brown,
  MD, FACS, FAANS, Neurosurgery Director, NYU-Winthrop
  Hospital CyberKnife® Program, Private Practice, Neurological
  Surgery, PC., Lake Success, New York Julie G. Pilitsis, MD, PhD,
  Chair, Department of Neuroscience & Experimental
  Therapeutics, Professor of Neurosurgery, Department of
  Neurosurgery, Albany Medical College, Albany, New York,
  Michael Schulder, MD, FAANS, Neurosurgery Program Director,
  and Vice Chair and Professor, Department of Neurosurgery,
  Donald and Barbara Zucker School of Medicine at Hofstra/
  Northwell, Hempstead, New York.
Description: First edition. | New York : Thieme, [2019] | Includes
  bilbiographical references and index. |
Identifiers: LCCN 2019021432 (print) | LCCN 2019021860 (ebook)
  | ISBN 9781626237759 (e-book) | ISBN 9781626237742 (print)
Subjects: LCSH: Nervous system–Surgery.
Classification: LCC RD593 (ebook) | LCC RD593 .B76 2019 (print)
  | DDC 617.4/8–dc23
LC record available at https://lccn.loc.gov/2019021432

Copyright © 2020 by Thieme Medical Publishers, Inc.

Thieme Publishers New York
333 Seventh Avenue, New York, NY 10001 USA
+1 800 782 3488, customerservice@thieme.com

Thieme Publishers Stuttgart
Rüdigerstrasse 14, 70469 Stuttgart, Germany
+49 [0]711 8931 421, customerservice@thieme.de

Thieme Publishers Delhi
A-12, Second Floor, Sector-2, Noida-201301
Uttar Pradesh, India
+91 120 45 566 00, customerservice@thieme.in

Thieme Publishers Rio de Janeiro, Thieme Publicações Ltda.
Edifício Rodolpho de Paoli, 25º andar
Av. Nilo Peçanha, 50 – Sala 2508,
Rio de Janeiro 20020-906 Brasil
+55 21 3172-2297 / +55 21 3172-1896
www.thiemerevinter.com.br

Cover design: Thieme Publishing Group
Typesetting by DiTech Process Solutions
Typesetting by Thomson Digital, India

Printed in the United States of America
by King Printing Co., Inc.   5 4 3 2 1

ISBN 978-1-62623-774-2

Also available as an e-book:
eISBN 978-1-62623-775-9

Important note: Medicine is an ever-changing science undergoing continual development. Research and clinical experience are continually expanding our knowledge, in particular our knowledge of proper treatment and drug therapy. Insofar as this book mentions any dosage or application, readers may rest assured that the authors, editors, and publishers have made every effort to ensure that such references are in accordance with **the state of knowledge at the time of production of the book**.

Nevertheless, this does not involve, imply, or express any guarantee or responsibility on the part of the publishers in respect to any dosage instructions and forms of applications stated in the book. **Every user is requested to examine carefully** the manufacturers' leaflets accompanying each drug and to check, if necessary in consultation with a physician or specialist, whether the dosage schedules mentioned therein or the contraindications stated by the manufacturers differ from the statements made in the present book. Such examination is particularly important with drugs that are either rarely used or have been newly released on the market. Every dosage schedule or every form of application used is entirely at the user's own risk and responsibility. The authors and publishers request every user to report to the publishers any discrepancies or inaccuracies noticed. If errors in this work are found after publication, errata will be posted at www.thieme.com on the product description page.

Some of the product names, patents, and registered designs referred to in this book are in fact registered trademarks or proprietary names even though specific reference to this fact is not always made in the text. Therefore, the appearance of a name without designation as proprietary is not to be construed as a representation by the publisher that it is in the public domain.

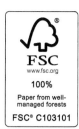

Acknowledgments/Dedication

To Brookes and Schuyler for special time gone by and to Rory for so many decades of love and support.

-Jeffrey A. Brown

To my mother for her unconditional love and support. To my husband Tim and children Ryan and Lauren who make it all worth it. To all my teammates in Neurosurgery and Neuroscience and Experimental Therapeutics, thank you for all you to do to care for existing patients and advance our field.

A special thank you to Pya Seidner who aided considerably with editing and communicating with the authors, editors and publishers.

-Julie G. Pilitsis

To my wife, Dr. Lu Steinberg, who believed in me and keeps me going.

-Michael Schulder

Contents

Contents

Preface

I attended college in the late 1960's-a revolutionary period. I had thought to study economics, but the mysteries of psychology drew me away from computer-programmed evaluations of the cost benefit of owning your own laundry machine instead of doing the job at a laundromat. This was the era of the mind-its "expansion," of LSD and a plethora of psychedelics. In 1968 Irving Cooper called a halt to any further functional cryoablation surgery for Parkinson's Disease. There were drugs to solve the problem now. In 1969 Jose Delgado published "Physical Control of the Mind: Toward a Psychocivilised Society." BF Skinner popularized his work on operant conditioning in 1971. The mind could be controlled by other means too, by other men, or by genetically embedded pleasure drives.

A year later, Michael Crichton, a Harvard Medical School graduate, published "Terminal Man," which brought to the forefront the dangers of surgical mind control. In 1973 I was at The University of Chicago as a first-year medical student. I approached Daniel X. Freedman, chair of the psychiatry department, to work in his research laboratory that summer. I was going to be a psychiatrist and focus on healing the complexities of the mind with empathy not surgery. When asked about my background, I mentioned my experience in college experimental psychology wherein I had spent time inserting electrodes into rat brains for behavioral experiments. Perfect. I was put to work doing just that-placing electrodes in the median midbrain raphe of rats to stimulate and compare the neurochemical effects to an intraperitoneal injection from a bottle of Sandoz Pure LSD. In 1973 this was the equivalent of being given responsibility for the keys to a nuclear power plant. I behaved and my move away from the mysteries of the talking profession had begun. Behavior could be modified electrically in a manner that would reproduce the chemical effects of a powerful mind-altering drug.

Then came "One Flew over the Cuckoo's Nest." It opened in theaters on November 19, 1975. The enduring image of big Chief Bromdon smashing his way to freedom from the horror of the lobotomized emptiness in the eyes of Randall Patrick McMurphy abruptly arrested the development of the burgeoning field of functional neurosurgery. L-Dopa was here. Surgery for mind and body control was grinding to a halt. The State of California outlawed it.

Seven years later, Lars Leksell visited the University of Chicago while I was finishing my residency training and spoke of his frame and his Gamma Knife. Our program acquired a Leksell stereotactic frame and we began using it. This is the way information was transmitted forty years ago. Meetings were meant to be just that-opportunities to meet with others, learn what they were doing in the field, perhaps spend a day with them in the operating room observing them and judging whether what they did was something you could do when the time was appropriate.

Leksell, after all, as Dr. Lunsford notes in his opening essay on the history of stereotactic neurosurgery, did just that. He spent time with Spiegel and Wycsis in Philadelphia, evaluated their work with the device they designed, then designed his own. In the last year of my training I visited L'Hopital Foche outside of Paris to learn from Gerard Guiot and years later from Peter Jannetta in Pittsburgh and Takanori Fukushima in Tokyo. Would it have been easier for Leksell or I had we been able to read a textbook on the subject? A textbook can serve as an introduction and a reference. It does not replace the active work of becoming a surgeon.

The purpose then of this effort by my co-editors and the authors of 41 chapters in the field is to provide a readable introduction to a fascinating field, and which will remain a reference for future reflection during the course of one's training or practice.

Readable is a key element. The editors and publisher have struggled to make these chapters concise, comprehendible and communicative. Every statement need not be matched with a reference number, but the essential references for the topic will have been listed for those who wish to dig deeper into the subject. This text is a companion to Starr, Barbaro, and Larson's "Neurosurgical Operative Atlas." Its intent is not to provide detailed operative nuances.

Several years ago my young daughter picked up an article I was writing, read through it, and declared it wordy and confusing and boring. I was embarrassed into learning how to write to communicate and joined a group of crime fiction writers determined to publish their stories. Take the opportunity to read something you have written aloud to even a small group and you will realize the point at which attention is lost. Try to find a way to stop that and you become a writer. A textbook may not be a crime mystery story, but it should keep you interested. Stereotactic neurosurgery is after all fascinating enough to use it repeatedly as a subject in iconic movies.

"Can a computer infer human intention or perception?" This is the opening question of the chapter on neuroprosthetics. How can one not be motivated to read on to find the answer? A good story asks a question, answers it, asks another, answers it and moves on in that way. What is the difference between the uses of a powered and an augmentative exoskeleton? What is the role of the nucleus accumbens in the treatment of medically refractory depression? What is the target in the functional treatment of Alzheimer's disease and why? Reduced mobility, depression and Alzheimer's disease in the elderly-these are huge worldwide challenges for the next generation to solve. Stereotactic neurosurgeons are positioned to be closely involved.

This textbook owes its origins to the confidence of Laligam Sekhar, master neurosurgeon, philosopher and innovator and I am grateful to him for the introduction to Timothy Hiscock to make it happen. Without my co-editors, Julie Pilitsis and Michael Schulder, it would not have been completed. The contribution of a chapter in a textbook does little to advance the academic career of those busy neurosurgeons who made the effort to communicate the essence of their sub specialized knowledge. I thank them for doing so. It is the essence of their well-deserved titles as Doctors of Medicine that they do so. After all, the word "doctor" means "teacher."

Throughout this text you will read the recommendations that a committee review each patient before a definite decision is made to proceed with surgery. Protocols are presented for the approach to that evaluation. There is comfort in the groupthink of protocol and committee decision approval. Neurosurgery, however, is a remarkable profession in which the operation is ultimately the responsibility of only one individual.

Once, before the ritual of a pre-incisional "time out" had been incorporated into surgical routine, I watched my chair step quietly away from the operating table after donning his gown and gloves, ready to clip a complex aneurysm, bow his head, close his eyes and remain silent for just a moment. What was he doing, I wondered?

We have a stunning responsibility as neurosurgeons. We hold a human life in our hands each time we operate. What these 41 chapters cannot address is that protocols and committees can be blankets of comfort, but they do not remove the final responsibility of our position. I hope that each of you will take a moment to reflect on that as you make use of the breadth of knowledge transmitted through the authors of these chapters. Be thankful for having been granted the privilege of service, and humbly ask for the guidance to perform it well.

Jeffrey A. Brown, MD, FACS

Contributors

Aviva Abosch, MD, PhD
Vice Chair for Research, Department of Neurosurgery
Professor of Neurosurgery and Neurology
Director of Stereotactic and Epilepsy Surgery
University of Colorado School of Medicine
Aurora, Colorado

Leonardo Almeida, MD
Assistant Professor
Department of Neurology
University of Florida College of Medicine
Gainesville, Florida

Jeffrey E., MD, PhD
Associate Professor of Neurosurgery
Harvard Medical School
Boston, Massachusetts

Marat V. Avshalumov, PhD, DABNM, CNIM
Chief Neurophysiologist
Neurological Surgery P.C.
Rockville Centre, New York
Adjunct Professor
Department of Neurosurgery
NYU School of Medicine
New York, New York

Gordon H. Baltuch, MD, PhD
Professor
Department of Neurosurgery
University of Pennsylvania
Philadelphia, Pennsylvania

Carolina Benjamin, MD
Clinical Instructor
Skull Base and Radiosurgery Fellow
Department of Neurosurgery
NYU Langone Medical Center
New York, New York

Stephan Bickel, MD, PhD
Department of Neurology
Northwell Health
Manhasset, New York

Aaron E. Bond, MD
Neurosurgeon
Semmes-Murphy Clinic
Memphis, Tennessee

Peter Brunner, PhD
Associate Professor
Department of Neurology
Albany Medical College
Albany, New York

Jeffrey A. Brown, MD, FACS, FAANS
Neurosurgery Director
NYU-Winthrop Hospital CyberKnife® Program
Private Practice
Neurological Surgery, PC
Lake Success, New York

Oguz Cataltepe, MD
Professor
Department of Neurosurgery
University of Massachusetts
Worcester, Massachusetts

Jason L. Chan, MD
Resident
Department of Clinical Neurosciences
University of Calgary
Calgary, Alberta, Canada

Robert F. Dallapiazza, MD, PhD
Assistant Professor
Department of Clinical Neurological Surgery
Tulane University School of Medicine
New Orleans, Louisiana

Chen-Chen Deng, MD
Department of Functional Neurosurgery
Ruijin Hospital
Shanghai Jiao Tong University School of Medicine
Shanghai, China

Lisa Deuel, MD
Fellow in Movement Disorders
University of Colorado Anschutz Medical Campus
Aurora, Colorado

W. Jeffrey Elias, MD
Professor of Neurological Surgery
University of Virginia
Charlottesville, Virginia

Dario Englot, MD, PhD
Assistant Professor of Neurological Surgery and Electrical
  Engineering, Radiology and Radiological Sciences, and
  Biomedical Engineering
Surgical Director of Epilepsy
Department of Neurological Surgery
Vanderbilt University Medical Center
Nashville, Tennessee

Pouya Entezami, MD
Resident
Department of Neurological Surgery
Albany Medical Center
Albany, New York

Walid I. Essayed, MD
Clinical Fellow
Department of Neurosurgery
Harvard Medical School
Brigham and Women's Hospital
Boston, Massachusetts

Zachary Fitzgerald, MD
Epilepsy Center
Neurological Institute
Cleveland Clinic
Cleveland, Ohio

Alexandra J. Golby, MD
Professor of Neurosurgery
Professor of Radiology
Harvard Medical School
Brigham and Women's Hospital
Boston, Massachusetts

Joshua L. Golubovsky, BS
Student
Lerner College of Medicine of Case Western Reserve
  University
Cleveland Clinic
Cleveland, Ohio

Jorge Gonzalez-Martinez, MD
Epilepsy Center
Cleveland Clinic
Cleveland, Ohio

Clement Hamani, PhD
Associate Professor
Department of Surgery
Affiliate Neuroscientist
Division of Neurosurgery
University of Toronto
Toronto, Ontario, Canada

Era Hanspal, MD
Assistant Professor of Neurology
Movement Disorders
Albany Medical Center
Albany, New York

David Harter, MD
Associate Professor
Department of Neurosurgery
NYU Langone Health
New York, New York

Travis W. Hassell, MD, PhD
Assistant Professor
Movement Disorders Division
Department of Neurology
Vanderbilt University Medical Center
Nashville Tennessee

Kathryn L. Holloway, MD
Professor
Department of Neurosurgery
Virginia Commonwealth University Health System
and
McGuire VAMC SE PADRECC
Richmond, Virginia

John Honeycutt, MD
Medical Director of Pediatric Neurosurgery
Cook Children's Hospital
Fort Worth, Texas

Roy S. Hwang, MD
Neurosurgeon
St. Luke's University Health Network
Bethlehem, Pennsylvania

Ronak H. Jani, BS
Department of Neurosurgery
University of Pittsburgh School of Medicine
Pittsburgh, Pennsylvania

Joohi Jimenez-Shahed, MD
Associate Professor
Department of Neurology
Baylor College of Medicine
Houston, Texas

Tyler J. Kenning, MD, FAANS
Associate Professor
Director, Pituitary and Cranial Base Surgery
Department of Neurosurgery
Albany Medical Center
Albany, New York

Ryan B. Kochanski, MD
Resident
Department of Neurosurgery
Rush University
Chicago, Illinois

Peter Konrad, MD PhD
Professor, Neurosurgery and Biomedical Engineering
Vanderbilt University Medical Center
Nashville, Tennessee

Cynthia S. Kubu, PhD, ABPP-CN
Professor
Center for Neurological Restoration
Cleveland Clinic
Cleveland, Ohio

Aaron Kucyi, MD
Fellow
Neurology and Neurological Sciences
Stanford University
Stanford, California

Steven M. Lange, MD
Department of Radiology
Thomas Jefferson University Hospital
Philadelphia, Pennsylvania

Eric C. Leuthardt, MD
Professor of Neurological Surgery, Neuroscience,
    Biomedical Engineering, and Mechanical Engineering
    & Materials Science
Director, Center for Innovation in Neuroscience and
    Technology
Director, Brain Laser Center
Department of Neurological Surgery
Washington University School of Medicine
St. Louis, Missouri

Dian-You Li, MD
Department of Functional Neurosurgery
Ruijin Hospital
Shanghai Jiao Tong University School of Medicine
Shanghai, China

Guo-Zhen Lin, MD
Department of Psychiatry
Ruijin Hospital
Shanghai Jiao Tong University School of Medicine
Shanghai, China

Nir Lipsman, MD, PhD
Scientist
Sunnybrook Health Sciences Centre
Toronto, Ontario, Canada

Andres Lozano, MD, PhD, FRCSC, FRSC, FCAHS
University Professor
Department of Surgery
 University of Toronto
Toronto, Ontario, Canada

L. Dade Lunsford, MD, FACS, FAANS
Lars Lekell and Distinguished Professor
Department of Neurological Surgery
University of Pittsburgh
Pittsburgh, Pennsylvania

Andre G. Machado, MD, PhD
Chairman
Neurological Institute
Cleveland Clinic
Cleveland, Ohio

Andres L. Maldonado-Naranjo, MD
Neurosurgery Resident
Department of Neurological Surgery
Cleveland Clinic Foundation
Cleveland, Ohio

Kevin Mansfield, MD
Neurosurgeon
Mercy Clinic Springfield
Springfield, Missouri

Nicole C.R. McLaughlin, PhD
Assistant Professor (Research)
Department of Psychiatry and Human Behavior
Alpert Medical School of Brown University
Providence, Rhode Island

Jonathan Melius, PA
Department of Neurosurgery
Albany Medical College
Albany, New York

Jonathan P. Miller, MD
George R. and Constance P. Lincoln Professor and
    Vice Chairman
Director, Functional and Restorative Neurosurgery Center
Department of Neurological Surgery
University Hospitals Cleveland Medical Center
Case Western Reserve University School of Medicine
Cleveland, Ohio

Alon Y. Mogilner, MD, PhD
Associate Professor
Departments of Neurosurgery and Anesthesiology
New York University Medical Center
New York, New York

Eric S. Molho, MD, FAAN, FANA
Professor of Neurology
Riley Family Chair in Parkinson's Disease
Department of Neurology
Albany Medical College
Albany, New York

Shayan Moosa, MD
Resident Physician
Department of Neurosurgery
University of Virginia
Charlottesville, Virginia

Denmark Mugutso, MS, MCN, CNIM
Neurophysiologist
Department of Neurophysiology
Neurological Surgery, PC
Rockville Centre, New York

Joseph S. Neimat, MD
Professor and Chairman
Department of Neurological Surgery
University of Louisville
Louisville, Kentucky

Ajay Niranjan, MD, MBA
Professor
Department of Neurological Surgery
University of Pittsburgh
Pittsburgh, Pennsylvania

Ika Noviawaty, MD
Assistant Professor
Department of Neurology and Neurosurgery
University of Massachusetts Medical School
Worcester, Massachusetts

Michael S. Okun, MD
Adelaide Lackner Professor and Chair of Neurology
Executive Director, Norman Fixel Institute for Neurological
  Diseases
University of Florida Health
Gainesville Florida

Alp Ozpinar, MD
Department of Neurosurgery
University of Pittsburgh Medical Center
Pittsburgh, Pennsylvania

Josef Parvizi, MD
Professor
Department of Neurology
Stanford University Medical Center
Stanford, California

Fenna T. Phibbs, MD, MPH
Associate Professor
Department of Neurology
Vanderbilt Medical Center
Nashville, Tennessee

Julie G. Pilitsis, MD, PhD
Chair, Department of Neuroscience & Experimental
  Therapeutics
Professor of Neurosurgery
Department of Neurosurgery
Albany Medical College
Albany, New York

Ashwin Ramayya, MD, PhD
Resident
Department of Neurosurgery
University of Pennsylvania
Philadelphia, Pennsylvania

Adolfo Ramirez-Zamora, MD
Associate Professor
Department of Neurology
University of Florida
Gainesville, Florida

Richard A. Rammo, MD
Chief Resident
Department of Neurosurgery
Henry Ford Health System
Detroit, Michigan

Wilson Z. Ray, MD
Associate Professor of Neurological and Orthopedic Surgery
Neurosurgery Residency Associate Director
Co-Director, Spinal Oncology
Washington University School of Medicine
Department of Neurological Surgery
St. Louis, Missouri

Gaddum Duemani Reddy, MD, PhD
Assistant Professor
Department of Neurosurgery
Upstate Medical University
Syracuse, New York

Anthony L. Ritaccio, MD
Senior Associate Consultant
Department of Neurology
Mayo Clinic
Jacksonville, Florida

David W. Roberts, MD
Professor of Surgery (Neurosurgery)
Geisel School of Medicine
Adjunct Professor of Engineering
Thayer School of Engineering at Dartmouth
Hanover, New Hampshire

Jarod L. Roland, MD
Resident
Department of Neurosurgery
Washington University School of Medicine
St. Louis, Missouri

Jeffrey V. Rosenfeld, MBBS, MD, MS, FRACS, FACS,
    FRCS(Edin.), IFAANS
Professor
Department of Surgery
Monash University
Senior Neurosurgeon
The Alfred Hospital, Melbourne
Victoria, Australia

Sepehr Sani, MD
Associate Professor
Department of Neurosurgery
Rush University
Chicago, Illinois

Gerwin Schalk, PhD
Research Scientist
National Center for Adaptive Neurotechnologies
Wadsworth Center, New York State Department of Health
Albany, New York

Michael Schulder, MD, FAANS
Neurosurgery Program Director, and Vice Chair
    and Professor
Department of Neurosurgery
Donald and Barbara Zucker School of Medicine at Hofstra/
    Northwell
Hempstead, New York

Jason M. Schwalb, MD, FAANS, FACS
Clinical Professor of Neurosurgery, Wayne State University
Surgical Director, Movement Disorder & Comprehensive
    Epilepsy Centers
Henry Ford Medical Group
Detroit, Michigan

Raymond F. Sekula, Jr., MD
Department of Neurosurgery
University of Pittsburgh Medical Center
Pittsburgh, Pennsylvania

Hamid Shah, MD
Assistant Professor
Department of Neurosurgery
Vanderbilt University
Nashville Tennessee

Jugal Shah, MD
Resident
Department of Neurosurgery
NYU Langone Health
New York, New York

Jessica Shields, MD, PhD
Resident
Department of Neurosurgery
LSU Health Sciences Center
New Orleans, Louisiana

Lauren L. Spiegel, MD
Movement Disorders Fellow
Department of Neurology
University of California San Francisco
San Francisco, California

Michael D. Staudt, MD
Resident
Department of Clinical Neurological Sciences
The University of Western Ontario
London, Ontario, Canada

Bo-Min Sun, MD, PhD
Deputy Director
Professor of Neurosurgery
Ruijin Hospital
Shanghai Jiao Tong University School of Medicine
Shanghai, China

Vishad Sukul, MD
Department of Neurosurgery
Albany Medical Center
Albany, New York

Jennifer A. Sweet, MD, FAANS
Assistant Professor of Neurosurgery
Case Western Reserve University
University Hospitals Cleveland Medical Center
Cleveland, Ohio

Ashesh A. Thaker, MD
Assistant Professor
Division of Neuroradiology
Department of Radiology
University of Colorado School of Medicine
Aurora, Colorado

Jamie Toms, MD
Resident
Department of Neurosurgery
Virginia Commonwealth University
Richmond, Virginia

Prashin Unadkat, MBBS
Resident Physician, Department of Surgery
Research Fellow, Departments of Neurosurgery
  and Radiology
Brigham and Women's Hospital
Harvard Medical School
Boston, Massachusetts

Tao Wang, MD
Department of Functional Neurosurgery
Ruijin Hospital
Shanghai Jiao Tong University School of Medicine
Shanghai, China

Tony R. Wang, MD
Resident Physician
University of Virginia
Charlottesville, Virginia

Charles Warnecke, BS, CNIM
Neurophysiologist
Neurological Surgery, P.C.
Rockville Centre, New York

Yan Wong, PhD
Senior Lecturer
Departments of Electrical and Computer Systems
  Engineering
Monash University
Clayton, Australia

David S. Xu, MD
Assistant Professor
Department of Neurosurgery
Baylor College of Medicine
Houston, Texas

Shikun Zhan, MD
Department of Functional Neurosurgery
Ruijin Hospital
Shanghai Jiao Tong University School of Medicine
Shanghai, China

1 History of Innovation in Stereotaxy/Functional Neurosurgery

David W. Roberts

Abstract

Neurosurgery has long led the surgical specialties in the development of innovative clinical applications of technique and technology, and the subspecialty of stereotactic and functional surgery has stood at the vanguard of such creativity.

Keywords: neurosurgery, stereotaxy, functional

1.1 Early Years and the Concept of Co-registration

Before Francis Gall and the much-maligned field of phrenology, the brain was thought to be a holistic organ. Gall, underappreciated as a neuroanatomist, pioneered the concept of localizing cerebral activity to varied brain regions. Fritsch and Hitzig identified circumscribed cortical sties in the brain that elicited contralateral limb movement. Ferrier followed this work by using stimulation and ablation to demarcate the primary sensory and motor cortices, further confirming the legitimacy of this new paradigm of cerebral functional identity. Modern stereotaxy then began with the work of two men, Sir Victor Horsley and Robert Clarke, at what was then known then as the National Hospital for Diseases of the Nervous System including Paralysis and Epilepsy at Queen Square in London, UK.

Horsley used electrical stimulation to identify then excise a cortical epileptic focus but struggled with imprecise cerebellar localization efforts. Clarke, a physiologist, devised a head-mounted instrument for accurate placement of a needle-like probe to minimize brain injury and improve precision. Instruments for cranial measurement and for localization on the scalp or cranium had been developed by others, including Bridges and Morgan, Broca, Kocher, Zernov, and Rossolimo, but "Clarke's instrument," as Horsley himself referred to it, was a three-dimensional digitizer, defining a coordinate space and capable of reliably directing a relatively atraumatic probe to target addresses within that space (▶ Fig. 1.1).[1,2,3] Substructures, like the dentate nucleus, could then be identified. Uniquely, the instrument used co-registration of that surgical space, combining the cranial features of the inferior orbital rim and the external auditory canals, with an atlas comprised of anatomic slices of the brain related to the same external landmarks.

From this founding principle, the defining concept of stereotactic surgery was born.

The variability of both the larger human forebrain and its relationship to external cranial features precluded the translation of the Horsley-Clarke instrument to clinical use. Spiegel and Wycis devised a frame that merged loci of the foramen of Monro and pineal gland obtained from pneumoencephalography into coordinates in a stereotactic device. They used it for thalamic ablations as a less invasive option to frontal leukotomy. Their work spawned the development of innumerable, ingenious stereotactic frames. Surgeons such as Leksell, Reichert and Mundinger, Talairach, and Narabayashi, among many others, designed devices.[4,5] The advent of computed tomography and magnetic resonance imaging brought new clinical capabilities and needs. Tumors could now be readily seen. How could they be safely reached to biopsy or remove? The ability to do so had been restricted to a subset of neurosurgeons who could, for example, interpret Leksell's spiral diagram to deal with radiologic parallax. By simplifying the co-registration process, the field was widely opened.

1906: Horsley and Clarke create the first stereotactic frame, co-registering the external auditory canal and inferior orbital rim with an anatomic atlas of the brain. Sachs brings it to the U.S. three years later, and the innovation is largely ignored.

1947: Spiegel-Wycis-Leksell introduce devices based at first on encephalographic landmarks.

1979: Brown, with Roberts, and Wells introduce computational elements of transformational equations with computed tomography to stereotaxy.

1986: Roberts proposes a frameless neuronavigational system integrated with the operating microscope.

1.2 The Computational Era

Computational co-registration underlays the design of a new stereotactic frame, the Brown-Roberts-Wells frame. More significant was the extension of stereotaxy to craniotomy and volumetric resection. Sheldon and Jacques adapted a tulip-retractor to a stereotactic frame for tumor resection, but it was Kelly who promoted the computer as a surgical tool by which multiple imaging data sets could be compiled into a single database, which could then be co-registered with the surgical field using an operating microscope attached to the guiding arc of an enlarged stereotactic frame.[6,7] Whereas early stereotaxy relied upon a surgeon's calculation of frame coordinates for a point selected within an atlas or tomographic image, the early computers of the 1980s could readily calculate the transformation required to move in either direction between large sets of points in a preoperative image and in the operative field.

Computational resources advanced the field dramatically, introducing what was initially called frameless stereotaxy, then neuronavigation, and now image-guidance. The functions of a stereotactic frame were to define an operative coordinate space, enable co-registration with preoperative coordinate spaces, and render that information useful to guide an instrument to its deep-seated target. Now this could be improved upon computer-based systems. It was now possible to eliminating the need even for the frame. The concept of stereotaxy was now projected beyond intracranial space. Non-contact digitizers based upon sonic, mechanical arm, optical, and electromagnetic

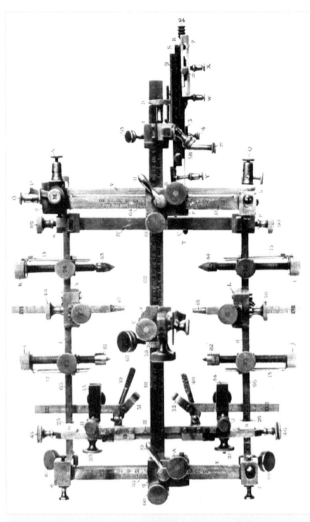

Fig. 1.1 Clarke's instrument, the stereotactic apparatus developed by Robert Clarke and Sir Victor Horsley.[3]

technologies defined a coordinate space and tracked instruments within that space (▶ Fig. 1.2).[8,9,10,11] Rapid computation of coordinate transformations correlating the surgical field with sets of fiducial points, surfaces, or volumes in imaging studies replaced human-scale point calculations relying upon super-structures attached to frame bases. Graphic displays that could indicate instrument location and project them onto appropriate radiologic image slices or superimpose it into heads-up displays in operating microscopes along with other relevant information as augmented reality radically advanced effector bandwidth and stereotaxic utility. Dozens of such systems created in individual laboratories made for an exciting, disruptive era that soon matured, coalescing into the handful of systems in use today. Without need of a frame, stereotaxy's co-registration principle now extends to much of general neurosurgery and increasingly to other surgical fields.

Stereotactic principles moved from burr holes with guidance to craniotomies with guidance. Now, the dilemma of intraoperative data degradation needed to be addressed. What was co-registered before surgery could change mid surgery. Intraoperative MRI and CT machines that can acquire new, updated radiologic images have proliferated. Such implementation and the optimization of its surgical application is ongoing.[12,13,14] Whether alternative approaches that rely on more easily acquired sparse data, such as that provided by the image of the surgical field through the operating microscope or intraoperative ultrasound to shift and deform preoperative images, proves more cost-effective and less cumbersome remains an open question.[15,16]

1.3 Effector Technologies

Horsley and Clarke's seminal contribution also included new instruments for consistent and reliable electrical stimulation and electrolysis of neural tissue (▶ Fig. 1.3). The history of the tool, or effector, enabled by stereotactic systems is one of equally striking innovation. Early lesioning techniques variously

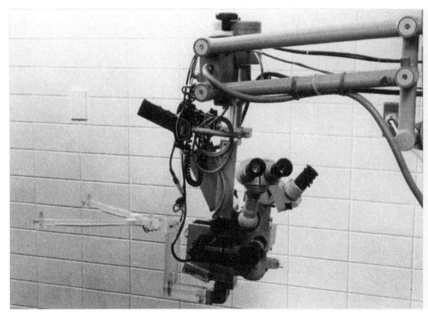

Fig. 1.2 The Dartmouth frameless stereotactic system, with the operating microscope tracked by a sonic digitizer[8] (used with permission of the Journal of Neurosurgery).

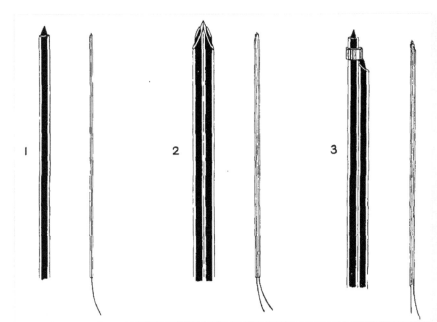

Fig. 1.3 Stereotactic needles developed by Horsley and Clarke for electrical stimulation and electrolysis.[3]

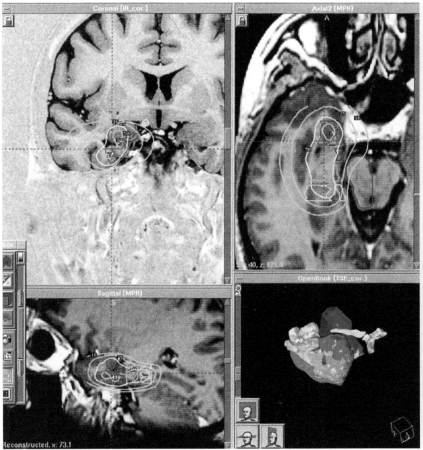

Fig. 1.4 Gamma Knife radiosurgery dose plan for treatment of right mesial temporal lobe epilepsy[21] (from J. Régis et al and used with permission of Thieme).

used anodal electrolysis, chemical approaches by alcohol injection, mechanical devices with rotating wire loops, extreme cold from cryoprobes primed with liquid nitrogen, radioactive isotopes with Yttrium, and heat from radiofrequency probes.[90] The need for reliability, consistency, safety, ease of use, and expense drove some of these choices, and although all have

been employed clinically, today temperature-monitored radiofrequency systems are the most widely used.

Leksell's innovation was the most radical. He saw the potential of coupling his stereotactic frame with ionizing radiation (▶ Fig. 1.4). After an earlier integration of his frame with proton beam radiation, he used multiple Cobalt-60 sources collimated by a helmet and radially focused on a selected target. The approach was facilitated by his arc-centered frame. Today it has been commercialized worldwide as the Gamma Knife (Elekta Instruments, Stockholm).[17] Adaptations of linear accelerators by others have flourished, as has proton beam radiation that finely contours its Bragg peak of energy to the target. High cost has limited its general distribution.[18,19,20]

Technologies enabling non-ablative modulation of neural tissue currently dominate functional applications today. Refinement of electrical stimulation from the nineteenth century laboratory to a stereotactically delivered, chronically implantable, programmable clinical device has produced an attractive alternative to destructive lesioning, and this innovation has become the dominant practice. The translation of non-human investigative electrical stimulation into clinical practice and the application in psychiatric disorders, pain, epilepsy and tremor have been pioneered by Heath, Delgado, Bechtereva, Cooper, Adams, Siegfried, Benabid, and many others.[22,23,24,25,26,27,28] Subsequent miniaturization and battery refinement reduced some of the burdens of clinical use and facilitated still wider clinical adoption. The full potential of this technology has not yet been realized, but some pioneering entrepreneurial projects have excited the field. The introduction of a responsive stimulator by NeuroPace (Mountain View, CA) for the treatment of intractable epilepsy–a system capable of continuous electroencephalographic monitoring, algorithmic seizure activity detection, and a programmable "counter-stimulus" effector response—illustrate that potential (▶ Fig. 1.5).[29] Closed-loop systems that monitor and modulate not only electrical, but in some implementations, neurochemical activity have demonstrated proof of concept in the laboratory and are being investigated.[30] The role of other translatable, emerging technologies including transplantation, infusion, and optogenetics invigorate the field.

Stereotaxy's accurate co-registration of surgical space has become an infrastructure on which additional innovations are being layered. Robotic arms with bushing guides for needle or probe trajectories were integrated with stereotactic frames early on, as in the implementations of Young, Kwoh, and Drake.[31,32,33] When multiple depth electrodes need to be implanted, as they often are in the investigation of epilepsy, the efficiencies of robotics become significant.

The digitization of the operative field provides opportunity for other functionalities as well. Image-guidance joined with seamless telecommunications invites teleconsultation or, with robotics, telesurgery. Technologically closely linked, educational and training opportunities abound. Simulators using generic or individual patient's imaged neuroanatomy and pathology afford practice opportunities analogous to those in aeronautical aviation.

1.4 Clinical Innovation

Innovation characterizes the clinical applications of this technology. In the1940s, stereotactic instrumentation was used to intervene in psychiatric illnesses, movement disorders, and chronic pain. It was not an accident that Spiegel and Wycis's first cases were for psychiatric disorders although their 1947 paper discussed potential applications in pain, movement disorders, trigeminal neuralgia, and cystic tumors. Leksell shared this orientation as did Talairach and Narabayashi. Interestingly, each of them was also trained in psychiatry, yet all of them recognized the technology's wider application.

With advances in neuroimaging and neuroscience and better understanding of anatomic and pathophysiologic substrates, a broad range of neurological disorders has become treatable. Interventions for movement disorders, pain, and epilepsy are now more effective. Most exciting, however, is the expansion of the field into the new areas of psychiatric illness, headache, eating disorders, addiction, vegetative state, memory, and the machine-brain interface.

These latter activities, initiated in a manner acceptable to our modern society, also expose a new horizon of neural augmentation, with all its associated ethical issues. Just as the innovative spirit of stereotactic and functional neurosurgery has realized remarkable therapeutic benefit, that innovative drive now demands new awareness, discussion, and responsibility.

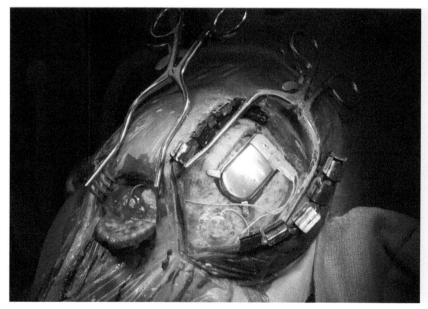

Fig. 1.5 Intraoperative image of an implanted NeuroPace responsive neural stimulation system, with the generator/battery component mounted cranially and bilateral hippocampal electrodes placed through occipital burr holes.

1.5 Conclusions

The dual identities of stereotactic and functional neurosurgery —a methodological technology and a clinical orientation centered on neurological function—underlie innovations in the field. The concept of spatial registration, foundational to the former, is a mathematical one, and seminal advances including the stereotactic frame, the registration algorithms, image-guidance, and updated registration represent applied geometric and algebraic mathematics. The clinical domain rests on neurophysiology, and it was apt that the specialty's journal for a time was *Applied Neurophysiology*. As that neuroscience discipline has advanced our understanding of how the brain is organized and functions, our ability to intervene is empowered.

References

[1] Critchley M. The Divine Banquet of the Brain. New York: Raven Press; 1979

[2] Serletis D, Pait TG. Early craniometric tools as a predecessor to neurosurgical stereotaxis. J Neurosurg. 2016; 124(6):1867–1874

[3] Horsley V, Clarke RH. The structure and functions of the cerebellum examined by a new method. Brain. 1908; 31(1):45–124

[4] Picard C, Olivier A, Bertrand G. The first human stereotaxic apparatus. The contribution of Aubrey Mussen to the field of stereotaxis. J Neurosurg. 1983; 59(4):673–676

[5] Spiegel EA, Wycis HT, Marks M, Lee AJ. Stereotaxic Apparatus for Operations on the Human Brain. Science. 1947; 106(2754):349–350

[6] Shelden CH, McCann G, Jacques S, et al. Development of a computerized microstereotaxic method for localization and removal of minute CNS lesions under direct 3-D vision. Technical report. J Neurosurg. 1980; 52(1):21–27

[7] Kelly PJ, Alker GJ , Jr, Goerss S. Computer-assisted stereotactic microsurgery for the treatment of intracranial neoplasms. Neurosurgery. 1982; 10(3):324–331

[8] Roberts DW, Strohbehn JW, Hatch JF, Murray W, Kettenberger H. A frameless stereotaxic integration of computerized tomographic imaging and the operating microscope. J Neurosurg. 1986; 65(4):545–549

[9] Watanabe E, Watanabe T, Manaka S, Mayanagi Y, Takakura K. Three-dimensional digitizer (neuronavigator): new equipment for computed tomography-guided stereotaxic surgery. Surg Neurol. 1987; 27(6):543–547

[10] Bucholz RD, Greco DJ. Image-guided surgical techniques for infections and trauma of the central nervous system. Neurosurg Clin N Am. 1996; 7(2):187–200

[11] Goerss SJ, Kelly PJ, Kall B, Stiving S. A stereotactic magnetic field digitizer. Stereotact Funct Neurosurg. 1994; 63(1–4):89–92

[12] Black PM, Moriarty T, Alexander E , III, et al. Development and implementation of intraoperative magnetic resonance imaging and its neurosurgical applications. Neurosurgery. 1997; 41(4):831–842, discussion 842–845

[13] Schulder M, Sernas TJ, Carmel PW. Cranial surgery and navigation with a compact intraoperative MRI system. Acta Neurochir Suppl (Wien). 2003; 85:79–86

[14] Nimsky C, Ganslandt O, von Keller B, Fahlbusch R. Preliminary experience in glioma surgery with intraoperative high-field MRI. Acta Neurochir Suppl (Wien). 2003; 88:21–29

[15] Roberts DW, Miga MI, Hartov A, et al. Intraoperatively updated neuroimaging using brain modeling and sparse data. Neurosurgery. 1999; 45(5):1199–1206, discussion 1206–1207

[16] Fan X, Roberts DW, Olson JD, et al. Image Updating for Brain Shift Compensation During Resection. Neurosurgery. 2017

[17] Leksell L. Stereotaxis and Radiosurgery: An Operative System. Springfield, Illinois: Charles C. Thomas; 1971

[18] Colombo F, Benedetti A, Pozza F, et al. Stereotactic radiosurgery utilizing a linear accelerator. Appl Neurophysiol. 1985; 48(1–6):133–145

[19] Adler JR , Jr, Chang SD, Murphy MJ, Doty J, Geis P, Hancock SL. The Cyberknife: a frameless robotic system for radiosurgery. Stereotact Funct Neurosurg. 1997; 69(1–4 Pt 2):124–128

[20] Kjellberg RN, Koehler AM, Preston WM, Sweet WH. Stereotaxic instrument for use with the Bragg peak of a proton beam. Confin Neurol. 1962; 22:183–189

[21] Régis J, Bartolomei F, Chauvel P. Radiosurgery. In: Baltuch G, Villemure J-G, eds. Operative Techniques in Epilepsy Surgery. New York: Thieme; 2009:188

[22] Heath RG. Electrical Self-Stimulation of the Brain in Man. Am J Psychiatry. 1963; 120:571–577

[23] Delgado JM, Hamlin H, Chapman WP. Technique of intracranial electrode implacement for recording and stimulation and its possible therapeutic value in psychotic patients. Confin Neurol. 1952; 12(5–6):315–319

[24] Bechtereva N, Bondartchuk A, Smirnov V, et al. Therapeutic electrostimulation of the brain deep structure. Vopr Neirokhir. 1972; 1:7–12

[25] Cooper IS, Amin I, Gilman S. The effect of chronic cerebellar stimulation upon epilepsy in man. Trans Am Neurol Assoc. 1973; 98:192–196

[26] Adams JE, Hosobuchi Y, Fields HL. Stimulation of internal capsule for relief of chronic pain. J Neurosurg. 1974; 41(6):740–744

[27] Siegfried J. Sensory thalamic neurostimulation for chronic pain. Pacing Clin Electrophysiol. 1987; 10(1 Pt 2):209–212

[28] Benabid AL, Pollak P, Louveau A, Henry S, de Rougemont J. Combined (thalamotomy and stimulation) stereotactic surgery of the VIM thalamic nucleus for bilateral Parkinson disease. Appl Neurophysiol. 1987; 50(1–6):344–346

[29] Morrell MJ, RNS System in Epilepsy Study Group. Responsive cortical stimulation for the treatment of medically intractable partial epilepsy. Neurology. 2011; 77(13):1295–1304

[30] Lee KH, Lujan JL, Trevathan JK, et al. WINCS Harmoni: Closed-loop dynamic neurochemical control of therapeutic interventions. Sci Rep. 2017; 7:46675

[31] Young RF. Application of robotics to stereotactic neurosurgery. Neurol Res. 1987; 9(2):123–128

[32] Kwoh YS, Hou J, Jonckheere EA, Hayati S. A robot with improved absolute positioning accuracy for CT guided stereotactic brain surgery. IEEE Trans Biomed Eng. 1988; 35(2):153–160

[33] Drake JM, Joy M, Goldenberg A, Kreindler D. Computer- and robot-assisted resection of thalamic astrocytomas in children. Neurosurgery. 1991; 29(1):27–33

2 A Brief History of Brain Stereotactic Frames

L. Dade Lunsford and Ajay Niranjan

Abstract

The first guiding devise was used by Dittmar in 1870s in an animal model. The first 3-dimensional targeting technique for human neurosurgery was described in 1908 by Victor Horsley and Robert Clarke. The collaborative effort of Spiegel and Wycis from the 1930s to 1950s, led to significant advances in the development of stereotactic devises. Extraordinary contributions by pioneers in neurosurgery throughout the world led to the development of currently used stereotactic guiding devises. Stereotactic head frames are now widely used for brain biopsy, radiosurgery, electrodes placement, and management of brain tumors, vascular malformations, and functional brain disorders. This article discusses the contribution of pioneers in the field and the development of brain stereotactic guiding device.

Keywords: stereotaxic, stereotactic, guiding device, head frame, stereotactic neurosurgery

"Old men should read new books and young men should read old books".

-Advice given by Peter Jannetta to Jeff Brown

In the history of medicine and neurosurgery the story of how stereotactic instruments were developed is extraordinary. That era now spans more than 150 years and it has led to the worldwide adoption of stereotactic technologies for the diagnosis and treatment of cranial, spinal and corporeal disease.

The term "stereotaxic" derives from the Greek root for "three-dimensional system" and is the correct spelling based on the Greek past participle. In 1973 the International Society for Research in Stereoencephalotomy, forerunner of the World Society of Functional and Stereotactic Surgery, described the word "stereotactic" as a combination of the Greek for "stereo," or three dimensional, with the Latin "tactus," meaning to touch. It was an equally appropriate origin of the word and the preferred spelling.[1] The range and diversity of devices developed during this 150 year interval are a testament to the ingenuity of surgeons and engineers who labored to build reliable and accurate image-guided ways to reach brain targets with the least risk.

2.1 The 19th Century

The gradual recognition that brain functions are localized led to the use of guiding devices to explore deep-seated regions of the brain in animals. In 1873 Dittmar, in Germany, described the use of a guiding device to make incisions in the medulla oblongata of rabbits.[2] A decade and a half later St. Petersburg physicians conceived a cranial localization tool to be fixed to the patient's skull to investigate function based on the concepts of phrenology- the idea that function is linked to external skull morphology.[3]

2.2 The 20th Century

Sir Victor Horsley and Robert Clarke are appropriately given credit for the development of the first stereotactic guiding device, which they described in the journal **Brain** in 1906.[4] The instrument could reliably direct a probe for the study of cerebellar physiology in cats. This first rectilinear system used an X-Y-Z axis to specify the target of a probe inserted through a holder mounted to the frame. It became the prototype for subsequent generations of stereotactic devices (▶ Fig. 2.1). Aubrey Mussen, a disciple of Clarke's, subsequently created a device patterned after the Horsley–Clarke frame.[5] As reported by Phil Gildenberg, this device was potentially applicable to human brain surgery.[6] Clarke apparently spent time in both London and Montreal, where this device was left at the Montreal Neurological Institute. It is not clear whether any patients were treated.

Stereotactic devices reliably permit selection of a safe passage route, creation of a cranial opening, and placement of a probe into an intracranial target that has been detected by imaging. In 1918, Capt. Aubrey Ferguson published a description of the removal of intracranial bullets using a guiding device (▶ Fig. 2.2).[7] This report appears to be the first publication of the actual human use of such a technology – an external guiding device with a mounted instrument (an extended pituitary forceps) directed to a target seen on X-ray imaging. Considering that x-ray visualization of the body had only recently been described, this was a remarkable, pioneering, but little recognized contribution.

During the 1930's Kirschner described the use of a cranial guiding device designed to facilitate transovale placement of a lesioning electrode to treat trigeminal neuralgia (▶ Fig. 2.3).[8] The 1940's were dominated by the collaborative development of a number of stereotactic devices patterned after the original Horsley-Clarke concept. Ernst Spiegel, an Austrian neurologist who emigrated to Philadelphia to escape the Nazi Anschluss,

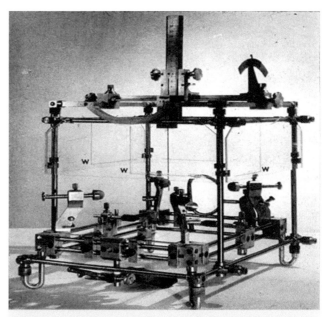

Fig. 2.1 Horsley-Clark system was the earliest recognized stereotactic guiding device, and was designed to reliably place a probe in the cerebellum of cats in order to study the physiology of the cerebellum.

teamed up with Henry Wycis a neurosurgeon working at Temple University to develop a practical stereotactic guiding system for use in human surgery.[9,10] This device, which they called the

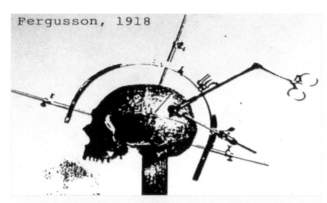

Fig. 2.2 Aubrey Ferguson developed perhaps the first human use guiding device to assist in the removal of intracranial bullet fragments in soldiers of the World War I. Reprinted with permission from Fergusson J. A preliminary note. A new system of localization and extraction of foreign bodies in the brain. *Br J Surg.* 1918;6:409-417.

stereoencephalotome, was the first to use internal brain landmarks shown by encephalography (▶ Fig. 2.4). As described by Gildenberg, the first device had only translational movements of the probe or electrode. When the carrier was positioned above the target a probe could be directed to the target. In later versions, the devices were mounted to plaster casts fixed to patient's heads. Some were rigidly fixed to the patient's cranial vault and were simply aiming devices. Additional devices were designed to have angular adjustments of the probe trajectory in order to match the angles of lines directed to the target based on AP and lateral x-rays. The same concerns of stability, rigidity, and reproducibility of device fixation present 75 years ago remain for the current generation MRI compatible devices. Even minimal movements can distort the target position and the probe trajectory. Spiegel and Wycis focused on movement and refractory behavioral disorders so as to minimize the surgical risk involved in its treatment. In the 1940s and 1950s the widely performed operation of frontal leucotomy was done by the more invasive craniotomy until Freeman began the practice of transorbital lobotomy.[11,12] Thousands of patients underwent such procedures in an era devoid of psychotherapeutic drugs.

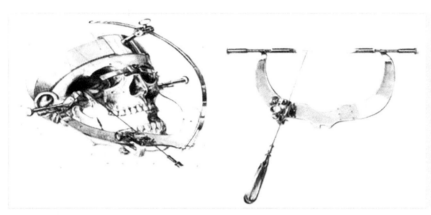

Fig. 2.3 Kirschner developed a stereotactic device in the 1930's for placement of a lesioning electrode in the foramen ovale to treat patients with trigeminal neuralgia (Reprinted with permission from Kirschner M. Die Punktionstechnik und die Elektrokoagulation es Ganglion Gasseri. *Arch Klin Chir.* 1933;176:581–620.)

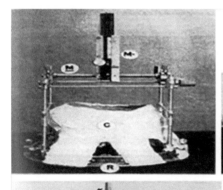
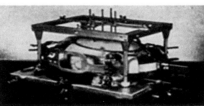
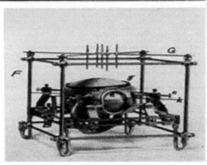

Fig. 2.4 The Spiegel-Wycis guiding device, also called the stereoencephalotome, was the first stereotactic device to use internal brain landmarks shown by encephalography (Reprinted with permission from Spiegel EA, Wycis HT. [Principles and applications of stereoencephalotomy]. *Acta Neurochir (Wien).* 1950;1(2–3):137–153.)

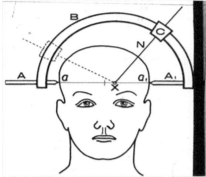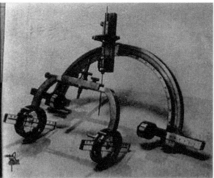

Fig. 2.5 The Leksell stereotactic system consists of rectilinear coordinate frame and a semicircular arc which is attached to the frame at chosen x,y,z coordinates of the target. The arc has a sliding probe carrier that allows the probe to move in left –right and antero-posterior angles.

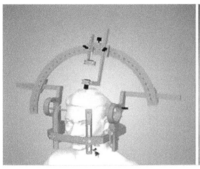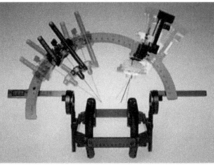

Fig. 2.6 The Leksell model G frame was designed to facilitate MRI targeting for both open as well as closed (radiosurgical) stereotactic procedures. This system allowed movement of the probe in multiple angles but always keeps the target at the center of the arc, whose radius is 19 cm.

Lars Leksell had been trained as a neurophysiologist and was largely responsible in the 1930's for the descriptions of the Gamma motor postural tone system. His collaborator, Ragnar Granit, later shared the 1967 Nobel Prize in Physiology or Medicine with George Wald and Keffer Hartline for his work on vision and retinal cones. Leksell went on to be concerned with what he considered to the poor neurosurgical outcomes of patients who underwent brain surgery in his home country of Sweden. Yet, his clinical mentor, Herbert Olivecrona, was the acknowledged Northern European master of neurosurgery, with a large experience in brain tumors and vascular malformations. Leksell, however, was convinced that less invasive and more accurate methods were needed to allow surgeons to reach deep-seated brain sites.

In 1947 Leksell traveled to Philadelphia for fellowship training with Spiegel and Wycis. When he returned to Stockholm, he submitted his landmark paper in which he described the prototype of a rectilinear coordinate system that bears his name (▶ Fig. 2.5).[13] The targeting was accomplished by direct imaging, when, for example, a calcified tumor capsule could be seen by skull x-ray. Otherwise, encephalography, with lateral and AP X-ray imaging, identified stable landmarks such as the anterior and posterior commissures. Targets in the internal capsule, globus pallidus or specific nuclei of the thalamus were found relative to these reliable points. Leksell's concept was that these devices should be simple enough that even a neurosurgeon could master their use!

Leksell was a restless and often unsatisfied inventor and he needed his device to be optimized to the last little screw. As imaging evolved from x-rays and encephalography, Leksell evaluated the use of ultrasound, computed tomography, and magnetic resonance imaging. The frame needed to be redesigned in order to accommodate these imaging changes so as to maintain reliability and imaging compatibility. New devices included the standard frame of the 1950s, the D frame of the 1970s introduced after the early development of CT, and eventually the G frame which was redesigned to facilitate MRI targeting for both open as well as closed (radiosurgical) stereotactic procedures (▶ Fig. 2.6). The target is positioned at the center of two arcs. The arcs allowed movement of the probe on the head from side to side and anterior to posterior while the target and probe tip remained at the X, Y and Z intersection. This is the arc-centered principle of localization. The angular adjustments of the probe trajectory optimized the trajectory so that the target was always reached when the probe was advanced the distance of the radius of the arc (19 cm).

Other devices were developed at many U.S. and European centers during the 1950s. These included in the United States the Todd-Wells device that translated the target to the intersection of the arcs and the Richert-Mundinger system (Freiburg, Germany), which used polar coordinates to place the target at the center of a base coordinate head ring (▶ Fig. 2.7). A phantom simulator was created to adjust the arc system, or target bow, so that the arc would facilitate placement of the probe at the target. The arc system was then transferred to the patient's base ring secured to the head, and the procedure began after appropriate burr hole placement. Tailarach and various students working in France used his apparatus to deliver multiple electrodes to targets selected for epilepsy surgery or implantation of radioactive isotopes for tumor management.

The eras of the 1950s and 1960s saw considerable stereotactic activity fostered by an immense interest in surgical options for behavioral, movement, and epileptic disorders. Multiple individual stereotactic devices were constructed depending on the interest of the stereotactic surgeon and then used at other centers when their students moved to new sites. For example, Irving Cooper in New York performed thousands of ablative procedures using his device. Edward Hitchcock, working in

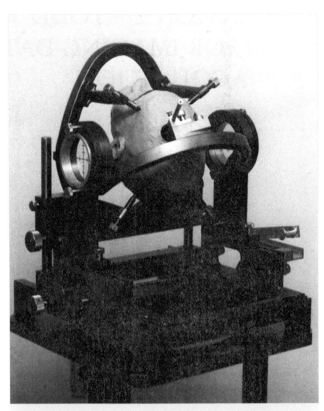

Fig. 2.7 The Todd-Wells system employs the arc-quadrent principle. The patient's head is fixed in a rigid holder that can be moved with three orthogonal degrees of freedom to position an intracranial target at the focal point of a fixed sphere defined by the arc quadrant.

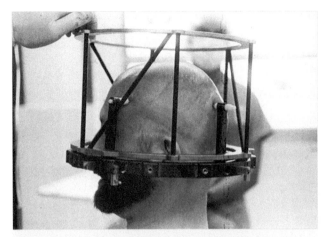

Fig. 2.8 The Brown-Roberts-Wells (BRW) was a CT compatible stereotactic system developed as a result of collaboration between a medical student, a neurosurgeon at the University of Utah, and the biomedical engineer Trent Wells.

Birmingham, England developed a base square device that could be used for functional as well as morphological surgery.

In 1977 Russ Brown described the use of the N localizer to define targets in computed tomography stereotactic space.[14,15] Subsequent collaboration with manufacturer Trent Wells and neurosurgeon Ted Roberts led to the commercial sale and use of the Brown-Roberts-Wells (BRW) device (▶ Fig. 2.8). The target coordinates were determined using a computer system relative to a base ring after determination of the target in stereotactic space. The probe was adjusted using four angular measurements to reproduce a preoperatively chosen trajectory. Using similar principles, the team of John Perry, Arthur Rosenbaum, and Dade Lunsford developed a similar CT compatible guiding device under the auspices of Pfizer Pharmaceuticals, which at the time had a significant interest in imaging technologies (▶ Fig. 2.9).[16]

Eric Cosman modified the BRW frame to facilitate imaging compatible functional and tumor surgery. The frame was then marketed as the Cosman-Roberts-Wells (CRW) device. Pat Kelly modified the original Todd Wells device to create his Kelly Stereotactic system. It incorporated CT imaging with laser and radiofrequency ablative technologies. His stereotactic operating suites at the Mayo Clinic and later at New York University became the most advanced neurosurgical operating rooms developed of the era. They combined advanced targeting imaging with precision CO_2 lasers to vaporize deep-seated brain tumors. His functional neurosurgical practice also used radiofrequency ablation to create thalamic lesions for movement disorders.

In the 1980s modifications of these original devices continued. Lauri Laitinen in Finland described the Laitinen Stereoguide, consisting of an oval shaped base ring with rigid skull fixation and an attached arc to house the probe (▶ Fig. 2.10).[17] Various adapters were used to define the target based on the imaging modality selected – plain X-rays, MRI, or CT.[18]

Most stereotactic devices were made from radiopaque metals. These required reengineering as imaging evolved to the use of CT and MRI. With CT scanning, dense metal could obscure the target or trajectory. With MRI, magnetic susceptibility artifacts became an issue. In response, a variety of aiming devices made of plastic or other imaging neutral compositions emerged in the 1980s. For example, Arun-Angelo Patil designed a device made of composite material that had a base platform and the now-standard detachable arc delivery system.[19]

During this interval from 1977- 2000 most neurosurgical training sites instructed residents on the safe and appropriate use of frame based technologies. The American Society of Testing and Manufacturing (ASTM) required that such devices be able to reliably place a probe at the target with an accuracy of +/– 1 mm. Device accuracy however is dependent on the accuracy and reliability of the imaging used to define the target. By using digital subtraction angiography with a 1024 × 1024 grid, theoretical mechanical accuracy can approach 0.1 mm. Of course, this disregarded brain or target-shift during open stereotactic procedures. Using a 512x 512 grid during CT imaging, accuracy approaches 0.5 mm. For most MRI units, the grid size is 256 × 256, such that accuracies of 1 mm are the maximum that can be obtained. For MRI based stereotactic surgery it is critical that magnetic susceptibility artifacts not distort the target position and imaging. The magnets must be properly shimmed and maintained, and regular verification studies with phantoms must be done to verify continued stereotactic compatibility.

2.3 The 21st Century

It is said that neurosurgery is a field where rediscovery occurs every 25 years. New pioneers never look at the literature more

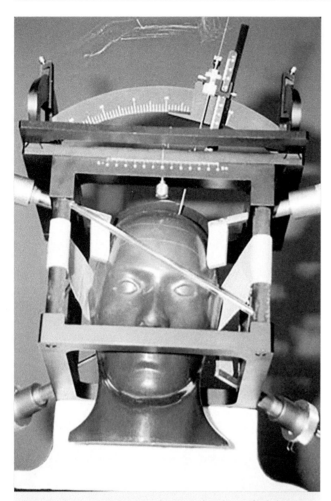

Fig. 2.9 John Perry, Arthur Rosenbaum, and Dade Lunsford also developed a CT compatible guiding device (the Pfizer frame) in 1978. The surgical procedure was performed within the CT scanner itself and led to the creation of the first dedicated intraoperative CT scanner installed at Presbyterian University Hospital, Pittsburgh, in 1982.

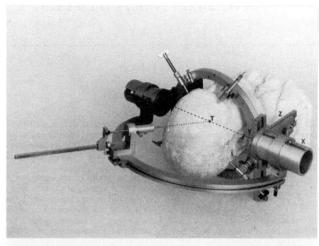

Fig. 2.10 The Laitinen system consists of the Stereoguide (oval base ring, two symmetrical cylinder components and a semicircular arc) and the CT/MRI adapter.

The migration to stereotactic technologies reduced the nearly 30% mortality rate seen with freehand brain tumor biopsy in the 1950's to a simple complication rate of requiring additional surgery of 0.1%.

than 25 years old, and are therefore prone to develop devices as if they were unique. The current emphasis on burr hole mounted probe aiming devices compatible with intraoperative CT or MRI is problematic from several viewpoints. Current neurosurgery trainees are no longer being taught frame based stereotactic techniques. The proponents of these aiming devices have neglected to give credit to the real pioneers such as Spiegel and Wycis who tried and largely abandoned these burr hole mounted systems because of concerns related to accuracy and reliability. Finally, being able to image the brain while passing a probe into it provides no reason for comfort. Repeated probes passes through delicate brain parenchyma increase the risk of hemorrhage with each pass. Note that freehand *mortality* rates in the 1950's during that era of freehand brain tumor biopsies approached 30%. Now, by using special software, a surgeon can plan the probe trajectory to a defined target before passing the needle. In a study of over 2500 frame-based stereotactic patient interventions during a 30-year experience at the University of Pittsburgh, the risk of a complication requiring further surgery was 0.1%.

Over the last 30 years frame-based techniques for target localization and immobilization have greatly enhanced the field of stereotactic radiosurgery. The Leksell Gamma knife alone has been used in more than one million patients. Closed skull obliteration of tumors, vascular malformations, and functional brain targets has revolutionized brain surgery worldwide. The range of applications for radiosurgery has greatly expanded the number and type of cases for which neurosurgeons can provide meaningful minimally invasive assistance to patients. The recent emergence of transcranial focused ultrasound techniques requires continued use of accurate frame based techniques. Similarly, the general field of radiation oncology has been altered by the realization that cranial, spinal, and other targets throughout the body can be reliably targeted using stereotactic methods for the delivery of focused radiation in single or multiple sessions. The "shot in the dark," of the past has given way to the benefits of highly conformal and selective radiation delivery methods that are only possible because of stereotactic principles.

I should conclude with a discussion of robotics. My 1988 textbook *Modern Stereotactic Neurosurgery* described the use of a new stereotactic system designed and built by Y S. Kwoh and colleagues in 1985.[20] Three decades later modifications have culminated in such devices as the ROSA robot. In theory, haptic technologies are able to duplicate the "feel" a brain surgeon develops while working in brain tissue. The role of a robot in brain surgery is evolving, but to paraphrase the "Steve Haines second law of statistics," a difference to be a difference must make a difference. It is incumbent on current and future generations to demonstrate value in the technologies that are being marketed and blithely bought by partially trained surgeons and unknowing hospital executives.

> For an innovation to truly be "significant" it must be more than a statistical parameter, it must make a difference in the lives of our patients. The significance of robots in neurosurgery has yet to be clarified.

References

[1] Gildenberg PL. Stereotactic versus stereotaxic. Neurosurgery. 1993; 32(6): 965–966

[2] Blomstedt P, Olivecrona M, Sailer A, Hariz MI. Dittmar and the history of stereotaxy; or rats, rabbits, and references. Neurosurgery. 2007; 60(1):198–201, discussion 201–202

[3] Zernov D. Encephalometer: Device for estimation of parts of the brain in humans. [in Russian]. Proc Soc Physicomed Moscow Univ.. 1889; 2:70–80

[4] Horsley V, Clarke RH. The structure and functions of the cerebellum examined by a new method. Brain. 1908; 31:45–124

[5] Picard C, Olivier A, Bertrand G. The first human stereotaxic apparatus. The contribution of Aubrey Mussen to the field of stereotaxis. J Neurosurg. 1983; 59(4):673–676

[6] Gildenberg PL. The history of stereotactic neurosurgery. Neurosurg Clin N Am. 1990; 1(4):765–780

[7] Fergusson J. A new system of localization and extraction of foreign bodies in the brain: A preliminary note. Br J Surg. 1918; 6(23):409–417

[8] Kirschner M. Die Punktionstechnik und die Elektrokoagulation des Ganglion Gasseri. Arch Klin Chir. 1933; 176:581–620

[9] Spiegel EA, Wycis HT, Marks M, Lee AJ. Stereotaxic Apparatus for Operations on the Human Brain. Science. 1947; 106(2754):349–350

[10] Spiegel EA, Wycis HT. [Principles and applications of stereoencephalotomy]. Acta Neurochir (Wien). 1950; 1(2–3):137–153

[11] Freeman W, Watts JW. Prefrontal lobotomy; survey of 331 cases. Am J Med Sci. 1946; 211:1–8

[12] Freeman W. Transorbital lobotomy; survey after from 1 to 3 years. Dis Nerv Syst. 1949; 10(12):360–363

[13] Leksell L. The stereotaxic method and radiosurgery of the brain. Acta Chir Scand. 1951; 102(4):316–319

[14] Brown RA. A stereotactic head frame for use with CT body scanners. Invest Radiol. 1979; 14(4):300–304

[15] Brown RA. A computerized tomography-computer graphics approach to stereotaxic localization. J Neurosurg. 1979; 50(6):715–720

[16] Perry JH, Rosenbaum AE, Lunsford LD, Swink CA, Zorub DS. Computed tomography/guided stereotactic surgery: conception and development of a new stereotactic methodology. Neurosurgery. 1980; 7(4):376–381

[17] Laitinen L. A new stereoencephalotome. Zentralbl Neurochir. 1971; 32 (1):67–73

[18] Laitinen LV, Liliequist B, Fagerlund M, Eriksson AT. An adapter for computed tomography-guided stereotaxis. Surg Neurol. 1985; 23(6):559–566

[19] Patil AA. Compute tomography-oriented stereotactic system. Neurosurgery. 1982; 10(3):370–374

[20] Kwoh YS, Hou J, Jonckheere EA, Hayati S. A robot with improved absolute positioning accuracy for CT guided stereotactic brain surgery. IEEE Trans Biomed Eng. 1988; 35(2):153–160

3 Frameless Navigation

Richard Rammo and Jason M. Schwalb

Abstract

Frameless navigation is an easy to use alternative to traditional frame-based stereotactic methods and has become an important neurosurgical tool. There had been concerns about its accuracy. However, advances in technology have improved it to the point that it is as accurate or even more accurate than frame-based techniques. This chapter will first review the principles of stereotactic neurosurgery, then discuss the varieties of frameless navigation devices that are available and their advantages and disadvantages.

Keywords: frameless, stereotaxy, navigation, imaging, fiducials, skull-mounted, arm-based

3.1 Principles of Stereotaxis

Stereotaxis tells us where a surgical instrument is in space. It allows one to limit surgical exposure because adjacent localization landmarks are not needed. Accuracy is the crucial element of functional neurosurgery. By improving accuracy, surgical risk is reduced. While target inaccuracy of 3–4 mm is of little consequence during exposure of a 4 cm tumor, greater precision is needed in functional neuromodulation.[1]

Originally, stereotactic neurosurgery simply involved registration and guidance of a probe to a specific point in space. Contemporary techniques of surgical navigation, or frameless sterotaxy, rely instead on registration of volumes, thereby increasing the method's versatility. An instrument's location is now known in real time and can be tracked relative to known points in the patient's anatomy, either with a traditional frame, optical tracking devices or with magnetic fields.[2]

3.2 Error

While stereotactic accuracy was at first thought to be only a characteristic of the frame used, Maciunas demonstrated that this was one of many factors.[3] Others include the accuracy of the imaging modality, the weight-bearing status of the frame, and patient position.[4] For instance, the prone position is less accurate. It results in a mean error of 2.8 mm in a traditional frame.[4]

CT is generally more accurate than MRI since MRI is subject to field inhomogeneity.[5] As described in the previous chapter, this can be minimized with appropriate quality control and phantom testing. Often, commercial software is used to merge the images from MRI and CT. However, these software packages use proprietary algorithms that are not transparent to the user. They should be used with caution.[3] For lesion generation or placement of electrodes for deep brain stimulation, many have felt that microelectrode recording, macroelectrode recording or, at least intraoperative testing is needed to counteract the inherent inaccuracies of stereotactic surgery with a traditional frame.[6,7]

3.3 Frameless Stereotaxis

Because of its ease of use and patient comfort the field has been moving towards frameless stereotaxy. With frameless surgery, the burden of frame placement, stereotactic planning and imaging while the patient is still wearing the frame is obviated. The fixed head can be referenced to a previously obtained MRI or CT with surface contours, landmarks, adhesive scalp fiducials or bone screws that were inserted before surgery. Imaging can be done at varied times before surgery. A wand can then be tracked relative to a reference arc using either optical or magnetic guidance.[8,9,10] A bulky stereotactic frame is not in the way of the approach and there is greater airway access. Finally, the added time needed to input the coordinates into a stereotactic frame is avoided.

For biopsies or depth electrode placement for epilepsy monitoring, an articulated arm can be attached to the head holder in a fixed relationship to the skull. Software can help the surgeon line up a trajectory to use a twist drill and then a biopsy needle or electrode by progressive adjustment of the articulating arm.

While the accuracy of these techniques has been criticized as being inadequate for many functional procedures (see previous section), the accuracy can be improved with different registration techniques. Not surprisingly, less mobile fiducials yield greater registration precision. Mascott et al., showed that skull-based fiducials are more accurate than non-implanted methods (1.7 ± 0.7 mm vs 4.0 ± 1.7 mm).[11] Thompson et al., also found that bone fiducials yield a lower registration error when compared to skin-based fiducials (1.35 mm versus 1.85 mm).[12]

If greater accuracy or multiple trajectories are needed, robotic systems such as ROSA (Zimmer Biomet, Warsaw, IN) are an option. Planning can be done in advance. Instead of making multiple joint adjustments along an articulated arm, the robot is connected to the head and "drives" to each trajectory. The ROSA robot has an accuracy of 1.59 mm when using a 3 T MRI scan with frameless registration on a phantom.[13] With CT-based imaging this decreases to 0.3 mm.[13] The increased speed that the ROSA provides makes it most useful in stereotactic EEG (sEEG) in which 10–15 different trajectories are needed during depth electrode placements.[14] At our center, we can place a depth electrode every 6 minutes with this device.

> **Potential advantages of frameless over frame-based techniques**
>
> - Frameless is more comfortable
> - No frame movement when using a prone position
> - No loss of accuracy because of the weight of the head
> - The frame is not in the way of the approach

3.4 Skull-mounted Frames

One concern with both the articulated arm and the ROSA is that each device can move relative to the head. They are not fixed to the skull. A skull-mounted frame can reduce this risk.

There are two different skull-mounted frames that have been used in stereotaxy – the NexFrame (Medtronic, Minneapolis, MN) and STarFix (FHC, Bowdoin, ME). NexFrame mounts over a pre set burr hole. It has a central element with limited rotation and translation. The trajectory can be varied without needing a cumbersome frame.[15] However, there are increased disposable costs per case since the skull-mounted frames cannot be reused. The accuracy of this device is 0.6–2.2 mm, which is comparable to that in both the Leksell and CRW frames.[9,16,17,18]

The STarFix, which stands for Surgical Targeting Fixture, is built using 3D printing technology and mounts onto pre-placed bone fiducials. These bone fiducials are inserted a week before surgery. Data from a subsequent high-resolution CT scan is relayed to the manufacturer who creates a disposable sterile frame that connects to the bone fiducials. The frame is mounted in the OR and the stereotactic trajectory is calculated. The accuracy of StarFix is 1.99 mm. This is similar to that obtained with the NexFrame.[19] StarFix, however, has the disadvantage of requiring the bone fiducials to be inserted days in advance of the planned procedure. Also, the use of a custom, pre-fixed frame limits trajectory variation. Two constructed frames are delivered by the manufacturer, but, if both are contaminated, the case must be aborted.

A third skull-mounted stereotactic guide is known as the Renaissance Guidance System (Mazor Robotics, Caesarea, Israel). The system includes a workstation with which trajectories are planned before surgery and uploaded to a robot. The robot is mounted on the skull, and the cylindrical device changes its conformation to align its guidance channel with the planned trajectory. A biopsy needle, RF probe, or other instrument is inserted through the channel to reach the desired target.

> Intraoperative re-registration and accuracy confirmation can with frameless systems yield even greater precision than can be achieved with traditional frame-based systems.

3.5 Intraoperative Reregistration and Confirmation of Accuracy

Even with a system that is fixed to the skull and yields accurate registration, intraoperative brain shift can affect probe placement accuracy. The brain will move relative to the skull during tumor removal or simply from CSF egress and air ingress.[20,21,22] Intraoperative reregistration with MRI, CT or ultrasound can adjust for this error.[15,23,24] Initial registration occurs before the incision, then re-registration with a repeat scan is done just before the critical portion of the operation. By adding this extra step one can reduce inaccuracies caused by parenchymal shift.

Intraoperative imaging can also be used to confirm accurate placement of a probe or electrode before completion of surgery. These methods use anatomic accuracy to determine the target instead of the more traditional MER. Burchiel et al., described the use of an intraoperative CT that is done after placement of the DBS electrode.[23] This scan is then merged with the

Table 3.1 Sources of inaccuracy in frameless stereotaxis and potential remedies

Source of Inaccuracy	Potential Remedy
Accuracy of instrument holder	Minimize number of joints
Accuracy of imaging modality, e.g., ventricuography, CT, MRI	CT has greater accuracy than MRI Decrease distance between slices
Accuracy of registration method	Less mobile bone screws are generally more accurate than surface landmarks or adhesive fiducials
Movement of the patient relative to the frame or fiducial	Strong fixation Bone screws
Brain shift	Minimize opening: twist drill rather than burrhole Avoid traversing the ventricular system Fibrin glue to prevent air entry and CSF loss Reregistration with intraoperative ventriculography, ultrasound CT or MRI
Deviation of the instrument	Stiffer cannulae Avoid collisions with adjacent bone
Surgeon error	Multiple people checking calculations Checklist use

preoperative imaging and analyzed for any deviation from the target. With efficient electrode placement or with a smaller dural opening, risk of shift can be minimized.

An alternate method to counteract brain shift uses the MRI scanner and recursive imaging. The ClearPoint system was developed specifically for intraoperative MRI (iMRI). It uses a modified frameless skull-mounted frame, adapted from the NexFrame, as the stereotactic guide (SMARTFrame).[9] The target is reassessed before a parenchymal pass is done and changes are made to account for brain shift. Accuracy is confirmed before skin closure. ClearPoint has a mean radial error that ranges from 0.5 ± 0.3 mm (in initial phantom studies) to 0.8 mm ± 0.3 mm with in-vivo GPi targets.[9,25] The two main disadvantages of this system are the high cost of its disposables and the need to perform the procedure inside an MRI scanner.

3.6 Conclusion

Frameless neuronavigation is complicated by errors that are similar to frame-based stereotaxis (▶ Table 3.1). However, in many cases frameless systems have the advantages of ease of usage and patient comfort. Under certain circumstances, frameless systems can yield more precise probe placement than traditional stereotactic frames.

References

[1] Ellis T-M, Foote KD, Fernandez HH, et al. Reoperation for suboptimal outcomes after deep brain stimulation surgery. Neurosurgery. 2008; 63(4): 754–760, discussion 760–761

[2] Grunert P, Darabi K, Espinosa J, Filippi R. Computer-aided navigation in neurosurgery. Neurosurg Rev. 2003; 26(2):73–99, discussion 100–101

[3] Maciunas RJ, Galloway RL , Jr, Latimer JW. The application accuracy of stereotactic frames. Neurosurgery. 1994; 35(4):682–694, discussion 694–695

[4] Rohlfing T, Maurer CR , Jr, Dean D, Maciunas RJ. Effect of changing patient position from supine to prone on the accuracy of a Brown-Roberts-Wells stereotactic head frame system. Neurosurgery. 2003; 52(3):610–618, discussion 617–618

[5] Langlois S, Desvignes M, Constans JM, Revenu M. MRI geometric distortion: a simple approach to correcting the effects of non-linear gradient fields. J Magn Reson Imaging. 1999; 9(6):821–831

[6] Gross RE, Krack P, Rodriguez-Oroz MC, Rezai AR, Benabid A-L. Electrophysiological mapping for the implantation of deep brain stimulators for Parkinson's disease and tremor. Mov Disord. 2006; 21 Suppl 14:S259–S283

[7] McClelland S , III, Ford B, Senatus PB, et al. Subthalamic stimulation for Parkinson disease: determination of electrode location necessary for clinical efficacy. Neurosurg Focus. 2005; 19(5):E12

[8] Hemm S, Wårdell K. Stereotactic implantation of deep brain stimulation electrodes: a review of technical systems, methods and emerging tools. Med Biol Eng Comput. 2010; 48(7):611–624

[9] Larson PS, Starr PA, Bates G, Tansey L, Richardson RM, Martin AJ. An optimized system for interventional magnetic resonance imaging-guided stereotactic surgery: preliminary evaluation of targeting accuracy. Neurosurgery. 2012; 70(1) Suppl Operative:95–103, discussion 103

[10] McInerney J, Roberts DW. Frameless stereotaxy of the brain. Mt Sinai J Med. 2000; 67(4):300–310

[11] Mascott CR, Sol J-C, Bousquet P, Lagarrigue J, Lazorthes Y, Lauwers-Cances V. Quantification of true in vivo (application) accuracy in cranial image-guided surgery: influence of mode of patient registration. Neurosurgery. 2006; 59(1) Suppl 1:ONS146–ONS156, discussion ONS146–ONS156

[12] Thompson EM, Anderson GJ, Roberts CM, Hunt MA, Selden NR. Skull-fixated fiducial markers improve accuracy in staged frameless stereotactic epilepsy surgery in children. J Neurosurg Pediatr. 2011; 7(1):116–119

[13] Lefranc M, Capel C, Pruvot AS, et al. The impact of the reference imaging modality, registration method and intraoperative flat-panel computed tomography on the accuracy of the ROSA® stereotactic robot. Stereotact Funct Neurosurg. 2014; 92(4):242–250

[14] Alomar S, Jones J, Maldonado A, Gonzalez-Martinez J. The Stereo-Electroencephalography Methodology. Neurosurg Clin N Am. 2016; 27(1):83–95

[15] Starr PA, Martin AJ, Larson PS. Implantation of deep brain stimulator electrodes using interventional MRI. Neurosurg Clin N Am. 2009; 20(2):193–203

[16] Bot M, van den Munckhof P, Bakay R, Sierens D, Stebbins G, Verhagen Metman L. Analysis of Stereotactic Accuracy in Patients Undergoing Deep Brain Stimulation Using Nexframe and the Leksell Frame. Stereotact Funct Neurosurg. 2015; 93(5):316–325

[17] Kelman C, Ramakrishnan V, Davies A, Holloway K. Analysis of stereotactic accuracy of the cosman-robert-wells frame and nexframe frameless systems in deep brain stimulation surgery. Stereotact Funct Neurosurg. 2010; 88(5):288–295

[18] Sharma M, Rhiew R, Deogaonkar M, Rezai A, Boulis N. Accuracy and precision of targeting using frameless stereotactic system in deep brain stimulator implantation surgery. Neurol India. 2014; 62(5):503–509

[19] Konrad PE, Neimat JS, Yu H, et al. Customized, miniature rapid-prototype stereotactic frames for use in deep brain stimulator surgery: initial clinical methodology and experience from 263 patients from 2002 to 2008. Stereotact Funct Neurosurg. 2011; 89(1):34–41

[20] Halpern CH, Danish SF, Baltuch GH, Jaggi JL. Brain shift during deep brain stimulation surgery for Parkinson's disease. Stereotact Funct Neurosurg. 2008; 86(1):37–43

[21] Ivan ME, Yarlagadda J, Saxena AP, et al. Brain shift during bur hole-based procedures using interventional MRI. J Neurosurg. 2014; 121(1):149–160

[22] Wirtz CR, Tronnier VM, Bonsanto MM, et al. Image-guided neurosurgery with intraoperative MRI: update of frameless stereotaxy and radicality control. Stereotact Funct Neurosurg. 1997; 68(1–4 Pt 1):39–43

[23] Burchiel KJ, McCartney S, Lee A, Raslan AM. Accuracy of deep brain stimulation electrode placement using intraoperative computed tomography without microelectrode recording. J Neurosurg. 2013; 119(2):301–306

[24] Riva M, Hennersperger C, Milletari F, et al. 3D intra-operative ultrasound and MR image guidance: pursuing an ultrasound-based management of brainshift to enhance neuronavigation. Int J CARS. 2017; 12(10):1711–1725

[25] Sidiropoulos C, Rammo R, Merker B, et al. Intraoperative MRI for deep brain stimulation lead placement in Parkinson's disease: 1 year motor and neuropsychological outcomes. J Neurol. 2016; 263(6):1226–1231

4 MRI and CT Imaging with Stereotactic Neurosurgery

Ashesh Thaker and Aviva Abosch

Abstract

Computed tomography (CT) and magnetic resonance imaging (MRI) are critical to stereotactic neurosurgery, and advances in imaging techniques have improved patient selection, anatomic targeting, and intraoperative trajectory planning. An understanding of the principles of frame-based and frameless imaging, basic CT and MRI imaging techniques, and MRI safety is indispensable for practitioners of stereotactic and functional neurosurgery.

Keywords: computed tomography (CT), magnetic resonance imaging (MRI), stereotactic frame, MRI safety

4.1 Introduction

Advances in modern neurosurgery have been synchronous with advances in neuroimaging. Roentgen's X-rays in 1895, Dandy's pneumoencephalography in 1918 and Moniz's angiography in 1927 each provided a stepping-stone for neurosurgical progress. CT and MRI imaging techniques and subsequent refinements in its diagnostic equipment have since led to dramatic improvements in neurosurgery, and to the patients served by it. Such benefits include improved diagnosis, more appropriate patient selection, enhanced target resolution, and optimized trajectory planning—all crucial to the field of stereotactic neurosurgery. This chapter will focus on current techniques for CT and MRI imaging in stereotactic neurosurgery, with an emphasis on imaging of the basal ganglia for the surgical treatment of movement disorders.

4.2 Imaging in Frames

In 1908 Horsley and Clarke established the principles of stereotactic technique for vertebrates. Their guiding device provided accurate localization of feline intracranial structures by ascertaining three-dimensional target coordinates with reference to skull landmarks and an external coordinate system.[1] In the 1940s, Spiegel and Wycis developed a skull-mounted rigid stereotactic frame and used contrast ventriculography with it to identify cerebral landmarks. The anterior and posterior commissural coordinates (AC-PC) are acquired by imaging the brain while the patient wears an applied frame. These points are correlated with stereotactic atlases to define spatial relationships (▶ Fig. 4.1). Important to movement disorders are the identifiable targets: ventrointermediate nucleus of the thalamus (Vim), subthalamic nucleus (STN), and the globus pallidum pars interna (GPi). *Indirect targeting* is a technique that makes use of consensus coordinates for the location of each target structure. Stereotactic atlases based on neural landmarks do not eliminate the problem of anatomic variability in patients, and either microelectrode recording or macrostimulation must be used to confirm the functional target. *Direct targeting* uses MRI and/or CT-MRI fusion to identify brain targets based on direct visualization of the target on MRI.

Indirect targeting: target localization based on consensus coordinates.

Direct targeting: target identification using MRI and or CT-MRI fusion with direct visualization of the target on the MRI.

Visualization of the Vim, the target for the treatment of tremor, is not possible using available MRI sequences at 3-Tesla, requiring indirect targeting with physiological confirmation techniques. 7-Tesla MRIs can visualize internal thalamic nuclei, and hold promise for improving anatomic-based targeting in DBS surgery.[2]

Modern stereotactic frames are MRI compatible and safe within MRI systems, with minimal distortion of the magnetic field. Still, even slight geometric distortion can be an issue, particularly close to the base of the frame, which therefore is positioned as far away from the target region as possible. Frames with smaller fiducial indicator boxes,such as the Laitinen and Leksell systems, produce less geometric distortion than their larger counterparts.[1]

4.3 Frameless Imaging

While rigid head frames have been essential to the origin of stereotactic technique, they have disadvantages. Frames simplify targeting of a single point in space with a probe. They are not designed to localize an instrument on an image.[3] Also, the physical frame itself is a constraint during surgery. It is uncomfortable

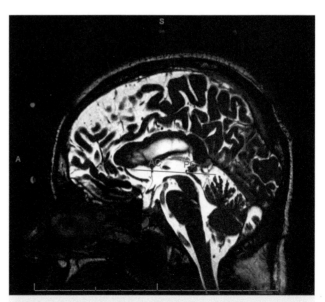

Fig. 4.1 Sagittal CISS sequence obtained with a rigid head frame, prior to DBS surgery for Parkinson's disease. The AC-PC line is indicated in red.

for patients to wear them. Large head circumferences may make them difficult to apply. In awake patients frameless stereotaxy can be combined with microelectrode recording and with macro-stimulation to verify correct placement. In asleep patients intra-operative MRI imaging alone can be used with a frameless system.

4.4 CT Imaging Techniques

CT provides excellent spatial and temporal resolution with superior delineation of bony anatomy and landmarks compared with MRI. CT is less prone to motion degradation and artifacts from the magnetic field inhomogeneity that may be present on MRI when metallic implants are used. However, CT as a sole imaging modality lacks sufficient soft tissue contrast for most stereotactic neurosurgery applications. The AC-PC line is difficult to identify if the head is not precisely aligned in the CT gantry. Deep gray structures are not well delineated by CT, particularly when a stereotactic frame is present. For this reason, images from CT scans are often fused with those from MRI, to combine advantages in both modalities (▶ Fig. 4.2).[4] CT protocols compatible with commercial surgical navigation software require contiguous (no gap or overlap) slices of 1–2 mm, axial (not helical) acquisition, no gantry tilt, and coverage of the entire head to include the hard palate, tip of the nose, both ears, the top of the head, and all fiducial markers. See Table 4-1 for the DBS planning CT protocol at our institution.

Table 4.1 Typical CT protocol for surgical planning prior to DBS electrode placement at our institution.

Scan type/gating	Axial	RECONSTRUCTIONS
Scan direction	Caudo-cranial	
Scan start	Skull base	3 mm x 3 mm CEREBRUM (230 mm FOV)
Scan stop	Through top of frame	1 mm x 1 mm CEREBRUM (300 mm FOV)
Breath hold	None	3 mm x 3 mm BONE (230 mm FOV)
IV contrast/saline	None	

4.5 MRI Imaging Techniques

MRI is the main imaging modality in stereotactic neurosurgery. However, low image quality on traditional 1.5 tesla (T) machines and antiquated pulse sequences that do not provide adequate contrast at the level of the globus pallidus interna (GPi) and subthalamic nucleus (STN) have limited the movement to direct targeting in some centers. At higher field strengths, image distortion may be unacceptable. Traditional stereotactic head frames and localizers are usually too bulky to permit the use of high-quality, multichannel MRI head coils.[5] High field strength scanners and new pulse sequences have, however, improved image quality. Advances in the technique and equipment used with intraoperative MRI, have led to increased adoption of direct targeting of the GPi and STN. However, adjuncts such as MRI-to-CT image fusion and intraoperative electrophysiology still play an important role in these surgeries at most institutions.

Standard MRI sequences for targeting the globus pallidus interna (GPi) and subthalamic nucleus (STN) include T1, SWI, T2*WI, phase-sensitive inversion recovery (PSIR), and IR-FSE. Trajectory planning is done with volumetric gadolinium-enhanced T1 images. They offer high spatial resolution and large vessel visualization. Targeted high-resolution axial fast spin echo (FSE) T2-weighted images are used to localize the target and show the electrode tip. SWI and IR sequences help to localize STN and identify the GPi and GPe border (▶ Fig. 4.3). These same sequences may be used intra-operatively to guide electrode placement. Specific protocols and parameters vary by institution, but a review of common sequences and image acquisition parameters can be found in the article by Starr et al., (Table 4-1).[6]

4.6 MRI Safety

Postoperative MRI is standard after DBS surgery to determine whether the implanted lead is positioned appropriately and to look for evidence of surgical hemorrhage. When imaging DBS leads, there are safety concerns from overheating of the lead with radiofrequency induced current. FDA-approved guidelines for DBS system imaging include: 1.5 Tesla magnet strength, a limitation on the applied head specific absorption rate (SAR) to 0.1 W/kg, and the use of a transmit/receive head coil only. This

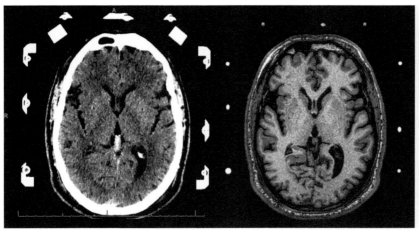

Fig. 4.2 Axial CT (left) and axial 3D T1 SPGR (right) performed with a stereotactic head frame, at the level of the basal ganglia in a patient with Parkinson's disease.

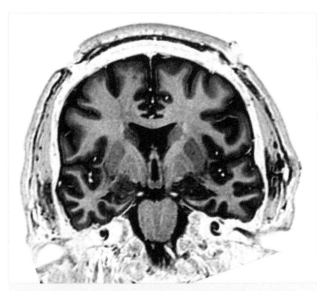

Fig. 4.3 Coronal IR-TSE sequence demonstrates excellent contrast between the striatum and pallidum.

limits the energy that can be delivered with the RF pulse.[7,8] With proper precautions, however, MRI can be performed safely in patients with implanted DBS devices.[9] Furthermore, with more than 150,000 DBS devices implanted worldwide, there is an expanding population of patients in whom the need for MR imaging is the same as all other patients.

4.7 Conclusion

High quality CT and MRI is critical to frame-based and frameless stereotactic neurosurgery. It improves patient selection and optimizes anatomic targeting, and trajectory planning. Future advances in neuroimaging techniques will further the preoperative and intraoperative evaluation of stereotactic and functional neurosurgical patients.

References

[1] Zrinzo L. The role of imaging in the surgical treatment of movement disorders. Neuroimaging Clin N Am. 2010; 20(1):125–140

[2] Abosch A, Yacoub E, Ugurbil K, Harel N. An assessment of current brain targets for deep brain stimulation surgery with susceptibility-weighted imaging at 7 tesla. Neurosurgery. 2010; 67(6):1745–1756, discussion 1756

[3] McInerney J, Roberts DW. Frameless stereotaxy of the brain. Mt Sinai J Med. 2000; 67(4):300–310

[4] Risholm P, Golby AJ, Wells W , III. Multimodal image registration for preoperative planning and image-guided neurosurgical procedures. Neurosurg Clin N Am. 2011; 22(2):197–206, viii

[5] Chandran AS, Bynevelt M, Lind CRP. Magnetic resonance imaging of the subthalamic nucleus for deep brain stimulation. J Neurosurg. 2016; 124(1):96–105

[6] Starr PA, Martin AJ, Larson PS. Implantation of deep brain stimulator electrodes using interventional MRI. Neurosurg Clin N Am. 2009; 20(2):193–203

[7] Larson PS, Richardson RM, Starr PA, Martin AJ. Magnetic resonance imaging of implanted deep brain stimulators: experience in a large series. Stereotact Funct Neurosurg. 2008; 86(2):92–100

[8] Dormont D, Seidenwurm D, Galanaud D, Cornu P, Yelnik J, Bardinet E. Neuroimaging and deep brain stimulation. AJNR Am J Neuroradiol. 2010; 31(1):15–23

[9] Chhabra V, Sung E, Mewes K, Bakay RA, Abosch A, Gross RE. Safety of magnetic resonance imaging of deep brain stimulator systems: a serial imaging and clinical retrospective study. J Neurosurg. 2010; 112(3):497–502

5 Functional Neuroimaging I: fMRI and Resting State fMRI

Aaron Kucyi, Jason L. Chan, Stephan Bickel and Josef Parvizi

Abstract

Functional magnetic resonance imaging (fMRI) is a useful strategy for presurgical planning and operative guidance in neurosurgery. This chapter will review what fMRI measures, applications of presurgical fMRI for localizing individual-specific functional anatomy, and methodological issues that should be considered when interpreting functional neuroimaging data in individual cases. The focus will be on planning for tissue resection in epilepsy and tumor surgery. The current applications and potential uses of functional neuroimaging for guiding deep-brain stimulation implantation in movement disorders, chronic pain and psychiatric disorders will also be described.

In the common "task-based" fMRI approach, brain activity is measured while a patient performs tasks that involve sensorimotor, language and memory functions to localize eloquent cortex. Recent developments suggest that "resting-state" fMRI, in which spontaneous brain activity is measured while a patient is in a task-free state, is a feasible, and potentially more useful, alternative for presurgical mapping of a broader range of functional regions. In both approaches, due to low signal-to-noise, data analysis issues, and the correlational nature of the approach, fMRI data in individual cases must be interpreted with caution. Ongoing research efforts are leading to increased sensitivity and specificity of functional neuroimaging, which may enable more effective and broader applications for personalized functional neurosurgery in the future.

Keywords: epilepsy, functional connectivity, presurgical mapping, fMRI, resting state, eloquent cortex, language

Task-based fMRI measures brain activity during instructed task performance.

Resting state fMRI measures spontaneous brain activity in a task free state.

The human brain is composed of local regions that have specialized functions in sensation, movement, and cognition. Yet, a survey map of anatomical landmarks is often unable to provide accurate inference about the functional importance of a given brain region, and the potential impact of injury to it. Thus, noninvasive functional neuroimaging has emerged as an attractive strategy for surgical guidance.

Functional neuroimaging methods, including functional magnetic resonance imaging (fMRI) and positron emission tomography (PET), involve indirect measures of neural activity, relying on changes in cerebral blood flow or metabolic activity that reflect the electrophysiological signaling of neuronal populations.[1] Blood-oxygen-level dependent (BOLD) fMRI, which is sensitive to the magnetic properties of deoxyhemoglobin in blood, is the most popular approach. In BOLD fMRI, with standard scanners of 1.5–3 Tesla strength, whole-brain activity is sampled every 2–3 seconds in spatial units of cubic voxels that are 2–4 mm³. New advances enable higher resolution.[2] Thus, in gray matter locations, voxel-level activity may reflect the pooled activity of hundreds of thousands of neurons. The BOLD response is said to be 'sluggish' in that it begins several seconds after an increase in neuronal activity, and plateaus after 6–12 seconds.[1] The BOLD signal is partly contaminated with non-neuronal 'noise.' Examples of such contamination include scanner-related and head-motion artifacts, respiratory and cardiac signals. Care must then be taken in data acquisition and its analysis.

fMRI is predominantly a research tool. Presurgical mapping is its most common clinical application. It is most often used for epilepsy surgery and tumor resections, but its role is expanding to involve planning for implanted electrodes in the treatment of movement disorders, chronic pain, and psychiatric disorders. The goal of presurgical fMRI, is to locate eloquent cortex such as in primary sensory, motor and language-dominant regions. Another application that has been used with limited success is fMRI for localization of epileptic tissue (see also Chapter 20 for discussion of EEG and imaging).[3] The relative effectiveness of fMRI may vary depending on the specific goal and case.

In presurgical fMRI, a "task-based" approach is used in which patients may perform such tasks as finger-tapping, over multiple time blocks that are interspersed with task-free periods. These tasks have not been standardized. Importantly, task-based fMRI is a correlational approach. For example, increased motor cortex activation during tongue movement does not indicate that the activated region is necessary and sufficient for tongue movement. Thus, since the earliest applications of presurgical fMRI, results have been verified using the effects of electrical cortical stimulation following neurosurgical implantation of electrode contacts.[4] For example, does stimulation of the BOLD-active region cause tongue movement? While there is often good overlap between fMRI results and electrical stimulation mapping of early sensory areas, the correspondence is not always straightforward. The fMRI results can also be compared to those from the more invasive intracarotid amobarbital procedure, or "Wada" test, in which a barbiturate is injected into the right or left internal carotid artery to inactivate one hemisphere. Results of task-based fMRI often show correspondence with the Wada test for mapping language- and memory-related functions. Results are more reliable for language than for memory testing. Currently, the American Academy of Neurology recommends that presurgical task-based fMRI for certain epilepsy subtypes be considered for lateralizing language, and in limited cases, memory functions, in place of the Wada test.[5]

Task-based fMRI requires time for instruction and training, expertise to conduct, and patient cooperation and compliance. Furthermore, the benefit of functionally localizing sensorimotor areas is often unclear, as they can be broadly identified anatomically with structural MRI. A distinct approach, known as "resting-state" (rs-fMRI, has been developed as a clinically feasible and potentially more effective approach for mapping a broader range of functional regions.[6] In rs-fMRI, the patient is instructed to *not* think about anything in particular for several minutes. Spontaneous brain activity is analyzed with correlations of BOLD time series among remote regions of the brain.

Regions that have synchronized activity are said to exhibit "functional connectivity," denoting integration into a network. Each brain region can be classified according to the network(s) to which it belongs. Research in healthy adults has revealed that segregated networks throughout the brain, including those related to sensorimotor, language, and memory processes, are readily identifiable and are reproducible in rs-fMRI.[7] Moreover, presurgical rs-fMRI functional connectivity of sensorimotor regions has been shown to correspond with the results of intracranial cortical stimulation better than with task-based activation.[8]

The rs-fMRI method is attractive both because of its demonstrated effectiveness and because of the ease of implementation. It requires little active participation from the patient. Additionally, theoretical concepts from basic neuroscience support the use of rs-fMRI. Converging evidence suggests that spontaneous correlated activity, when considered over at least several minutes, reflects the 'intrinsic' organization of the brain that is partly constrained by anatomical connectivity and that is predictive of functional co-activation during tasks.[9] Spontaneous activity is continuous and thus its study is not limited to the resting-state context. Indeed, task-based fMRI lasting several minutes can be analyzed with both task-based activation and spontaneous functional connectivity approaches. In a new development, the combination of these two analyses outperformed individual analysis of identifying sensorimotor regions that correspond with the output of direct cortical stimulation.[10]

However, several issues in functional connectivity analysis remain unresolved. Compared to task-based fMRI, the analysis is more error prone from non-neural noise factors such as head motion. Special care is needed in data preprocessing, although no consensus has yet been reached on best practices.[11] Moreover, the ideal scan duration remains unknown. Scans longer than six minutes or multiple scans are known to produce more reliable results but may not always be clinically feasible.[12] In both task-based and rs-fMRI, the data processing strategies and statistical thresholds used are variable. Standards for general fMRI data analysis are beginning to emerge,[13] and some such practices could be adopted clinically.

Although less common in practice, task-based and functional connectivity approaches to functional neuroimaging have been applied to psychiatric disorders.[14] In treatment-resistant major depressive disorder, PET and fMRI have been used to identify mood circuitry to target with deep brain stimulation.[15] In addition, there is evidence that intrinsic rs-fMRI networks have relevance for personalized targeting of regions related to cognitive and affective dysfunctions. For example, intracranial stimulation of a mid-cingulate cortex region that was individually mapped to the rs-fMRI "salience network" caused a stereotyped cognitive and affective experience that could be described as a "will to persevere."[16]

Future such research may lead to a broader range of applications for personalized functional neurosurgery.

References

[1] Heeger DJ, Ress D. What does fMRI tell us about neuronal activity? Nature Reviews Neuroscience. 2002;3(2):142-151.

[2] Feinberg DA, Setsompop K. Ultra-fast MRI of the human brain with simultaneous multi-slice imaging. Journal of magnetic resonance. 2013;229:90-100.

[3] Stufflebeam SM, Liu H, Sepulcre J, Tanaka N, Buckner RL, Madsen JR. Localization of focal epileptic discharges using functional connectivity magnetic resonance imaging. Journal of neurosurgery. 2011;114(6):1693-1697.

[4] Jack CR, Jr., Thompson RM, Butts RK, et al. Sensory motor cortex: Correlation of presurgical mapping with functional MR imaging and invasive cortical mapping. Radiology. 1994;190:85-92.

[5] Szaflarski JP, Gloss D, Binder JR, et al. Practice guideline summary: Use of fMRI in the presurgical evaluation of patients with epilepsy: Report of the Guideline Development, Dissemination, and Implementation Subcommittee of the American Academy of Neurology. Neurology. 2017;88(4):395-402.

[6] Zhang D, Johnston JM, Fox MD, et al. Preoperative sensorimotor mapping in brain tumor patients using spontaneous fluctuations in neuronal activity imaged with functional magnetic resonance imaging: initial experience. Neurosurgery. 2009;65(6 Suppl):226-236.

[7] Yeo BT, Krienen FM, Sepulcre J, et al. The organization of the human cerebral cortex estimated by intrinsic functional connectivity. Journal of neurophysiology. 2011;106(3):1125-1165.

[8] Wang D, Buckner RL, Fox MD, et al. Parcellating cortical functional networks in individuals. Nature neuroscience. 2015;18(12):1853-1860.

[9] Fox MD, Raichle ME. Spontaneous fluctuations in brain activity observed with functional magnetic resonance imaging. Nature Reviews Neuroscience. 2007;8(9):700-711.

[10] Fox MD, Qian T, Madsen JR, et al. Combining task-evoked and spontaneous activity to improve pre-operative brain mapping with fMRI. NeuroImage. 2016;124(Pt A):714-723.

[11] Power JD, Schlaggar BL, Petersen SE. Recent progress and outstanding issues in motion correction in resting state fMRI. NeuroImage. 2015;105C:536-551.

[12] Laumann TO, Gordon EM, Adeyemo B, et al. Functional System and Areal Organization of a Highly Sampled Individual Human Brain. Neuron. 2015;87 (3):657-670.

[13] Nichols TE, Das S, Eickhoff SB, et al. Best practices in data analysis and sharing in neuroimaging using MRI. Nature neuroscience. 2017;20(3):299-303.

[14] Dyster TG, Mikell CB, Sheth SA. The Co-evolution of Neuroimaging and Psychiatric Neurosurgery. Frontiers in neuroanatomy. 2016;10:68.

[15] Mayberg HS. Targeted electrode-based modulation of neural circuits for depression. The Journal of clinical investigation. 2009;119(4):717-725.

[16] Parvizi J, Rangarajan V, Shirer WR, Desai N, Greicius MD. The will to persevere induced by electrical stimulation of the human cingulate gyrus. Neuron. 2013;80(6):1359-1367.

6 Functional Neuroimaging II

Walid I. Essayed, Prashin Unadkat and Alexandra J. Golby

Abstract

Functional neuroimaging is a constantly evolving and increasingly important tool for modern neurosurgery including preoperative and intraoperative surgical guidance. With the development of these modern techniques, frontiers between anatomical, microstructural, metabolic, and functional imaging have become blurred. In this chapter, we review the state of the art of currently available methods, while emphasizing advantages and limitations of each technique, The chapter is structured around the physiological basis of the modalities: metabolic for fMRI, PET and indirectly tractography, versus electrophysiological for TMS and MSI.

Keywords: functional neuroimaging, fMRI, positron emission tomography, PET, tractography, DTI, transcranial magnetic stimulation, nTMS, magnetic source imaging, MEG

Functional neuroimaging is a continuously evolving and increasingly important tool for modern neurosurgery including preoperative and intraoperative surgical guidance. In this chapter, we will review the state of the art of currently available methods, while emphasizing advantages and limitations of each technique, understanding of which is imperative for judicious use and interpretation.

With the development of these modern techniques, frontiers between anatomical, microstructural, metabolic, and functional imaging have become blurred. Techniques such as fMRI (functional Magnetic Resonance Imaging) and PET (Positron Emission Tomography) are directly based on metabolic underpinnings of the biological function, while tractography is based on the structural substrate of the function, specifically water molecule distribution along myelinated white matter fibers axons. Other modalities such as TMS (Transcranial Magnetic Stimulation) and MSI (Magnetic Source Imaging) are founded on the electromagnetic properties associated with the electrical neuronal function. We limit our review to these techniques and will not include other methods such as perfusion-MR, MR spectroscopy, and EEG. The chapter is structured around specific imaged function: metabolic for fMRI, PET, and indirectly tractography, versus electrophysiological for TMS and MSI.

Metabolic Function Functional Magnetic Resonance Imaging is the most popular modality used to understand the functional neuroanatomy of the the cortex, and is clinically used to understand the relationship of functional areas with respect to some lesion or underlying pathology. The growing popularity of clinical fMRI is in part due to the increasing availability of high field strength magnets at most centers, relatively short scan time, non-invasiveness, and the absence of any known side effects.

Direct Methods The physiological basis of fMRI is the blood oxygen level dependent (BOLD) signal. Principally based on the phenomenon of neurovascular coupling, task related neuronal activity within specific areas of the cortex leads to a greater increase in cerebral blood flow (CBF) as compared to the increased cerebral metabolic rate of oxygen ($CMRO_2$) within that region.

fMRI Specifically, deoxyhemoglobin is used as an endogenous paramagnetic contrast agent, leading to a drop in the fMRI signal. In the region of neuronal activation, dilution of paramagnetic substance by a relative increase in oxyhemoglobin, which is diamagnetic, leads to an overall increase in the fMRI signal on the $T2^*$-weighted images, which forms the basis of BOLD fMRI. Gradient-echo fMRI is the most widely used sequence for clinical applications due to its high sensitivity. High resolution fMRI is heavily dependent on a favorable signal to noise ratio.

6.1 Artifacts and Limitations

Several imaging artifacts can adversely impact the quality of fMRI. Motion related artifacts, caused by voluntary movement or breathing can compromise results. Susceptibility artifacts from prior surgeries or tissue interfaces can lead to signal dropout. BOLD signal from large venous structures may give false-positive results and do not represent true neuronal activity. The neurovascular decoupling that occurs due to abnormal hemodynamic autoregulation around tumors, can lead to false negative results. Lastly, although fMRI has excellent spatial resolution, the delayed hemodynamic response to neuronal activity reduces the temporal resolution compared to electrophysiologic brain mapping techniques like Magnetoencephalography (MEG).

6.2 Task Paradigm Selection

Since its advent, fMRI has been increasingly useful to guide medical and surgical care in different brain pathologies. While multiple functions have been mapped, commonly tested in presurgical evaluations are motor, sensory, language, vision and occasionally memory.

Depending on the function of interest, the patient performs a specific task paradigm with a "block" or "event-related" design. Patient preparation with pre-exam explanation and assessment of the ability to follow task instructions reduces false-positive and false-negative results. Careful adjustment of task paradigms depending on patient age or pre-existing neurological deficit may be warranted to insure adequate task performance.

6.3 Key Applications

- Motor, sensory, and language mapping for risk stratification and surgical planning in tumor resection and epilepsy surgery (▶ Fig. 6.1).[1,2]
- Validation and guidance of other techniques: preoperative white matter tractography, intraoperative direct cortical stimulation guidance, decreasing the risk of induced seizures and patient fatigue during awake surgery (▶ Fig. 6.1).[2]
- Assessment of neuroplasticity and its prognostic correspondences.[3]

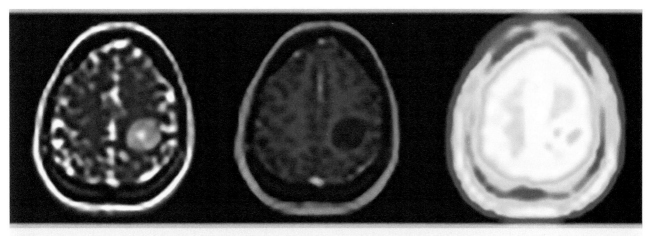

Fig. 6.1 30 y.o. female with a left W.H.O grade III oligodendroglioma in the motor cortex. The lesion has a relatively homogenous hypo T1 and hyper T2 signal, without any contrast enhancement. The PET study (F-18 fluroethyltyrosine) shows areas of high uptake within the lesion. These results directed the focused histopathological assessment, confirming the anaplastic nature of this lesion.

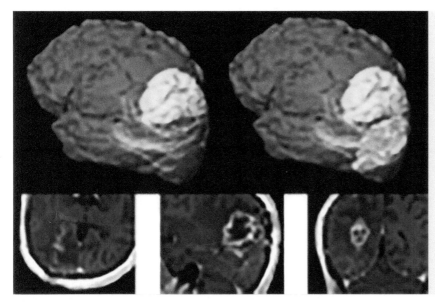

Fig. 6.2 49 y.o. male with a recurrent right parietooccipital recurrent glioblastoma. Tractography shows a downward displacement of the optic radiation fibers. The cortical activation detected on the functional MRI (blue) confirms the tractography results, showing cortical activation only under the cortical portion of the tumor. Axial, sagittal, and coronal views of the lesion displacing the optical radiation caudally without clear invasion. Pre-and post- resection visual fields were normal.

6.4 PET

Positron Emission Tomography (PET) is the tomographic acquisition of annihilation photons released by positron emitting radiotracers, which is frequently integrated with computed x-ray tomography (CT) providing the basis for structural imaging. Cellular uptake of the positron emitting tracers can be highly variable but is usually measurable in hours, leading to low temporal resolution. This represented the major limitation for the use of PET as a method of normal brain functional imaging. Recently promising amino acid uptake-based radiotracers have been developed, particularly for brain imaging. These radiotracer advances associated with development of acquisition methods are progressively opening major diagnostic, therapeutic, and prognostic applications for the use of PET in brain tumor management.

6.4.1 Diagnostic Applications

- Assessment of tumor grade in newly diagnosed tumors (▶ Fig. 6.2).[4]
- PET-guided biopsy.[5]
- Differentiation between tumor and inflammatory tissue.[6]

6.4.2 Therapeutic Applications

- PET guided surgical resection and radiation therapy.[7]
- Early assessment of treatment response in gliomas and primary CNS lymphoma.[8]
- Post-treatment evaluation and restaging.[5,9]

6.4.3 Prognostic Value

PET can provide useful prognostic information in multiple brain neoplastic pathologies including gliomas, metastasis, and primary CNS lymphomas.[10,11]

6.5 Indirect Methods

6.5.1 Tractography

White matter tractography is based on the diffusion of water molecules in the brain providing the unique possibility of *in vivo* non-invasive assessment of the orientation, location, and integrity of important white matter tracts. Tractography is currently the only available method for non-invasive *in vivo* assessment of white matter tracts. The ever-growing technical complexities and nuances of acquisition, processing, and tract identification methods can be challenging, however successive clinical studies confirmed promising correlations between tractography results and patient outcomes, in both retrospective and prospective studies.[12,13] The development of methods able to identify even thin tracts though regions of complex crossing fibers and peritumoral edema,[14] and the integration of these tractography results with other functional techniques such as fMRI and nTMS,[15] will help extend the spectrum of applications of tractography in functional neurosurgery.

6.5.2 Key Applications

Pre-surgical and Surgical Management

Tractography allows the non-invasive spatial analysis of brain's white matter, establishing it as a major tool for the pre-operative risk stratification and resection planning of any intra-axial lesion. Multiple reports presently corroborate the preoperative assessment to function preservation in neoplastic, vascular, and epilepsy surgery.[16,17] Multiple teams have demonstrated the usefulness of white matter spatial analysis for intraoperative guidance by integrating tractography data with the operative microscope.[18]

Deep Brain Stimulation (DBS)

The progressive development of DBS as a major tool to treat various pathologies ranging from Parkinson's disease to resistant depression disorders, brought to light the complexity of DBS actual functioning mechanisms of DBS, which is currently understood to be based on local, regional, and sometimes distal circuitry, hence the value of white matter tractography as a method for understanding its efficacy and to explain stimulation's adverse effects. Retrospective studies and direct tract targeting reports are progressively establishing the full reach of tractography in DBS.[19]

Prognostic Value

White matter tractography is an invaluable tool for the assessment and monitoring of major tract involvement in hemispheric, brainstem, and spine pathologies: traumatic, neoplastic, and degenerative.[20,21]

6.6 Electrophysiological Function

6.6.1 Navigated Transcranial Magnetic Stimulation (nTMS)

The use of Transcranial Magnetic Stimulation for brain mapping is becoming increasingly popular because of the ability to navigate the location of stimulation points on an individual's MRI. Analogous to direct cortical stimulation, albeit non-invasive, nTMS is based on the principle of inducing electric currents within underlying brain tissue via a magnetic field generated from a coil over the skin surface. The secondary electric current is proportional to the strength of the magnetic field and is set based on the individual's Resting Motor Evoked Potentials. Its use for motor mapping has shown good correlation with DCS. nTMS is showing promise for language mapping and has advantages over fMRI with a better temporal resolution along with the advantage of a direct causal relationship with function.[22] nTMS-defined cortical regions can be used to guide white matter tractography.[15] Further research will assess the possible application and real potential for this technique including its integration with other cortical mapping approaches.

6.6.2 Magnetic Source Imaging (MSI)

MSI is a method of brain mapping using MEG data coregistered with anatomical data from MRI. MEG is based on the principle of detecting magnetic fields produced as a result of spontaneous or task related brain electrical activity using a super conducting interference device (SQUID). MEG has several advantages. Firstly, it has excellent temporal resolution, which is on the order of milliseconds. Another advantage is that it directly measures brain activity as opposed to the BOLD signal in fMRI. So far, MEG has been used for motor, language, visual and auditory mapping as well as localizing seizure activity.[23] As of now, high cost and siting requirements have significantly limited its more widespread use, but multiple clinical applications will be possible in the future.

6.7 Conclusion

The array of functional imaging techniques will continue to improve in sensitivity and specificity. A thorough understanding of the advantages and limitations of each technique holds the keys for the pertinent indication and interpretation of its results.

References

[1] Holodny AI, Shevzov-Zebrun N, Brennan N, Peck KK. Motor and sensory mapping. Neurosurg Clin N Am. 2011; 22(2):207–218, viii

[2] Kekhia H, Rigolo L, Norton I, Golby AJ. Special surgical considerations for functional brain mapping. Neurosurg Clin N Am. 2011; 22(2):111–132, vii

[3] Robles SG, Gatignol P, Lehéricy S, Duffau H. Long-term brain plasticity allowing a multistage surgical approach to World Health Organization Grade II gliomas in eloquent areas. J Neurosurg. 2008; 109(4):615–624

[4] Hatakeyama T, Kawai N, Nishiyama Y, et al. 11C-methionine (MET) and 18F-fluorothymidine (FLT) PET in patients with newly diagnosed glioma. Eur J Nucl Med Mol Imaging. 2008; 35(11):2009–2017

[5] Farwell MD, Pryma DA, Mankoff DA. PET/CT imaging in cancer: current applications and future directions. Cancer. 2014; 120(22):3433–3445

[6] Juhász C, Bosnyák E. PET and SPECT studies in children with hemispheric low-grade gliomas. Childs Nerv Syst. 2016; 32(10):1823–1832

[7] Grosu AL, Weber WA, Franz M, et al. Reirradiation of recurrent high-grade gliomas using amino acid PET (SPECT)/CT/MRI image fusion to determine gross tumor volume for stereotactic fractionated radiotherapy. Int J Radiat Oncol Biol Phys. 2005; 63(2):511–519

[8] Suchorska B, Tonn JC, Jansen NL. PET imaging for brain tumor diagnostics. Curr Opin Neurol. 2014; 27(6):683–688

[9] Boellaard R, O'Doherty MJ, Weber WA, et al. FDG PET and PET/CT: EANM procedure guidelines for tumour PET imaging: version 1.0. Eur J Nucl Med Mol Imaging. 2010; 37(1):181–200

[10] Kamson DO, Mittal S, Robinette NL, et al. Increased tryptophan uptake on PET has strong independent prognostic value in patients with a previously treated high-grade glioma. Neuro-oncol. 2014; 16(10):1373–1383

[11] Li W, Ma L, Wang X, Sun J, Wang S, Hu X. (11)C-choline PET/CT tumor recurrence detection and survival prediction in post-treatment patients with high-grade gliomas. Tumour Biol. 2014; 35(12):12353–12360

[12] Winston GP, Daga P, White MJ, et al. Preventing visual field deficits from neurosurgery. Neurology. 2014; 83(7):604–611

[13] Zhu FP, Wu JS, Song YY, et al. Clinical application of motor pathway mapping using diffusion tensor imaging tractography and intraoperative direct subcortical stimulation in cerebral glioma surgery: a prospective cohort study. Neurosurgery. 2012; 71(6):1170–1183, discussion 1183–1184

[14] Chen Z, Tie Y, Olubiyi O, et al. Corticospinal tract modeling for neurosurgical planning by tracking through regions of peritumoral edema and crossing fibers using two-tensor unscented Kalman filter tractography. Int J CARS. 2016; 11(8):1475–1486

[15] Weiss C, Tursunova I, Neuschmelting V, et al. Improved nTMS- and DTI-derived CST tractography through anatomical ROI seeding on anterior pontine level compared to internal capsule. Neuroimage Clin. 2015; 7:424–437

[16] Bello L, Gambini A, Castellano A, et al. Motor and language DTI Fiber Tracking combined with intraoperative subcortical mapping for surgical removal of gliomas. Neuroimage. 2008; 39(1):369–382

[17] Chen Z, Tie Y, Olubiyi O, et al. Reconstruction of the arcuate fasciculus for surgical planning in the setting of peritumoral edema using two-tensor unscented Kalman filter tractography. Neuroimage Clin. 2015; 7:815–822

[18] Kuhnt D, Bauer MH, Becker A, et al. Intraoperative visualization of fiber tracking based reconstruction of language pathways in glioma surgery. Neurosurgery. 2012; 70(4):911–919, discussion 919–920

[19] Calabrese E. Diffusion Tractography in Deep Brain Stimulation Surgery: A Review. Front Neuroanat. 2016; 10:45

[20] Mickevicius NJ, Carle AB, Bluemel T, et al. Location of brain tumor intersecting white matter tracts predicts patient prognosis. J Neurooncol. 2015; 125(2):393–400

[21] Yao Y, Ulrich NH, Guggenberger R, Alzarhani YA, Bertalanffy H, Kollias SS. Quantification of Corticospinal Tracts with Diffusion Tensor Imaging in Brainstem Surgery: Prognostic Value in 14 Consecutive Cases at 3 T Magnetic Resonance Imaging. World Neurosurg. 2015; 83(6):1006–1014

[22] Lefaucheur JP, Picht T. The value of preoperative functional cortical mapping using navigated TMS. Neurophysiol Clin. 2016; 46(2):125–133

[23] Jung J, Bouet R, Delpuech C, et al. The value of magnetoencephalography for seizure-onset zone localization in magnetic resonance imaging-negative partial epilepsy. Brain. 2013; 136(Pt 10):3176–3186

7 Intraoperative CT Imaging

Jamie Toms and Kathryn Holloway

Abstract

Functional neurosurgery, be it epilepsy surgery, deep brain stimulation, or a lesioning procedure, involves precise target localization and modification. Both computed tomography (CT) and magnetic resonance imaging (MRI) can be used for intraoperative imaging in order to precisely plan, place, and confirm surgical locations. This chapter focuses on intraoperative CT imaging.[1]

Keywords: deep brain stimulation, functional neurosurgery, intra-operative imaging, target localization

7.1 Patient Selection

Intraoperative CT imaging serves two purposes. First, it is used to register and assess an implant location, as in the registration of a stereotactic frame or a bone fiducial. Second, it can act as a stereotactic device in conjunction with a frameless navigation system. For example, it can be used for O-arm navigation of pedicle screws, Vertek arm alignment, or a fiducial-less Nexframe case. The precise location of the positioned device can then be evaluated.

All stereotactic devices have a delivery error in the range of 2 mm as measured with current techniques. Thus, intraoperative imaging provides ongoing accuracy feedback and allows interpretation of physiologic data based on the actual location not the expected location. The intraoperative CT scanner can also be used to verify the correct delivery of a device to a location within the brain whether or not it was placed stereotactically. For example, it can identify the position of a shunt within the ventricles. Intraoperative CT imaging should therefore be performed when stereotactic guidance is required, or intraoperative verification of device location is desired.

7.2 Imaging Device Selection

What are the advantages of CT scans over MRI? CT scans have a high geometric accuracy, but they lack soft tissue contrast needed to identify particular brain structures.[2] One method to circumvent this problem is to merge the intraoperative CT images with a preoperative MRI. Doing this creates a risk of co-registration error. On the other hand, CT imaging does have some advantages. It can be performed on larger, heavier patients, those with pacemakers and other electronic implants, with patients awake or asleep, and with the head fixed or free.

Portable intraoperative CT imaging devices are being used more often. A fixed intraoperative diagnostic CT scanner is less commonly present. Portable technologies include O-arm (Medtronic, Inc., Minneapolis, MD), Ceretom (NeuroLogica Corporation Danvers, MA), BodyTom (NeuroLogica Corporation Danvers, MA), and Airo CT (Brainlab Munich Germany). By the time of publication, there may be additional choices as well. The main consideration in choosing an imaging device is its compatibility with other equipment, the level of image quality

sought, size limitations, field of view, and of course, availability. Earlier portable CTs had a limited field of view, but this has been corrected with the previously mentioned devices. The O-arm has a large bore to accommodate imaging of microelectrode tracks and the second iteration has a sufficiently large enough field of view to visualize a stereotactic frame localizer. It is also widely available since it is also used in spine surgery. The bore of the Ceretome, however, is much smaller than the others causing the patient to lay completely flat, and this creates limitations on positioning. Nonetheless, it is been put to excellent use during asleep deep brain stimulation (DBS) implantation surgery.[3] The BodyTom is large, which limits its portability. The Airo CT and O-arm can seamlessly integrate with commercially available navigation systems as a stereotactic device. As long as a reference arc is attached, the O-arm can be paired with the Stealth Station to provide registration with a scan. The Brain Lab and Airo CT are similarly connected. Each system has a unique work flow, but the principles are the same.

In this chapter we will describe the use of the O-arm for fiducial-less, frameless DBS placement as an example of using the scanner as a stereotactic device. The updated Stealth software package, Cranial 3.0 is required for this approach.

We will also discuss its use in the intraoperative identification of implant locations.

7.3 Operative Procedure

For DBS lead placement with an O-arm, patients are placed in a lounge chair position. Their head lies in a radiolucent head holder that has an anterior cervical collar restraint. The collar can help with airway management and act as a restraining device for emergence from sedation. It can be removed for greater comfort during intraoperative microelectrode recording functional testing.

The patient's head lies in the center of the O-arm ring. Three positions of the O-arm are programmed. In the "park" position the surgeon has maximum access to the patient's head. The "scan" position is best for imaging. It must have less than 15 degrees of tilt in order to be used as a registration or navigated scan. The "intermediate" position is a transition point that allows for the O-arm to move from "park" to "scan" without colliding with the bed, patient, or equipment. A FESS frame (▶ Fig. 7.1a) (a friction fit navigation head frame commonly used in nasal sinus surgery) with reference arc is applied to the patient s forehead with a silastic strap. Along with a reference arc, a silastic strap attaches it to the patient's forehead. The surgeon obtains a low dose O-arm image (standard mode = 0.6mSV) and that image is merged with the preoperative MRI images on the Stealth Station using the Cranial 3.0 software. The burr hole site is marked on the patient's scalp with the blunt navigation probe.

The FESS frame is removed, and the patient is then prepped and draped. The burr hole is made and the Stimloc and Nexframe (Medtronic, Inc., Minneapolis, MD) are secured to it and aligned to the target (▶ Fig. 7.1b). The center cannula is inserted

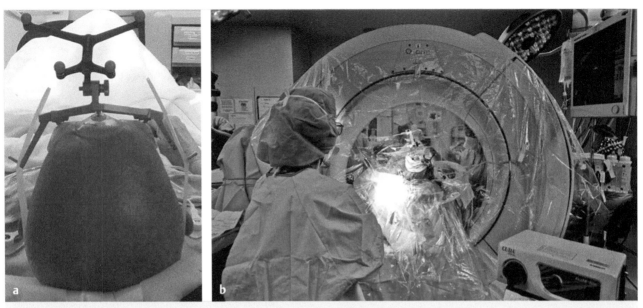

Fig. 7.1 (a) FESS frame placed on the patient's head for bur hole localization. **(b)** Fiducial-less O-arm set up with drapes and Nexframe device.

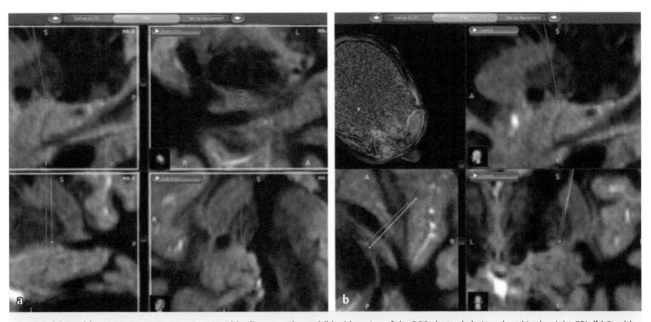

Fig. 7.2 (a) Stealth trajectory view comparing actual (red) versus planned (blue) location of the DBS electrode being placed in the right GPi. **(b)** Stealth anatomic view comparing actual (red) versus planned (blue) location of the deep brain stimulator electrode.

in the brain and another image is obtained. The more efficient workflow for transferring and merging O-arm images in Cranial 3.0 allows the new image to be transferred, merged, and analyzed while the microelectrode recording equipment is set up. The central cannula is then evaluated on the O-arm image for its location within the anatomy. The optimal second track is then chosen based on the location of the center cannula and is inserted. Once the microelectrode or deep brain stimulator lead has reached the target depth, the O-arm can be used to take an image of the implant location. The implants are imaged with the high definition mode. This mode takes more images per rotation, but the milliamperage (mA) is lowered so that the

radiation dose is roughly equivalent to the standard mode scan. Each of these images provides ongoing feedback on stereotactic accuracy and allows the physiologic data to be interpreted within the context of the anatomy and the actual implant location rather than its expected location (▶ Fig. 7.2). In a group of 32 patient's undergoing fiducial-less registration, the authors have found that there was no difference in the number of microelectrode tracks required as compared to the author's fiducial-based cases (unpublished data).

In the authors' experience, intraoperative CT can also be useful for placing difficult shunts or Ommaya reservoirs. An enhanced mode image (2.2 mSV) has the same dose as a

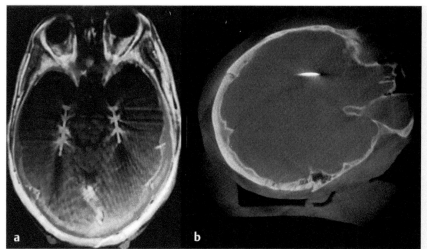

Fig. 7.3 Immediate post-lead placement O-arm scans showing lead placement. **(a)** Intraoperative merge of O-arm image and preoperative MRI showing placement of bilateral hippocampal depth electrodes in a responsive neurostimulator implantation. **(b)** Location of the metal probe during a laser ablation operation prior to merging with preoperative imaging.

diagnostic CT and will allow imaging of soft tissue. The ventricles can be visualized, but metal artifact can limit visualization. Even though in most cases the enhanced mode is sufficient for targeting the ventricles for shunt or Ommaya reservoir placement, the intraoperative images can be merged with preoperative ones if more clarity is desired. Intraoperative CT can also be used when placing a responsive neurostimulator for epilepsy patients and in laser ablation procedures (▶ Fig. 7.3). Additionally, detection of a large intraparenchymal hemorrhage on an enhanced mode O-arm image has been reported.[4]

7.4 Conclusion

Intraoperative CT scanning permits efficient and accurate intraoperative registration and implant location verification. This gives the surgeon the opportunity to recognize and correct any clinically relevant deviations from the plan before leaving the operating room.

References

[1] Burchiel KJ, McCartney S, Lee A, Raslan AM. Accuracy of deep brain stimulation electrode placement using intraoperative computed tomography without microelectrode recording. J Neurosurg. 2013; 119(2):301–306

[2] Holloway K, Docef A. A quantitative assessment of the accuracy and reliability of O-arm images for deep brain stimulation surgery. Neurosurgery. 2013; 72 (1) Suppl Operative:47–57

[3] Mirzadeh Z, Chapple K, Lambert M, et al. Parkinson's disease outcomes after intraoperative CT-guided "asleep" deep brain stimulation in the globus pallidus internus. J Neurosurg. 2016; 124(4):902–907

[4] Katisko JPA, Kauppinen MT, Koivukangas JP, Heikkinen ER. Stereotactic operations using the o-arm. Stereotact Funct Neurosurg. 2012; 90(6):401–409

8 Microelectrode Recordings in Deep Brain Stimulation Surgery for Movement Disorders

Adolfo Ramirez-Zamora, Leonardo Almeida and Michael S. Okun

Abstract

Deep Brain Stimulation (DBS) is a well-established treatment for medication-refractory Parkinson's disease, dystonia and essential tremor. Optimal placement of DBS leads within the targeted nuclei is a crucial factor for successful outcomes. Intra-operative neurophysiology facilitates localization of targeted regions known to produce positive responses. In this chapter, we will we will review the anatomy relevant to DBS surgery and discuss the basics of microelectrode recording (MER) techniques used to target varied basal ganglia nuclei and cerebral sites.

Keywords: deep brain stimulation, tremor, Parkinson's disease, dystonia, microelectrode recordings, MER, DBS surgery

8.1 Introduction

Deep brain stimulation (DBS) is a well-established therapy for a variety of medication refractory movement disorders. Successful DBS outcomes depend on appropriate patient selection, post-operative programming, management of non-DBS related issues, and recognition of potential complications of the therapy. Accurate electrode placement is a pivotal step to produce positive outcomes.

Accurate electrode placement depends on appropriate targeting combined with MER. The exclusive use of image-guided indirect stereotactic targeting may affect outcome because of poor image acquisition technique, brain shift and pneumocephalus. Judicious use of MER can precisely map the motor territory and identify target boundaries that in turn can be verified by macrostimulation through the DBS lead. The final position of the DBS lead can be selected by identification of intraoperative thresholds that optimize clinical benefit and limit unwanted side effects.

MER identifies neuronal action potentials and facilitates testing of kinesthetic cells, cells with movement-evoked neuronal responses. It can characterize the topography and territory within a specific nucleus or cerebral region and determine its boundaries. It is dependent on clinical expertise. There are three major elements to the recording technique:

- **Target verification**- pass a single microelectrode to verify that physiology matches the expected region based on imaging. This technique is the one most prone to error.
- **Ben Gun approach**- named after Professor Alim-Louis Benabid, this approach depends on passing multiple microelectrodes simultaneously and has the advantage of fixing brain tissue in place to avoid shift during a procedure. The technique depends on using the best of the five simultaneous penetrations. Several groups have modified this technique and use two or three MER passes instead of five.
- **MER mapping**- The most accurate and detailed of the approaches uses single MER passes and determines the next pass based on the previous pass. This allows the physician to map a structure in three dimensions and to choose the best site for the electrode. Although more accurate, this technique can be more time consuming and more vulnerable to brain shift. The benefits of additional MER passes, however should be weighed against the risk of injury, usually hemorrhage.

This chapter will review basic intraoperative MER and macrostimulation techniques for the treatment of movement disorders. It will focus on the most common conditions and targets, discuss anatomy, boundaries and tips for ideal target placement. ▶ Table 8.1 summarizes important principles for MER mapping and anatomic localization.

8.2 Subthalamic Nucleus

The subthalamic nucleus (STN) is a complex biconvex almond-shaped structure densely surrounded by fiber tracts. Successful treatment of Parkinson's Disease and tremor relies in accurate placement of a DBS lead in the vicinity of the sensorimotor territory and its surrounding structures (▶ Fig. 8.1).

Many centers use an oblique target trajectory to the STN to avoid the ventricular system and to maximize the length of the electrode within the nucleus. The lateral-to-medial orientation in the coronal plane requires an angle of 10–30 degrees with an orientation angle in the sagittal plane ranging from 40 to 90 degrees (45°– 60° being the most common range) to avoid the motor cortex. The MER track may arbitrarily commence at various distances from the STN target with most centers recording at 10–30 mm above the predetermined anatomical target. Goals of MER are to identify the characteristic spontaneous discharge patterns of the STN, to locate surrounding nuclei and uncover the motor territory that contains movement-related cells. Modulation of the motor region cells is appreciated by an audible change in the discharge frequency that is reproducible and synchronous with passive movement of contralateral and occasionally ipsilateral joints. Neuronal activity characteristic of the dorsal and ventral thalamus may be encountered along the trajectory leading toward the STN. Neuronal discharges are irregular, persistent, low to moderate in frequency and have a more tonically active pattern and firing between 28–40 Hz.[1] Approximately 1–2 mm above the STN and below the thalamic nuclei, the Zi is encountered. The Zi consists of irregular, transient and low-density neuronal discharges with low tonic firing rates and occasional bursting neurons (25–45 Hz).[2,3] There is an increase in background activity before the electrode enters STN. The characteristic STN neuronal firing has tonic but bursty, high frequency, high density, irregular discharge patterns with occasional bursts and mean firing rates in the 34- to 47-Hz range. Below the STN, SNr neuronal firing follows a more regular, sustained, high frequency, tonic pattern compared to STN, and there is a lack of bursting, tremor cells and movement related cells in SNr.[4]

Table 8.1 Suspected lead location based on recordings and effects of stimulation

	STN	GPi	VIM
Anterior	• STN identified higher than expected and may have a larger gap between STN and SNr. • Absent thalamic activity. • CS or CB side effects (Tonic muscle contractions) due to stimulation of the IC at similar voltage with most ventral and dorsal contacts. • Caution should be exercised as a long run of STN can be encountered on passes adjacent to the internal capsule.	• MER reveals absence of the GPi or kinesthestic cells. • Could also have a long run of GPi cells anteriorly. • Large portion of striatum might be encountered with long MER tracks. • Anteriorly located DBS leads may provide no observable acute effects at higher voltages.	• Absence of passive kinesthetic thalamic cells. • No adverse effects with high levels of stimulation. • Limited or no tremor control. • Possible mood changes or non-specific dizziness.
Posterior	• Prominent thalamic activity during MER depending on lead trajectory. • Potentially short STN run of physiology activity and encountered lower (more ventral) than expected. • Paresthesias due to stimulation of nearby medial lemniscus.	• Posterior tracks are recognized by the presence of CS or CB side effects due to stimulation of the IC. Thresholds for AE with most ventral contact is lower compared with dorsal contacts (Based on anterior DBS trajectory angle). • The location of the optic tract in relation to the lower border of the GPi might increase with more posterior and medial tracks. • Depending on mediolateral location there may be a ventrally located gap between GPi and OT.	• Tactile sensory cells on the border between Vc and VIM. • Prominent cutaneous receptive neurons activated by light touch on MER. • Persistent paresthesias at low thresholds following strict somatotopic organization.
Lateral	• Absent neuronal activity or short STN runs on MER (1–2 mm) depending on trajectory • Absence of SNr below STN. • CS or CB side effects (Tonic muscle contractions) due to stimulation of IC • Congruous and simultaneous eye deviation due to activation of the frontal eye field fibers traversing in the inner most location of the IC.	• MER typically reveals large segment of GPe and a small segment of GPi usually with a large lamina between them. • Possible border cells. • Absence of optic tract or IC during MER. • Absence of CS or CB side effects due to IC activation.	• Short VIM tracks noted on MER • CS or CB side effects (Tonic muscle contractions) due to stimulation of IC.
Medial	• MER findings suggestive of Rn. • Dizziness, nausea, or a "warm feeling due to stimulation of Rn. • Ipsilateral medial eye deviation and diplopia due to stimulation of oculomotor nerve fibers.	• MER typically reveals large segment of GPi and a small segment of GPe. • The location of the optic tract in relation to the lower border of the GPi increases with more medial tracks. • A comparable low threshold for side effects (muscle contractions) in all contacts is usually seen based on approach angles.	• Prominent jaw and perioral cutaneous receptive neurons activated by light touch on MER. • Marked orofacial paresthesias and dysarthria with stimulation
Dorsal	• Absence of adverse effects or improvement of symptoms.	• Dorsally located DBS leads may provide no observable acute effects at higher voltages.	• Limited or absent benefit on tremor control without sensory adverse effects
Ventral	• MER recordings consistent with Snr. • Potential sudden changes in effect. • Possible CS or CB side effects due to stimulation of IC.	• Optic tract stimulation may result in visual phosphenes. • CS or CB side effects due to stimulation of the IC. Thresholds for AE with most ventral contact is lower compared with dorsal contacts (Based on anterior DBS trajectory angle).	• Paresthesias affecting face arm and leg symmetrically due to stimulation Lm.

▶ Table 8.1 Suggested anatomical localization of electrode based on microelectrode findings and stimulation. Abbreviations: AE=Adverse effects, CS=corticospinal, CB=corticobulbar, IC=internal capsule, Lm=medial lemniscus, STN=subthalamic nucleus, Gpi=Globus Pallidus Internus, Gpe=Globu Pallidus Externa, SNr=Substancia nigra, VIM= ventral Intermediate nucleus, Rn=Red nucleus. Note that many of the above effects may be inconsistent due to trajectory.

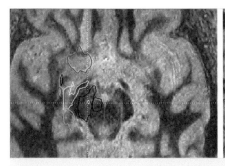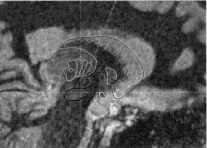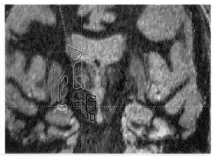

Fig. 8.1 Appropriate location of DBS lead within the subthalamic nucleus in relationship with surrounding structures in sagittal, coronal and axial view.

The use of micro-stimulation can complement MER. Microstimulation at 300 Hz, 200–300 sec pulse width, 1–2 second train duration, in biphasic pulses up to 100 microamps can be used to determine potential side effects and assist in delineating regional anatomy.[5] Hyperhydrosis is a common adverse effect of stimulation of dorsomedial, anteromedial, and posteromedial locations in the STN region.[6] Other visual disturbances such as gaze deviation are more difficult to localize to a single region or structure. Once a final trajectory has been identified, macrostimulation can be done with the uninsulated tip of the inner guide cannula used for the microelectrode, or with the DBS lead. Intraoperative test stimulation is done on each contact spanning the STN using a 60–90 millisecond pulse width and frequency of 130–180 Hz. If no reproducible adverse effect is elicited using stimulation up to 10V, the pulse width can be widened and the test repeated to exclude electrical malfunction. Each contact is tested in either monopolar or bipolar stimulation and lack of any side effects at a high voltage is an important clue that the lead is suboptimally placed (▶ Fig. 8.1).

8.3 Globus Pallidus Internus (GPi)

The sensorimotor region of the internal segment of the globus pallidus internus (GPi) can be the target for DBS in both PD and dystonia. The DBS lead is implanted in the ventral, posterior and lateral aspect of the GPi as this location maximizes effectiveness and limits the occurrence of intolerable side effects. The GPi is surrounded by the posteriorly and medially located internal capsule. The internal capsule fibers also project ventrally. The optic tract is located ventrally. The globus pallidus externa (GPe) lies laterally to the GPi. Compared to the STN target, typical stereotactic targeting of the GPi requires a less oblique or even strictly parasagittal (0°–15°) approach in reference to the coronal angle. This approach may help to avoid penetrating the ventricle though the GPi is usually sufficiently lateral that this is not an issue. The sagittal angle is anteriorly positioned both to avoid the motor cortex and to produce a trajectory sparing the internal capsule (approximately in the range from 40° to 60°angles with respect to the intercommissural plane.

A typical MER trajectory targeting the GPi region traverses the striatum, corona radiata, GPe, GPi and optic tract. More posterior MER tracks pass may traverse the internal capsule. Initially, MER tracts may reveal the presence of low frequency (4–6 Hz) low-density discharges with irregular neuronal activity characteristic of the striatum. Following striatal recordings

is a quiet background without discernable neuronal activity and this is usually consistent with passage through white matter tracts and the external medullary lamina surrounding the GPe. In the GPe region, neuronal activity is irregular with lower-frequency discharges (34 -19 Hz). MER may uncover two possible neuronal discharge patterns: higher-frequency units (50–21 Hz) that are tonically active but with frequent short pauses (pausers), and less commonly lower-frequency units (18–12 Hz) sometimes referred to as low frequency pausers.[7] Pausing cells may be interrupted by high-frequency burst (bursting cells) and the burst are typically faster than those encountered in the ventrolateral thalamus.[8] Another group of neuronal bodies located around the pallidum fire with moderate frequency and regularity. These cells are known as border cells and may be observed between GPe and GPi, and between GPi and the optic tract. Border cells may also be encountered on the posterior border of GPi or in the lamina separating the dorsal and ventral GPi. The overall background activity is elevated prior to entering GPi and it is reduced upon exiting the target with MER.

Within the sensorimotor (posteroventrolateral) region, passive and/or active limb movements, often by multiple joints, elicit driving of unit discharges more often contralaterally, but they can be ipsilateral. After traversing border cells at the ventral aspect of GPi and the fibers of the ansa lenticularis, the optic tract can be identified. The optic tract is typically 0.5–1.5 mm below the GPi border. Light flashes delivered to the eyes produce evoked discharges within the fibers of the optic tract that can be appreciated aurally more than by their visual representations on the oscilloscope. Microelectrode stimulation at this level can produce phosphenes. The goals of MER include identifying a track that is not too lateral and close to GPe, observing kinesthetic cells consistent with the posterolateral sensorimotor region, and defining a safe distance from the internal capsule, which is located posterior and medially. The lead should be placed adjacent to the optic tract but not in the optic tract (▶ Fig. 8.2). The placement of the final lead is highly dependent on the trajectory. More vertical trajectories, for example, would require a distance of 3 mm or more from the posterior capsular border and 2–3 mm from the presumed lateral border. Although the relative run length of GPi and GPe and the presence of somatotopic driving responses may yield clues to the location of the MER track, this information can be misleading especially if a target verification method of a single tract is employed. The best testing to look for benefit thresholds and side effects is with macrostimulation. It can be accomplished

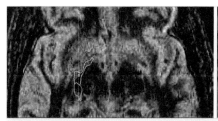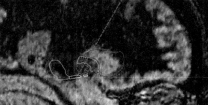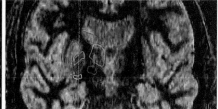

Fig. 8.2 Appropriate location of DBS lead within the Globus Pallidus Interna in relationship with surrounding structures in sagittal, coronal and axial view.

after the final lead is positioned. Testing is done with the same parameters used for chronic neurostimulation- a pulse with of 60–90 µs and a frequency of 130 or 180 Hz. One examines carefully for signs of facial pulling, speech difficulty or other evidence of muscle contraction.

Threshold is determined by the occurrence of side effects. An expected bipolar energy delivery of 4–5V or, if monopolar, 3–4V is recommended for potentially therapeutic contacts. The need to reposition a DBS lead depends on the thresholds at specific contacts. Increasing pulse width is recommended to induce capsular effects if no effect is seen during intraoperative testing. As noted above, regarding STN stimulation, a lack of side effects in the operating room suggests that there is a technical problem or a DBS lead failure.

In patients with dystonia, the transition from the external to internal pallidum is more difficult to distinguish by MER. In the dystonic GPi, the cells manifest a highly unusual discharge pattern, termed high frequency bursting or "packets of cells." These cells discharge in irregularly spaced bursts and do so on a relatively high background discharge rate.

8.4 VIM Nucleus of the Thalamus

The ventral intermediate nucleus (VIM) of the thalamus is the most common target for the treatment of medically refractory essential tremor, but is also frequently a target for other tremor disorders. Posterior to the VIM is the principal sensory thalamic nucleus that receives input from the medial lemniscal and spinothalamic sensory afferents, referred to as the ventral caudalis (Vc). Anterior to the VIM/Vop nuclei lies the region that receives afferents from the basal ganglia output nuclei (GPi, SNr), incorporating ventro–oralis anterior (Voa) and the ventral anterior nucleus (VA). Ventrally lies the medial lemniscus itself. Dorsally, the dorsal region of the ventral tier nuclei surrounds Vim. Medially, the VIM receives proprioceptive afferents with receptive fields including the face region. Finally, the posterior limb of the internal capsule borders Vim laterally. The trajectory of the DBS lead or MER pass is equally as importance for successful placement of a thalamic DBS. A more vertical VIM approach is preferred by most centers. The anterior/sagittal angle determines whether the more dorsal contacts would move anteriorly with respect to Vim. Moreover, a smaller angle in the sagittal plane may place the lead through the long axis of the VIM distributing the electrodes closer to the sensory thalamus and anterior nuclei respectively and potentially limiting its efficacy. For this reason, most centers attempt to implant the electrode in parallel with the border of Vim and Vop. Additionally, a more vertical AC-PC angle of the DBS lead trajectory has been associated with improved head tremor suppression.[9]

One of the goals of MER is to identify the anterior border of the sensory thalamus. Characteristic Vim discharges and passive motor somatotopic cells will aid in facilitating placement of the DBS lead 2–3 mm anterior to the Vc border and medial to the capsule border. Initial track recording 15–25 mm dorsal to the ventral border of the VIM target generally traverses first through the dorsal thalamus. This is followed by identification of tonically active units with a firing rate between 3–18 Hz, which are more characteristic of the Voa/Vop region. As the microelectrode passes ventrally towards the Vim, more higher frequency neuronal units are observed. Neuronal discharge density is low to moderate but synchronized by passive kinesthetic movements of the joints rather than by active movements. The strict somatotopy within the thalamus usually places the facial receptive fields medially, with the representation of the fingers lateral to face. Upper extremity representation is ventromedial and lower extremity dorsolateral. Ventromedial neurons respond to jaw opening and closing and tongue protrusions and retractions. Finally, ventrocaudal advance into sensory receptive neurons yields units with well-defined cutaneous receptive fields. These are activated by light touch within a narrow somatotopic region. Neuronal discharging frequency, density and background usually remain unchanged while the electrode advances.

As opposed to GPi and STN targeting, microstimulation can provide exquisite detail of the regional neuroanatomy surrounding the electrode and can facilitate mapping. Microstimulation in the sensory thalamus may produce marked paresthesias at very low current thresholds (e.g., 1–5 microA). If microstimulation produces widespread (face, arm and leg) paresthesias at relatively higher threshold (around 25 microA), this suggests stimulation of the medial lemniscus. Although one single track can provide much of the information required for implantation, most centers perform a posteriorly located track to ensure identification of the border of Vc. A perfect single track would be one that has hand passive motor cells followed by hand tactile, and finally by hand region light touch.

Final lead implantation is ideally located in the region containing neurons with kinesthetic receptive fields corresponding to the hand approximately 2 -3 mm anterior to the border of sensory thalamus at the intercommisural level or below, as some surgeons prefer to place the lead into the zona incerta (▶ Fig. 8.3). Macroelectrode stimulation following MER mapping, or in lieu of it in some centers, is performed routinely after DBS lead implantation to assess the voltage or current

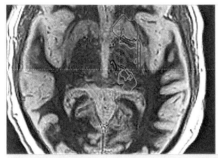 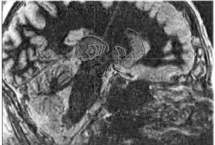 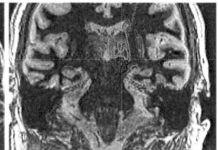

Fig. 8.3 Appropriate location of DBS lead within the VIM thalamic nucleus in relationship with surrounding structures in sagittal, coronal and axial view.

threshold for the suppression of tremor and side effects. Adverse effects will depend on the location of active electrodes with respect to the surrounding neuroanatomical structures. Orofacial transient paresthesias are common when stimulating with the most ventral and medial contact (which is closer to Vc). Transient paresthesias are common with successful lead placement (1–3 mA).

8.5 Tips for Good MER

Regardless of the technique implemented, the goal of MER is to assess neural activity (or the lack of it) to delineate an ana-tomo-physiological map prior to determining the final DBS lead position. Important considerations before MER include:
- the preoperative discontinuation of centrally active medications, adequate positioning, carefully-checked recording equipment, the elimination of electrical noise, and development of a stereotactic plan.
- Importance of finishing the anterior-posterior or lateral-medial plane and identifying boundaries one at a time, as the final electrode placement before macrostimulation will rely on a linear distance from these borders.
- Avoidance of pitfalls related to acute neurological changes (potential intracranial hemorrhage), influence of sedation on the recordings, and early identification of signs of brain shift.
- Clear understanding of the regional anatomy and effects of stimulation of the structures surrounding the basal ganglia are critical for successful DBS placement. A consistent and detailed approach to record and test neuronal activity along

with open communication amongst the participants in MERs is also imperative.

References

[1] Hutchison WD, Allan RJ, Opitz H, et al. Neurophysiological identification of the subthalamic nucleus in surgery for Parkinson's disease. Ann Neurol. 1998; 44(4):622–628

[2] Merello M, Tenca E, Cerquetti D. Neuronal activity of the zona incerta in Parkinson's disease patients. Mov Disord. 2006; 21(7):937–943

[3] Sterio D, Zonenshayn M, Mogilner AY, et al. Neurophysiological refinement of subthalamic nucleus targeting. Neurosurgery. 2002; 50(1):58–67, discussion 67–69

[4] Starr PA, Subramanian T, Bakay RA, Wichmann T. Electrophysiological localization of the substantia nigra in the parkinsonian nonhuman primate. J Neurosurg. 2000; 93(4):704–710

[5] Starr PA, Christine CW, Theodosopoulos PV, et al. Implantation of deep brain stimulators into the subthalamic nucleus: technical approach and magnetic resonance imaging-verified lead locations. J Neurosurg. 2002; 97(2):370–387

[6] Ramirez-Zamora A, Smith H, Youn Y, Durphy J, Shin DS, Pilitsis JG. Hyperhidrosis associated with subthalamic deep brain stimulation in Parkinson's disease: Insights into central autonomic functional anatomy. J Neurol Sci. 2016; 366:59–64

[7] Vitek JL, Bakay RA, Hashimoto T, et al. Microelectrode-guided pallidotomy: technical approach and its application in medically intractable Parkinson's disease. J Neurosurg. 1998; 88(6):1027–1043

[8] Lozano A, Hutchison W, Kiss Z, Tasker R, Davis K, Dostrovsky J. Methods for microelectrode-guided posteroventral pallidotomy. J Neurosurg. 1996; 84(2): 194–202

[9] Moscovich M, Morishita T, Foote KD, Favilla CG, Chen ZP, Okun MS. Effect of lead trajectory on the response of essential head tremor to deep brain stimulation. Parkinsonism Relat Disord. 2013; 19(9):789–794

9 Cortical and Subcortical Mapping

Anthony I. Ritaccio, Peter Brunner and Gerwin Schalk

Abstract

Electrical stimulation mapping (ESM) is the most common technique used to delineate functional cortex. It may be done in an epilepsy-monitoring unit using implanted electrodes, or in the operating room in either awake or anesthetized patients. The results guide strategies to minimize sensorimotor and linguistic injury from surgery. Increasingly, however other complementary methods, such as passive electrocorticographic (ECoG)-based functional mapping and cortico-cortical evoked potentials (CCEPs), are being used.

Keywords: functional mapping, electrocorticography, electrical stimulation

9.1 Introduction

9.1.1 Primary Concepts

Neurosurgical resections are done with two goals: (1) optimization of resection extent and (2) minimization of deficit extent, especially when eloquent cortex is at risk.[1] For epilepsy surgery, functional mapping allows the surgeon to maximize resection of the epileptogenic zone in order to eliminate seizures while minimizing the risk of functional loss. Surgical tumor resection, however, is done to increase survival. The purpose of functional mapping is to optimize the postoperative quality of life.[2]

9.1.2 Justification

Functional zones can be distorted or topographically obscured by a lesion or its associated edema. The epileptic zone or intra-axial tumor may be in eloquent cortex. Congenital abnormalities may obliterate conventional anatomic landmarks and the location, duplication, and anatomic extent of eloquent cortex is variable.[3] Also, lesion location and a patient's age at lesion onset leads to varied degrees of brain plasticity.

The focus of this chapter is the review of established functional mapping techniques such as ESM and somatosensory evoked potential (SSEP). However, emerging techniques and their clinical relevance will also be discussed.

9.2 Basic Physiological Principles of ESM

For mapping precision, bipolar stimulation is used when both cathode and anode touch target tissue. This may be accomplished either with subcortical grid electrodes or depth electrodes when mapping in an epilepsy monitoring unit or with a handheld stimulator during open surgery.

Modeling of current flow in a bipolar paradigm shows a sharp drop in current midway between electrodes (5 mm for 1 cm inter electrode designs).[4] The area stimulated depends on the distance from the stimulating electrode and the amount of current applied. Charge density is a function of charge and the cross-sectional area of the electrode surface in contact with the brain. Potential mechanisms of injury by charge transfer and electrolysis have been obviated by the use of stimulators that have a biphasic pulse and constant current. Chronaxie-convergent paradigms used for decades have prevented injury from thermal deposition.

ESM effects occur because of local electrical diffusion. The initial axon segments and nodes of Ranvier have the highest excitability to applied current, perhaps because they have the highest sodium channel concentration.

9.3 Patient Selection

Actionable mapping information is obtainable only on patients with intact linguistic and sensorimotor abilities. Stimulation trains for mapping are 1–2 seconds for somatosensory and motor cortex and ≤ 10 seconds for language identification. Any significant impairment in sensation, motor paresis, or speech hesitancy/anomia will prevent adequate testing within these temporal constraints.

9.4 Preoperative Evaluation

Functional magnetic resonance imaging (fMRI) and diffusion tensor imaging (DTI) help to locate linguistic and sensorimotor cortex. This additional data aides optimal placement of grid and strip electrodes for two-stage epilepsy surgery or best guides site selection for intraoperative ESM.

There is a no level IV data confirming the ability of fMRI and DTI to reduce morbidity and fMRI has poor temporal resolution. It is not sensitive and/or accurate enough to be used independently as a localization method.[5] fMRI is useful in language lateralization, but it characteristically identifies multiple contributing functional language regions. ESM "interference" mapping identifies critical or causal nodes. DTI has lower spatial resolution for motor function preservation study than direct electrical stimulation of white matter tracts.[6] Inaccurate correlations between DTI and ESM can be created by tumor invasion and intraoperative brain shift. Also, when imaging the arcuate fasciculus, recent DTI technology lacks end-to end-point tracking reliability, making localization of conventional frontal and temporal language termini inaccurate.

9.5 Operative Procedure

9.5.1 Medication and Anesthetic Considerations

Twenty mg/kg phenytoin or one gram of levetiracetam for parenteral anticonvulsant prophylaxis is given before surgery. Reduced doses of mannitol (0.5 g/kg of 20% mannitol) are recommended, since higher doses are associated with nausea and vomiting when the patient is awake. The most frequent strategy for awake craniotomy is the "asleep-awake-asleep" method. Rapidly reversible intravenous anesthesia, usually Propofol, is used initially. Dexmedetomidine is also commonly used. Inhalation anesthetics that suppress EEG signal and increase the latency or reduce the amplitude of SSEPs should be avoided.

9.5.2 Electrode and Stimulator Considerations

To perform ESM, electrodes are placed on the cortex and connected via a switch box to a cortical stimulator that delivers biphasic pulsed electrical charge to a pair of electrodes (▶ Fig. 9.1). For chronic mapping, cortical electrode grids composed of platinum-iridium discs (4 mm in diameter with 2–3 mm exposed) that are spaced 10 mm center-to-center and embedded in silicone to form grids and strips of various sizes (4 × 5 or 8 × 8 electrode arrays) are placed. Grids can be trimmed to match the shape of the craniotomy or are preshaped to fit specific areas (for example, 35-contact grid in a dedicated 4 × 3 mesial flap). Strips with four to twelve contacts provide cortical coverage beyond the extent of the craniotomy. Depth electrodes (composed of 2- to 5-mm-long cylindrical platinum-iridium electrodes with a diameter of 1 mm and spaced 5–10 mm apart) may also be used. Intraoperatively, a handheld Ojemann probe, which has a pair of ball electrodes mounted 5 mm apart, is used to perform ESM throughout the awake resection process.

9.5.3 Stimulation Paradigms and Techniques

Extraoperative, chronic ESM is indicated for epilepsy surgery on candidates who have undergone implantation of subdural grid/strip electrodes or stereo-electroencephalographic (SEEG) depth arrays in or near eloquent cortex. This mapping is done in a monitoring unit. With SEEG stimulation mapping of conventionally inaccessible cortical regions such as the insula,

ventral, and medial cortex is possible. The disadvantage of SEEG mapping is that it has a limited sampling size compared to subdural grid coverage.

Epilepsy evaluations require electrocorticography (ECoG) to monitor for seizures and stimulus-induced after-discharges that may summate to seizures. Modern stimulator and switching boxes are often integrated into existing EEG video monitoring systems and provide an intuitive graphical user interface. Intraoperative ESM may be done at the time of tumor or epileptic focus resection. Grid, strip, depth or wand electrode interfaces can be used. Differences in cortical physiology, varied disc/sphere electrode configurations and electrode diameters, inter-electrode distance choices and current shunting through cerebrospinal fluid result in a wide variety of stimulation protocols. (▶ Fig. 9.1).[7] Intraoperative ESM may be done on an anesthetized patient to measure motor responses, but patients need to be awake for somatosensory, motor, or linguistic study. Cooperation or a subjective report is needed. Intraoperarative ESM provides localization guidance for both cortical grey matter and subcortical fiber tracts, as both may be stimulated. This "hodotopic" view considers both nodes and networks. It is superior to other available techniques in preserving function as has been shown in many large surgical studies, particularly in patient sundergoing glioma resection.[8,9]

Both positive responses (regional movement, dysesthesia, phosphenes) and negative responses (motor inhibition, speech arrest, anomia) may occur with stimulation. The effect of ESM is a complex amalgam of neuronal excitation and inhibition, interneuron and local fiber tract involvement.[10] Distinctions have been codified between eloquent cortex that is obtainable and eloquent cortex that is indispensable.[11] Indispensable cortex refers to primary motor cortex/pyramidal tracts, primary sensory cortex, primary visual cortex, Broca and Wernicke's regions, and the arcuate fasciculus. Indispensable regions are to be preserved in any resection strategy if possible. Basal temporal language or fusiform gyrus face recognition areas may be mapped. However, absolute avoidance is not necessary. These regions can be resected without significant morbidity.

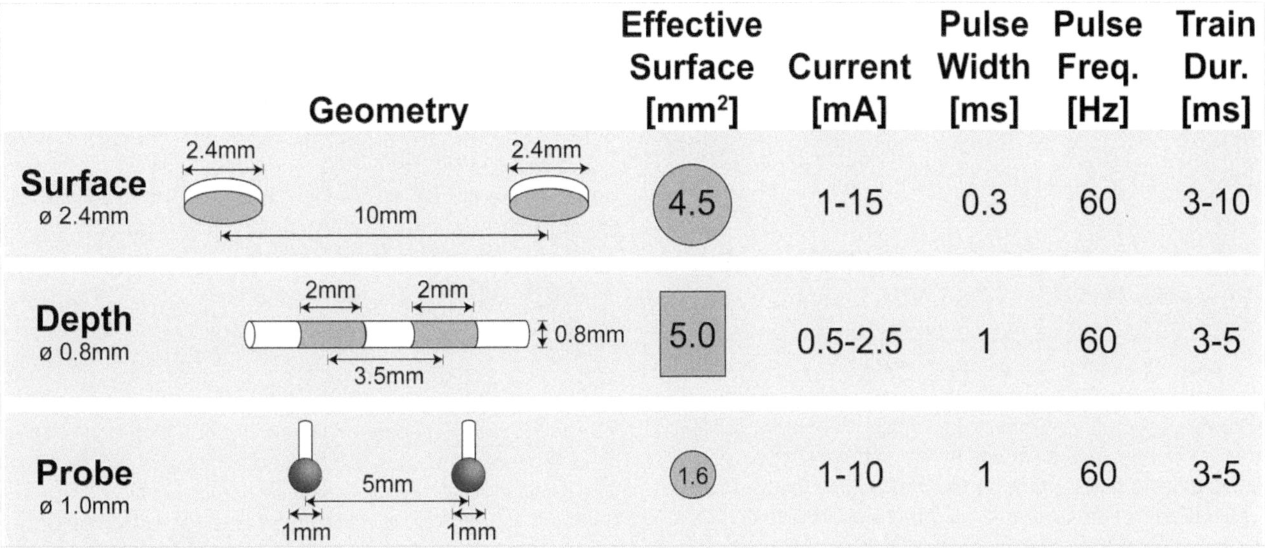

	Geometry	Effective Surface [mm²]	Current [mA]	Pulse Width [ms]	Pulse Freq. [Hz]	Train Dur. [ms]
Surface ø 2.4mm	2.4mm — 10mm — 2.4mm	4.5	1-15	0.3	60	3-10
Depth ø 0.8mm	2mm 2mm ↕0.8mm 3.5mm	5.0	0.5-2.5	1	60	3-5
Probe ø 1.0mm	5mm 1mm 1mm	1.6	1-10	1	60	3-5

Fig. 9.1 Common stimulation parameters for surface, depth, and intraoperative probe electrodes. Inter-electrode distances and exposed stimulation surfaces are illustrated to scale.

9.5.4 Mapping Methods

Somatosensory Mapping

Assessments in the postcentral gyrus require an awake, alert patient to describe or confirm localized paresthesias or dysesthesias. Stimulation is first applied suprasylvian with subsequent progression superiorly to activate orofacial, hand, brachial, truncal, and lower limb regions in sequence.

Motor mapping: Motor mapping may be done on either an awake or anesthetized patient. The mapping proceeds in a similar inferior-superior orientation, with an observer watching the contralateral side for any induced clonic activity.

Stimulator settings for sensorimotor mapping differ depending on whether one is using a commercially available handheld wand or stimulating directly through a subdural grid array placed on the pre/postcentral gyri (**Fig. 9.1**). Wand stimulation (with 5-mm electrode spacing) starts at 1–2 mA using a 60 Hz frequency and 1 msec pulse width. It proceeds in 1–2 mA increments up o a 10-mA maximum. If motor mapping is performed under anesthesia, initial current settings can start at 4–5 mA. If a grid with 1-cm center-to-center electrode spacing is used, common stimulation settings are 50 Hz and 50 msec pulse width with 1–15 mA. Stimulation trains of more than 2–3 seconds to elicit effect are not necessary

Language Mapping

Language mapping in awake patients is needed when the operative area of interest includes dominant hemisphere frontal and temporal language regions. Common tasks employed include number counting, sentence repetition, and object naming Frontal lobe language sites may induce language arrest and posterior superior temporal sites may induce a receptive deficit. Results, however, can be a combination of aphasia, anomia, or speech arrest depending on the stimulation site and applied current. Sites with any object-naming deficit, but with intact sentence repetition are considered to be anomic regions. Stimulator settings depend on the stimulation device but are similar to those used with somatosensory and motor assessments. Haglund et al., and others have established the concept of a "safety margin."[12,13] The distance of the resection margin from the nearest ESM language site is the most important variable in the duration and permanency of postoperative language deficits. A safety margin of 1 cm for frontal language sites and 2 cm for temporal naming sites has been codified based on observations of linguistic deficits that have occurred in violation of this strategy.[12]

White Matter Tract Mapping

ESM of subcortical white matter fascicles is feasible and is done to preserve function and maximize the extent of tumor resection. When mapping descending motor tracts, multichannel electromyography is used to facilitate detection of target muscle.[14] Awake stimulation of white matter pathways relevant to language systems, such as the arcuate fasciculus, uncinate fasciculus or the superior/inferior longitudinal fasciculi is valuable for the resection of deep lesions.[15] Stimulation parameters are the same as for cortical stimulation, but the level of anesthesia required can complicate motor tract mapping.

9.5.5 SSEPs to Define Central Sulcus

SSEPs are electrical responses to the stimulation of a peripheral nerve. SSEPs can be used to preserve motor and somatosensory function during surgery. With this technique the median nerve is electrically stimulated and SSEP responses are recorded from an ECoG grid that is positioned over the cortical surface. The location of the central sulcus is determined from the phase reversal of the N20/P20 component in the SSEP response. It denotes the transition from primary motor to sensory function.

9.5.6 Data Aggregation and Co-registration Strategies and Methods

In chronic mapping paradigms, the delineation of functional from dysfunctional cortex requires aggregation of the mapping data and available epilepsy monitoring results and their co-registration to the patient's anatomy/lesion. ECoG electrode locations are determined from a postoperative CT image that is co-registered to a preoperative structural MRI image. The aggregated and co-registered results are then visualized as overlays in a neuronavigation system that is used to plan and aid the surgical resection.

9.6 Perioperative Management (Including Complications)

9.6.1 Electrocorticography

ECoG is an essential component of operative stimulation paradigms. During stimulation it monitors local after-discharges (ADs) that may summate into seizures. ADs indicative a local convulsive threshold, which requires that stimulation begin at low amplitudes and increases in steps of 1–2 mA until effect is seen or an AD is produced. If ADs are known to be present, testing should be performed at 1–2 mA lower than AD threshold. If testing is negative, these higher current settings may be revisited cautiously, as there is often an accommodation effect over time and useful testing may not be possible. The presence of ADs needs to be known because they may produce false positive language arrests. Any clinical or subclinical seizures that are caused by stimulation can be quenched by lavage with iced Ringer's solution or, if needed, parenteral administration of midazolam or propofol.

9.7 Emerging Roles for Novel Techniques

9.7.1 Optical Imaging/MEG/TMS/CCEP/ Passive ECoG Summary

The technique of preoperative mapping has hardly unchanged since the seminal work of Penfield and his contemporaries eight decades ago.[16] Better understanding of brain physiology and technical sophistication of sensing, stimulation, and computing technology in recent years has changed this. A number of recent studies have evaluated the clinical applicability of passive ECoG-based functional mapping, cortico-cortical evoked potentials (CCEPs), transcranial magnetic stimulation (TMS), and magnetoencephalography (MEG).[17,18,19,20,21,22]

Passive functional mapping records electrical signals from the brain using the same electrodes that are placed for ESM. After signal amplification by a biosignal amplifier, a computer extracts ECoG features that are known to reflect brain activity underneath the electrode. By determining the locations that change this brain activity during a task such as motor movement or language reception, an algorithm can create a map of eloquent cortex. This passive ECoG-based functional mapping approach has been evaluated in different clinical scenarios and shows a strong relationship to ESM.[19,23]

CCEPs integrate aspects of ESM with passive functional mapping. CCEP evaluates ECoG responses to individual electrical stimuli and can thereby identify those cortical locations that are anatomically connected to the stimulation sites. For example, electrical stimulation of receptive language nodes can highlight expressive language locations in the inferior frontal lobe, presumably by communication through the arcuate fasciculus.[24]

Similar to ESM, TMS electrically interrupts brain function by applying magnetic pulses. Because it is noninvasive, its localization accuracy is limited, but it has particular use in evaluating language lateralization as a non-invasive alternative to the intracarotid amobarbital (WADA) test.[25]

MEG is a noninvasive method similar to scalp EEG, except that it is based on detection of magnetic instead of electric fields. For this reason, MEG has a higher spatial resolution than EEG. Though MEG is not widely available, a few studies have explored its value for presurgical functional mapping.[22]

9.7.2 Possible Integration of Novel Techniques into the Armamentarium

A growing number of centers have integrated the techniques described above into clinical practice. In time, passive ECoG mapping and CCEP techniques are likely to become fully integrated into the neurosurgical armamentarium, while the unreliability and expense associated with TMS and MEG, respectively, may limit their application to specific cases or to clinical research.

9.8 Conclusion

Localization of function through the use of ESM techniques has been established for decades. Abundant level IV evidence exists to document that common mapping methods preserve eloquence, shorten postoperative motor and linguistic deficits, and augment quality of life.[3,26] Alternative methods are evolving to complement these long-existing techniques.

References

[1] Gil-Robles S, Duffau H. Surgical management of World Health Organization Grade II gliomas in eloquent areas: the necessity of preserving a margin around functional structures. Neurosurg Focus. 2010; 28(2):E8

[2] Duffau H. Brain mapping in tumors: intraoperative or extraoperative? Epilepsia. 2013; 54 Suppl 9:79–83

[3] Ojemann G, Ojemann J, Lettich E, Berger M. Cortical language localization in left, dominant hemisphere. An electrical stimulation mapping investigation in 117 patients. J Neurosurg. 1989; 71(3):316–326

[4] Nathan SS, Sinha SR, Gordon B, Lesser RP, Thakor NV. Determination of current density distributions generated by electrical stimulation of the human cerebral cortex. Electroencephalogr Clin Neurophysiol. 1993; 86 (3):183–192

[5] Austermuehle A, Cocjin J, Reynolds R, et al. Language functional MRI and direct cortical stimulation in epilepsy preoperative planning. Ann Neurol. 2017; 81(4):526–537

[6] Ohue S, Kohno S, Inoue A, et al. Surgical results of tumor resection using tractography-integrated navigation-guided fence-post catheter techniques and motor-evoked potentials for preservation of motor function in patients with glioblastomas near the pyramidal tracts. Neurosurg Rev. 2015; 38(2):293–306, discussion 306–307

[7] Hamberger MJ, Williams AC, Schevon CA. Extraoperative neurostimulation mapping: results from an international survey of epilepsy surgery programs. Epilepsia. 2014; 55(6):933–939

[8] De Benedictis A, Duffau H. Brain hodotopy: from esoteric concept to practical surgical applications. Neurosurgery. 2011; 68(6):1709–1723, discussion 1723

[9] De Witt Hamer PC, Robles SG, Zwinderman AH, Duffau H, Berger MS. Impact of intraoperative stimulation brain mapping on glioma surgery outcome: a meta-analysis. J Clin Oncol. 2012; 30(20):2559–2565

[10] Ranck JB , Jr. Which elements are excited in electrical stimulation of mammalian central nervous system: a review. Brain Res. 1975; 98(3):417–440

[11] Zago S, Ferrucci R, Fregni F, Priori A. Bartholow, Sciamanna, Alberti: pioneers in the electrical stimulation of the exposed human cerebral cortex. Neuroscientist. 2008; 14(5):521–528

[12] Haglund MM, Berger MS, Shamseldin M, Lettich E, Ojemann GA. Cortical localization of temporal lobe language sites in patients with gliomas. Neurosurgery. 1994; 34(4):567–576, discussion 576

[13] Ojemann GA, Dodrill CB. Verbal memory deficits after left temporal lobectomy for epilepsy. Mechanism and intraoperative prediction. J Neurosurg. 1985; 62(1):101–107

[14] Keles GE, Lundin DA, Lamborn KR, Chang EF, Ojemann G, Berger MS. Intraoperative subcortical stimulation mapping for hemispherical perirolandic gliomas located within or adjacent to the descending motor pathways: evaluation of morbidity and assessment of functional outcome in 294 patients. J Neurosurg. 2004; 100(3):369–375

[15] Duffau H. Stimulation mapping of white matter tracts to study brain functional connectivity. Nat Rev Neurol. 2015; 11(5):255–265

[16] Penfield W, Boldrey E. Somatic motor and sensory representation in the cerebral cortex of man as studied by electrical stimulation. Brain. 1937; 60(4): 389–443

[17] Crone NE, Miglioretti DL, Gordon B, Lesser RP. Functional mapping of human sensorimotor cortex with electrocorticographic spectral analysis. II. Event-related synchronization in the gamma band. Brain. 1998; 121(Pt 12):2301–2315

[18] Leuthardt EC, Miller K, Anderson NR, et al. Electrocorticographic frequency alteration mapping: a clinical technique for mapping the motor cortex. Neurosurgery. 2007; 60(4) Suppl 2:260–270, discussion 270–271

[19] Brunner P, Ritaccio AL, Lynch TM, et al. A practical procedure for real-time functional mapping of eloquent cortex using electrocorticographic signals in humans. Epilepsy Behav. 2009; 15(3):278–286

[20] Matsumoto R, Nair DR, LaPresto E, et al. Functional connectivity in the human language system: a cortico-cortical evoked potential study. Brain. 2004; 127 (Pt 10):2316–2330

[21] Picht T, Schmidt S, Brandt S, et al. Preoperative functional mapping for rolandic brain tumor surgery: comparison of navigated transcranial magnetic stimulation to direct cortical stimulation. Neurosurgery. 2011; 69(3):581–588, discussion 588

[22] Cheyne D, Bostan AC, Gaetz W, Pang EW. Event-related beamforming: a robust method for presurgical functional mapping using MEG. Clin Neurophysiol. 2007; 118(8):1691–1704

[23] Korostenskaja M, Wilson AJ, Rose DF, et al. Real-time functional mapping with electrocorticography in pediatric epilepsy: comparison with fMRI and ESM findings. Clin EEG Neurosci. 2014; 45(3):205–211

[24] Tamura Y, Ogawa H, Kapeller C, et al. Passive language mapping combining real-time oscillation analysis with cortico-cortical evoked potentials for awake craniotomy. J Neurosurg. 2016; 125(6):1580–1588

[25] Pelletier I, Sauerwein HC, Lepore F, Saint-Amour D, Lassonde M. Non-invasive alternatives to the Wada test in the presurgical evaluation of language and memory functions in epilepsy patients. Epileptic Disord. 2007; 9(2):111–126

[26] Sanai N, Mirzadeh Z, Berger MS. Functional outcome after language mapping for glioma resection. N Engl J Med. 2008; 358(1):18–27

10 Parkinson Disease–Evaluation and Medical Treatment

Lisa Deuel and Eric S. Molho

Abstract

A diagnosis of Parkinson's disease (PD) is established by recognizing the core motor symptoms of bradykinesia, rigidity, gait impairment and, in some patients, the classically described resting tremor. Treatment of the classical motor features with levodopa remains the central management strategy in PD but there are now numerous options for minimizing motor fluctuations and non-motor features of PD. Drug regimens must be individualized to the patient's unique needs and propensity for side effects. There is no effective disease modifying treatment available that can slow or halt progression.

Keywords: Parkinson disease, motor fluctuations, levodopa, Lewy body, non-motor symptoms

10.1 Introduction

10.1.1 Epidemiology

Parkinson's disease (PD) is a progressive neurodegenerative condition that is characterized by the presence of bradykinesia and at least one of three additional features including resting tremor, postural instability, and rigidity.[1] It is primarily a disease of the elderly, affecting one percent of the population over the age of 60; however, young-onset cases diagnosed before the age of 40 years do occur and may be associated with certain genetic mutations. A male predominance exceeding 60% has been consistently noted. Whether there are racial differences, including the possibility that Caucasians are at greater risk than Asians and African Americans, is controversial.

PD is the result of the interaction amongst several genetic and environmental factors.[2] Epidemiological studies link pesticide exposure, well water consumption, welding, and military exposure to Agent Orange with an increased risk of developing PD. Less than 10% of cases are linked to a monogenetic cause. There are five identified autosomal dominant genetic inheritance patterns and five with autosomal recessive patterns. Beyond these rare disease-causing mutations, there are now several well-characterized risk modifying genes.[3] In 2010, the estimated economic burden of PD in the United States was $14.4 billion, and this burden likely will continue to increase.[4]

10.1.2 Pathology

PD is associated with a loss of dopaminergic cells and reduced pigmentation in the substantia nigra pars compacta of the midbrain. By the time the patient presents with initial motor features, 60–70% of these dopaminergic neurons have already been lost. Microscopy at autopsy shows the presence of Lewy bodies. These are round cytoplasmic inclusions containing pathological forms of the protein alpha-synuclein.

The classical description of PD as a pure motor disorder resulting from isolated dopaminergic cell degeneration has been substantially modified in recent years. According to the Braak hypothesis, first published in 2003, abnormal alpha-synuclein accumulates in a spreading geographic fashion. The olfactory bulbs and lower brainstem are affected early, followed by the midbrain, then the symptom onset advances rostrally to those caused sequentially by disease involving the subcortical regions and basal ganglia, and finally involving selected cortical regions.[5] This pattern may explain the timing and sequence of symptom onset, and why, for example, olfactory dysfunction may predate motor features, while cognitive impairment appears later in the disease course. Another important implication of this theory is that dopaminergic dysfunction is only a small part of a more complex disease process involving the serotonergic, noradrenergic, and cholinergic systems, giving rise to non-motor features such as autonomic, sleep, mood, and, of course, cognitive symptoms.

10.2 Diagnosis

Symptoms classically present asymmetrically. Unilateral onset is common. Further support of the diagnosis is garnered by observing the patient over time for persistent asymmetry and dramatic improvement after initiation of levodopa therapy. Levodopa-induced dyskinesias will eventually develop and the disease and disability will progress over ten or more years. Exclusion criteria, which may suggest a diagnosis of secondary parkinsonism or Parkinson-plus syndrome, include abnormal brain imaging, prior exposure to neuroleptic medications, or atypical findings such as supranuclear gaze palsy, cerebellar and long tract signs or early onset of dementia, frequent falls, or severe orthostatic hypotension. A suspected diagnosis of PD may take months or even years to confirm, since much of the supporting data is clarified as the disease unfolds in time.

10.2.1 Motor Features of PD

Bradykinesia is essential for the diagnosis of PD. It can manifest in many ways, including slowed movements, reduced amplitude or decrement with repetitive movements, diminished facial expression (hypomimia), soft speaking (hypophonia), or small handwriting (micrographia). Patients may also have asymmetric muscle rigidity, resting tremor, and postural abnormalities that manifest as a stooped and tilted trunk with flexion at the elbows and knees. Postural instability is the inability to recover balance once it is perturbed. A narrow stance, shuffling, short steps, reduced arm swing, and en-bloc turning are characteristic of a parkinsonian gait. Ambulation is further complicated by freezing (hesitations and sticking of the feet to the floor, particularly when walking through doorways or changing direction), and festination (increasing forward momentum as the center of gravity propels the body forward).

10.2.2 Non-motor Features of PD

Dopamine deficiency leads to the motor features of PD; however, dysfunction among other neurotransmitter systems results in several common and debilitating non-motor symptoms.[6,7] One of the early signs of PD, often noted in retrospect, is olfactory dysfunction. This has been explored as an early predictive marker in asymptomatic family members of affected individuals.[8]

Serotonergic dysfunction can manifest early in "pre-motor" PD, resulting in REM sleep behavior disorder that often predates classical motor symptoms, as well as causing mood disorders such as depression and anxiety. Patients may also experience sympathetic (noradrenergic) and parasympathetic (cholinergic) nervous system dysfunction. Symptoms of this are constipation, gastroparesis, urinary frequency and urgency, sexual dysfunction, and orthostatic hypotension. Other common non-motor symptoms are fatigue, daytime sleepiness, apathy and a variety of sensory complaints including pain. Any of these can profoundly impact quality of life. Cognitive decline and psychosis are late complications that will reduce quality of life and cause a loss of independence.[9,10]

10.3 Evaluation

There are no blood tests or imaging findings that are both sensitive and specific enough to confirm the diagnosis of idiopathic PD. The primary task of any diagnostic evaluation, therefore, is to rule out other neurodegenerative diseases and secondary causes of parkinsonism. Text box 1 (p. 37) presents the most important conditions in the differential diagnosis of PD, and Text box 2 (p. 37) presents the key history and exam findings that should alert the clinician to an alternative diagnosis.

Magnetic resonance imaging of the brain is generally unremarkable, though it may be useful in identifying secondary causes of parkinsonism. Similarly, blood testing is performed to screen for Wilson's disease, liver dysfunction, or hypothyroidism. A dopamine transporter imaging study is available (DaTscan®). This measures the functional integrity of the nigrostriatal neuron.[11] It can be used to distinguish idiopathic PD, which is characterized by reduced uptake, from drug-induced parkinsonism and other PD mimickers unrelated to dopaminergic dysfunction-essential tremor or normal pressure hydrocephalus. Unfortunately, DaTscan® is not specific enough to differentiate idiopathic PD from other degenerative forms of parkinsonism such as progressive supranuclear palsy or multiple system atrophy.

Differential diagnosis of PD in adults

- Other degenerative diseases
  - Dementia with Lewy bodies (DLB)
  - Multiple system atrophy (MSA)
  - Progressive supranuclear palsy (PSP)
  - Corticobasal degeneration (CBD)
- Secondary parkinsonism
  - Drug-induced parkinsonism (from neuroleptics, antiemetics)
  - Vascular parkinsonism
  - Post-encephalitic parkinsonism
  - Normal pressure hydrocephalus (NPH)
  - Autoimmune encephalitis
  - Wilson's disease
  - Structural brain injuries (stroke, tumor, bleed)
  - Toxic injuries (MPTP, carbon monoxide)
- Pseudoparkinsonism
  - Essential tremor
  - Dystonic tremor
  - Other gait disorders in elderly

When to suspect an atypical or secondary form of parkinsonism

- Strict hemiparkinsonism → structural brain lesions
- Lower body parkinsonism → NPH, vascular parkinsonism
- Early dementia → DLB, PSP, NPH
- Early falls/ataxia → PSP, MSA, CBD, NPH,
- Impaired saccades/diplopia → PSP
- Unilateral limb myoclonus, apraxia, cortical sensory loss → CBD
- Early dysautonomia (orthostatic fainting, impotence) → MSA
- Early urinary incontinence → MSA, NPH
- Poor or no response to L-dopa → all of the above

NPH = normal pressure hydrocephalus, DLB = dementia with Lewy bodies, PSP = progressive supranuclear palsy, MSA = multiple system atrophy, CBD = corticobasal degeneration

10.4 Management

Dopamine replacement with levodopa is the mainstay of treatment. Motor symptoms are expected to respond well, with the potential exception of tremor, which can be unresponsive to medications. Carbidopa is combined with levodopa to block its peripheral metabolism by dopa-decarboxylase. It improves bioavailability within the central nervous system and decreases peripheral side effects. It is an oral medication marketed in a variety of "immediate" release and longer acting formulations, and now as a gastrointestinal gel delivered directly to the duodenum through a battery-powered pump (Duopa®).[12] The most common dose related side effects include nausea, orthostatic lightheadedness, sedation and, in patients with cognitive impairment, hallucinations.

10.4.1 Long-term Response to Levodopa

Early in the disease course, levodopa three times daily is sufficient for a sustained response. This "long-duration response" relies on a residual population of functional neurons that can store levodopa and gradually release dopamine in a physiological manner. As the disease progresses, however, many factors contribute to a less predictable and less sustained medication response. Initially, fluctuations tend to be predictable "wearing off" episodes, but with advanced disease, the fluctuations become more severe and unpredictable, and can be associated with drug-induced hyperkinetic involuntary movements termed dyskinesia.

Several adjunctive treatments are available for use as monotherapy or in conjunction with carbidopa-levodopa. Synthetic dopamine agonists help in both early and advanced disease. These medications generally provide a less robust response and have a higher incidence of sudden daytime sleepiness, impulse control disorders, hallucinations, and orthostatic hypotension. Enzyme inhibitors including monoamine oxidase (MAO-B) inhibitors and catechol-O-methyltransferase (COMT) inhibitors, prolong levodopa effectiveness by blocking its metabolic degradation. Amantadine is an antiviral medication that can be used

Table 10.1 Medical treatment options for motor fluctuations

Mild to Moderate (simple wearing-off)	Severe (unpredictable or complicated by dyskinesia)
More frequent l-dopa doses	Add tolcapone (COMT inhibitor)
Controlled release l-dopa formulations	Add amantadine (dyskinesia)
Add COMT inhibitor (entacapone)	Apomorphine sq injections (rescue therapy)
Add dopamine agonist (ropinirole, pramipexole, rotigotine)	Carbidopa/levodopa intestinal gel infusion pump
Add MAO-B inhibitor (selegiline, rasagiline)	Deep brain stimulation (DBS)

as monotherapy for mild disease or as an adjunct to dopamine replacement therapy. In advanced disease, it can minimize disabling dyskinesia and provide some anti-parkinsonian effects. Anticholinergic agents have many side effects but may be used in patients with tremor-predominant PD.

10.4.2 Long-term Treatment Strategies

Strategies designed to delay the initiation of levodopa therapy or approximate "continuous dopaminergic stimulation" in early disease have not proven successful at preventing motor fluctuations or altering long-term outcomes.[13,14,15] Thus, adjunctive medications should be used in early disease to treat levodopa resistant symptoms or in patients who have trouble tolerating levodopa. In advanced disease they can help to minimize motor fluctuations. Treatment strategies need be individualized since symptom profiles, medication responsiveness and side effects can vary widely between patients. ▶ Table 10.1 summarizes the medication options for treating motor fluctuations.

10.4.3 Treatment of Non-motor Features

Non-motor features can contribute to morbidity. Depression and anxiety are common and can be difficult to manage with the conventional therapies. Cognitive decline is also common, often with progression to dementia in advanced disease.[9] Cholinesterase inhibitors, which were originally approved for treatment of Alzheimer's disease dementia, can be used in PD with modest and temporary benefits. In general, a useful initial strategy to treat the psychosis that develops in advanced disease is to reduce or eliminate adjunctive PD medication. This comes at a potential cost of worsening motor symptoms. When further PD medication reductions are no longer feasible, the antipsychotic medications clozapine (Clozaril) and quetiapine (Seroquel), can be added to treat hallucinations and delusions.[10,16] A novel serotonin 2A inverse agonist, pimavanserin (Nuplazid®), was recently approved by the FDA to target this unmet need.[17]

10.5 Conclusion

PD is a progressive neurodegenerative condition that is characterized by the presence of bradykinesia and at least one of the three additional features- resting tremor, postural instability, and rigidity. It is generally asymmetric. DaTscan® may help to confirm the diagnosis. Treatment options for motor and non-motor symptoms exist. Unfortunately, there are no known means to slow the inevitability of disease progression.

References

[1] Lang AE, Lozano AM. Parkinson's disease. First of two parts. N Engl J Med. 1998; 339(15):1044–1053

[2] Kieburtz K, Wunderle KB. Parkinson's disease: evidence for environmental risk factors. Mov Disord. 2013; 28(1):8–13

[3] Ferreira M, Massano J. An updated review of Parkinson's disease genetics and clinicopathological correlations. Acta Neurol Scand. 2017; 135(3):273–284

[4] Kowal SL, Dall TM, Chakrabarti R, Storm MV, Jain A. The current and projected economic burden of Parkinson's disease in the United States. Mov Disord. 2013; 28(3):311–318

[5] Braak H, Del Tredici K, Rüb U, de Vos RA, Jansen Steur EN, Braak E. Staging of brain pathology related to sporadic Parkinson's disease. Neurobiol Aging. 2003; 24(2):197–211

[6] Marras C, Chaudhuri KR. Nonmotor features of Parkinson's disease subtypes. Mov Disord. 2016; 31(8):1095–1102

[7] Martínez-Fernández R, Schmitt E, Martinez-Martin P, Krack P. The hidden sister of motor fluctuations in Parkinson's disease: A review on nonmotor fluctuations. Mov Disord. 2016; 31(8):1080–1094

[8] Siderowf A, Jennings D, Eberly S, et al. PARS Investigators. Impaired olfaction and other prodromal features in the Parkinson At-Risk Syndrome Study. Mov Disord. 2012; 27(3):406–412

[9] Barba AL, et al. Dementia, in Parkinson's Disease. In: Ebadi M, Pfeiffer RF, eds. Boca Raton, FL: CRC Press; 2013:413–433

[10] Molho ES, Factor SA. Psychosis, in Parkinson's Disease and Nonmotor Dysfunction, Pfeiffer RF, Bodis-Wollner I, eds. Totowa, NJ: Humana Press; 2013:63–90

[11] Cummings JL, Henchcliffe C, Schaier S, Simuni T, Waxman A, Kemp P. The role of dopaminergic imaging in patients with symptoms of dopaminergic system neurodegeneration. Brain. 2011; 134(Pt 11):3146–3166

[12] Olanow CW, Kieburtz K, Odin P, et al. LCIG Horizon Study Group. Continuous intrajejunal infusion of levodopa-carbidopa intestinal gel for patients with advanced Parkinson's disease: a randomised, controlled, double-blind, double-dummy study. Lancet Neurol. 2014; 13(2):141–149

[13] Fox SH, Lang AE. 'Don't delay, start today': delaying levodopa does not delay motor complications. Brain. 2014; 137(Pt 10):2628–2630

[14] Rascol O, Hauser RA, Stocchi F, et al. AFU Investigators. Long-term effects of rasagiline and the natural history of treated Parkinson's disease. Mov Disord. 2016; 31(10):1489–1496

[15] Gray R, Ives N, Rick C, et al. PD Med Collaborative Group. Long-term effectiveness of dopamine agonists and monoamine oxidase B inhibitors compared with levodopa as initial treatment for Parkinson's disease (PD MED): a large, open-label, pragmatic randomised trial. Lancet. 2014; 384(9949):1196–1205

[16] Miyasaki JM, Shannon K, Voon V, et al. Quality Standards Subcommittee of the American Academy of Neurology. Practice Parameter: evaluation and treatment of depression, psychosis, and dementia in Parkinson disease (an evidence-based review): report of the Quality Standards Subcommittee of the American Academy of Neurology. Neurology. 2006; 66(7):996–1002

[17] Cummings J, Isaacson S, Mills R, et al. Pimavanserin for patients with Parkinson's disease psychosis: a randomised, placebo-controlled phase 3 trial. Lancet. 2014; 383(9916):533–540

11 Surgery for Parkinson's Disease

Jessica Shields, Steven M. Lange, Julie G. Pilitsis

Abstract

Multiple studies have shown that deep brain stimulation (DBS) has been effective in reducing motor signs (tremor, bradykinesia, dystonia) and improving functionality and quality of life for patients with Parkinson's Disease (PD).[1,2,3] Compared with medical therapy alone, DBS has been associated with a greater quality of life, including improvement in mobility, activities of daily living, and emotional well-being, and has not been shown to produce worse outcomes in those with greater preoperative disease severity. Careful patient selection, intraoperative planning, and post-operative care is essential for good outcomes.

Keywords: deep brain stimulation, Parkinson's Disease, subthalamic nucleus, globus pallidus interna, tremor

11.1 Patient Selection

As in any operation, careful patient selection is paramount for best outcomes. A multidisciplinary approach including neurology, neurosurgery, and neuropsychology at a minimum is essential to success. Under current recommendations, patients should have had symptoms of Parkinson Disease (PD) for a minimum of 5 years. Candidates for surgery have symptoms that impede their quality of life despite optimal medical management.[4] The EARLY STIM trial compared DBS versus medical therapy in a cohort of early stage patients with PD (mean age 53 years with an eight year disease duration) and found significant improvement in quality of life, motor disability, and activities of daily living (ADL) subscales on the Unified Parkinson Disease Rating Scale (UPDRS).[5] There are no absolute guidelines in terms of age. In our practice, we have treated PD patients as young as 16 and as old as 80 years. In the aged population, comorbidities and complex medical conditions must be considered. Mostly important, the surgery should make a meaningful improvement in the patient's life that outweighs the risk of surgery.

Cardinal symptoms, including rigidity, bradykinesia, ON/OFF fluctuations and tremor, improve to the greatest extent. Postural instability and freezing of gait, which occur despite medication, are notoriously difficult to treat with DBS. Dementia and inability to participate in the process of DBS programming are contraindications to surgery. Up to 30% of DBS failures to relieve symptoms have been related to inappropriate indications for surgery.[6]

Pre-operative work up includes medical clearance, Core Assessment Program for Surgical Interventional Therapies in Parkinson's Disease (CAPSIT-PD) testing, a neuropsychological evaluation, and an MRI with fine cuts through the basal ganglia that are devoid of significant motion artifact. The CAPSIT includes UPDRS testing. The UPDRS-3, that is the motor section of the exam, is performed ON medications and OFF medications.[7] In general, good candidates for surgery have a greater than 30% improvement in UPDRS score with levodopa challenge; however, patients with isolated tremor symptoms or asymmetric disease may not have this 30% improvement and still have meaningful outcomes.

The neuropsychological battery generally includes the Mattis Dementia (MDRS) Rating Scale, Dementia Rating Scale (DRS), Stroop test (ST), Trail Making Test Part A and B (TMT A/B), Wisconsin Card Sorting Test (WCST), and the Parkinson Disease Questionnaire (PDQ-39). Screening for cognitive decline and independence in activities of daily living is vital for pre-operative evaluation because patients with concurrent cognitive decline may have this exacerbated, and the MDRS has been shown to decline over the course of 36 months in patients receiving DBS to the subthalamic nucleus (STN).[3] Psychiatric symptoms such as depression have also been reported to worsen with STN DBS, making it an important pre-operative consideration.[8]

11.2 Operative Procedure

PD medications are stopped 12 hours prior to the surgery to ensure accurate neurophysiological recording. Anesthesia is usually intravenous sedation combined with local anesthetic in cases where microelectrode recording (MER) will be performed. In MRI based cases, child dystonia cases and other rare indications, anesthesia is used. We prefer to have systolic blood pressure less than 140 mmHg and diastolic blood pressure less than 90 mmHg during the procedure and for 24 hours post-operatively.

Cases may be performed with a traditional frame based procedure (e.g. Leksell, Elekta; Cosman-Roberts-Wells, Integra) or with a "frameless" approach (e.g. Clearpoint, MRI Interventions; StarFix, Pacific Neuroscience). The accuracies between these two methods have been measured with phantoms or with patients undergoing DBS implantation and found to be similar.[9,10,11] Stereotactic planning is performed using MRI. Trajectories should avoid sulcal veins and extreme proximity to the ventricle to reduce risk of bleeding and deflection. Targets may be identified directly when using 3 T MRI or indirectly when using 1.5 T MRI. Indirect targeting is based off the anterior and posterior commissure. The surgeon's choice between the three possible targets (Vim of the thalamus, GPi, STN) depends largely on clinical characteristics. For patients with dystonia as a primary complaint or patients with neuropsychological issues, the GPi is typically chosen.[3] Several studies have found equivocal post operative effects when comparing the GPi and STN. For patients who have less cognitive reserve and have tremor as a primary complaint, the Vim may be selected after careful discussion with the patient that the other PD symptoms will not be treated.

A burr hole is then created with the 14 mm perforator drill bit for the insertion of microelectrodes. To minimize brain shift, fibrin sealant is used. Intraoperative electrophysiological via MER are used to reveal characteristic neuronal signals of the specific brain target.[12] Once the target is selected, the DBS lead is placed and macrostimulation is performed to test for benefit, but especially for stimulation induced side effects that may preclude programming post-operatively. Once tested, the lead is anchored and buried under the skin. At a separate sitting, on average one week later, a second surgery is performed to connect an extension lead from the DBS lead to the implantable pulse generator which is usually placed in the chest. Decisions for which target and whether to perform bilateral or unilateral operations are generally undertaken by the multidisciplinary team during their monthly meeting. Intraoperative MRI may also used by experienced centers in place of MER.[13]

11.3 Complications

Serious surgical complications following DBS tend to be rare, such that a 30-day perioperative mortality and permanent neurological morbidity has been reported to be close to 0.4% and 1.0%, respectively, according to multicenter studies.[14] Intracranial complications that may result from DBS surgery include intracranial hemorrhage (ICH), venous infarction, and peri-electrode edema. Though the etiology of ICH in DBS remains unclear, some hypothesized risk factors include: the number of electrodes used for intraoperative microelectrode recording (MER); added force needed to pass the cannula through the cortex; trajectory through or near the ventricle; and past use of microelectrodes with step-offs. Planning of entry points, repeated verification of coordinates, and systematic monitoring of systolic blood pressure are suggested in order to minimize the risk of peri- and post-surgical ICH. Treatment involves controlling blood pressure, stabilizing vital signs, maintaining euvolemia, avoiding hyperthermia, correcting coagulopathies, and mitigating seizure activity; resolution of symptoms is often witnessed in the postoperative period.

Systemic complications of DBS surgery include venous air embolism and seizures. The risk of seizures in DBS is low (0.2–2.3%), and is reportedly higher within the first 48 hours after DBS surgery. Seizures are most likely to occur in the setting of ICH, peri-electrode edema, or ischemia which increase the risk of postoperative seizures by 30- to 50-fold.[15]

Hardware-related issues comprise a considerable percent of DBS-related complications, though improved technologies and evolving surgical techniques have limited hardware-related issues.[16,17] Hardware complications are defined as those events related to implanted leads (fracture or migration), the extension wire (erosion, tightening, and fracture), or the IPG (malfunction, flipping) that required additional surgical intervention. Most common in our practice is erosion. To avoid this, we have begun drilling off some of the outer table both at the burr hole site and extension site to countersink the device and thus render it lower profile. Lead fracture may occur and the patient generally presents with shocking sensation. In some cases, the fracture can be determined through high impedances or abnormalities on x-ray. In other cases, the battery or extension site must be explored. Lead migration is rare and generally occurs in the immediate perioperative period. Suboptimal therapy is usually noted.

Infections remain the most common complication of DBS and may occur anywhere in the DBS system.[18] Many superficial infections can be treated with oral antibiotics, while deeper infections often require removal of the portion of the implanted hardware that is affected. Early surgical treatment with partial hardware removal and appropriate antibiotic prophylaxis is

considered in many cases to be effective conservative management for DBS-related infection, especially by *S. aureus*. Avoidance of wound complication is best correlated with a consistent surgical team, awareness of biofilm formation, strict enforcement of sterility, timeliness of the procedure, and use of prophylactic antibiotics perioperatively.

The synaptic connections found in the basal ganglia have implications on behavior due to their intimate relationships with limbic, subcortical, and prefrontal. Stimulation induced side effects may include: dyskinesia, diplopia, dysarthria, dysphagia, mania, apathy, and impulsivity and are largely reversible with decreased settings and medication adjustments.

11.4 Conclusion

DBS is a successful therapy for the treatment of PD and related movement disorders. Today, the STN and GPi are the most commonly used targets in PD. Acute and long-term results after DBS show a dramatic and stable improvement of a patient's clinical condition.

References

[1] Weaver FM, Follett KA, Stern M, et al. CSP 468 Study Group. Randomized trial of deep brain stimulation for Parkinson disease: thirty-six-month outcomes. Neurology. 2012; 79(1):55–65

[2] Deuschl G, Schade-Brittinger C, Krack P, et al. German Parkinson Study Group, Neurostimulation Section. A randomized trial of deep-brain stimulation for Parkinson's disease. N Engl J Med. 2006; 355(9): 896–908

[3] Follett KA, Weaver FM, Stern M, et al. CSP 468 Study Group. Pallidal versus subthalamic deep-brain stimulation for Parkinson's disease. N Engl J Med. 2010; 362(22):2077–2091

[4] Okun MS, Foote KD. Enough is enough: moving on to deep brain stimulation in patients with fluctuating Parkinson disease. Arch Neurol. 2009; 66(6): 778–780

[5] Schüpbach WM, Maltête D, Houeto JL, et al. Neurosurgery at an earlier stage of Parkinson disease: a randomized, controlled trial. Neurology. 2007; 68(4): 267–271

[6] Okun MS, Tagliati M, Pourfar M, et al. Management of referred deep brain stimulation failures: a retrospective analysis from 2 movement disorders centers. Arch Neurol. 2005; 62(8):1250–1255

[7] Defer GL, Widner H, Marié RM, Rémy P, Levivier M. Core assessment program for surgical interventional therapies in Parkinson's disease (CAPSIT-PD). Mov Disord. 1999; 14(4):572–584

[8] Berney A, Vingerhoets F, Perrin A, et al. Effect on mood of subthalamic DBS for Parkinson's disease: a consecutive series of 24 patients. Neurology. 2002; 59(9):1427–1429

[9] Henderson JM, Holloway KL, Gaede SE, Rosenow JM. The application accuracy of a skull-mounted trajectory guide system for image-guided functional neurosurgery. Comput Aided Surg. 2004; 9(4):155–160

[10] Maciunas RJ, Galloway RL , Jr, Latimer JW. The application accuracy of stereotactic frames. Neurosurgery. 1994; 35(4):682–694, discussion 694–695

[11] Holloway KL, Gaede SE, Starr PA, Rosenow JM, Ramakrishnan V, Henderson JM. Frameless stereotaxy using bone fiducial markers for deep brain stimulation. J Neurosurg. 2005; 103(3):404–413

[12] Gross RE, Krack P, Rodriguez-Oroz MC, Rezai AR, Benabid AL. Electrophysiological mapping for the implantation of deep brain stimulators for Parkinson's disease and tremor. Mov Disord. 2006; 21 Suppl 14:S259–S283

[13] Starr PA, Martin AJ, Ostrem JL, Talke P, Levesque N, Larson PS. Subthalamic nucleus deep brain stimulator placement using high-field interventional magnetic resonance imaging and a skull-mounted aiming device: technique and application accuracy. J Neurosurg. 2010; 112(3):479–490

[14] Voges J, Koulousakis A, Sturm V. Deep brain stimulation for Parkinson's disease. Acta Neurochir Suppl (Wien). 2007; 97(Pt 2):171–184

[15] Pouratian N, Reames DL, Frysinger R, Elias WJ. Comhensive analysis of risk factors for seizures after deep brain stimulation surgery. J Neurosurg. 2011; 115(2):310–315

[16] Kocabicak E, Temel Y. Deep brain stimulation of the subthalamic nucleus in Parkinson's disease: surgical technique, tips, tricks and complications. Clin Neurol Neurosurg. 2013; 115(11):2318–2323

[17] Joint C, Nandi D, Parkin S, Gregory R, Aziz T, Aziz T. Hardware-related problems of deep brain stimulation. Mov Disord. 2002; 17(3) Suppl 3: S175–S180

[18] Hariz MI. Complications of deep brain stimulation surgery. Mov Disord. 2002; 17(3) Suppl 3:S162–S166

12 Essential Tremor: Evaluation, Imaging and Medical Treatment

Lauren Len Spiegel and Joohi Jimenez-Shahed

Abstract

Essential tremor (ET) is a common movement disorder characterized by postural and action tremors of the hands, head and voice, often with a family history, that tends to improve with alcohol and worsens with stress or anxiety. It can typically be distinguished from other tremor types, including parkinsonian, dystonic, neuropathic, and drug-induced tremors. Symptoms are often symmetric and clinical progression is typically slow. The pathophysiology is thought to be mediated by abnormal output activity in the cerebello-thalamo-cortical pathways, and is supported by post-mortem and imaging studies. Medical treatments for ET include propranolol and primidone (amongst others) and may require polypharmacy in advanced cases.

Keywords: essential tremor, propranolol, primidone, diagnosis, pathophysiology, treatment

12.1 Introduction

Essential Tremor (ET) is one of the most common movement disorders with an estimated prevalence of 0.4%-3.9% with an even higher prevalence of 4.6% in those older than 65.[1,2] This disorder has a bimodal distribution of age at onset with a small peak in those individuals in their second and third decade with a larger incidence in individuals in their seventh and eight decades.[3]

12.1.1 Phenomenology and Family History

Essential Tremor is defined as a typically hereditary and predominantly postural and kinetic tremor syndrome affecting the hands. Tremor of other body parts (e.g., the head, voice and trunk) may also be present.[4] The characteristic 4–12 Hz postural tremor is typically bilateral and largely symmetric.[4,5] Approximately 60–70% of patients report improvement with alcohol, while anxiety, stress, and caffeine worsen tremor.[5] Half of ET patients have a family history, especially those with onset earlier in life.[6] Younger-onset ET patients perform similar to unaffected peers in education and working life while the older-onset patients may have dementia and increased mortality, though neither differs significantly in their level of response to oral medications.[6] A specific disease-causing gene(s) has not been identified.

12.1.2 Rating Scales

Symptom severity can be assessed in the research and clinical settings using clinical scales such as the Fahn-Tolosa-Marin Tremor Rating Scale (TRS) and the Tremor Research Group Essential Tremor Rating Assessment Scale (TETRAS). The TRS is a 5-point (0–4) scale with a maximum total score of 144[7] while the TETRAS was developed more recently and has a maximum score of 64.[8] Both clinical scales include assessment of tremor amplitude in different positions and tasks along with impact on activities of daily living.

12.1.3 Clinical Progression

Progression of ET is slow, especially earlier in the disease process. Patients with younger onset and family history may experience symptoms for over 40 years.[9] One study found four factors that significantly correlated with increased baseline tremor score: older age at first clinic visit, longer disease duration, use of drugs for movement disorders, and the presence of voice tremor. Three factors significantly correlated with faster tremor progression: unilateral or head or neck tremor at onset, asymmetrical disease, and longer duration between baseline and previous follow-up. In this study, the TRS score increased by less than 1 point per year prior to the first clinic visit and approximately 2 points per year during the observed study period (mean follow-up = 3.6 years).[10]

12.1.4 Differential Diagnosis

Differentiating tremor syndromes can be difficult given the overlap of rest, postural, and kinetic tremors in tremor disorders. Specific types of tremor are required for diagnosis of their tremor syndrome while other tremors are allowed for diagnosis (▶ Table 12.1). For instance, while action tremor is typically associated with ET and rest tremor with Parkinson's disease (PD), rest tremor can be seen in up to 30% of ET, but tends to

Table 12.1 Differentiation of tremor subtypes

Tremor	Frequency (Hz)	Rest	Postural	Kinetic	Dystonia
Essential	4–12	+	*	+	-
Parkinsonian	3–11	*	+	+	-
Dystonic	4–8	+	*	*	*
Neuropathic	4–11	-	*	+	-
Drug-induced	2–10	+	+	+	-

Data from Consensus Statement of the Movement Disorder Society on Tremor (1998).
* Required for Diagnosis, + May be present, - Almost always absent

Table 12.2 Medications for essential tremor

	Total Daily Doses (mg)	Level of Recommendation	Potential Side Effects
Primidone	250–750	A	Sedation, nausea, dizziness, ataxia, acute toxic reaction, bone marrow suppression
Propranolol	120–320	A	Bradycardia, syncope
Alprazolam	0.125–3	B	Sedation, abuse potential, withdrawal
Atenolol	50–200	B	Bradycardia, syncope
Gabapentin	1200–3600	B	Sedation
Sotalol	75–200	B	Bradycardia, syncope
Topiramate	200–400	B	Renal stones, glaucoma, word-finding difficulties, anorexia, paresthesias
Nadolol	40–80	C	Bradycardia, syncope
Nimodipine	120	C	Bradycardia
Clonazepam	0.5–6	C	Sedation, abuse potential, withdrawal
Botulinum Toxin	Variable	C	Muscle weakness, dysphagia, hoarseness
Lyrica	150 mg-600 mg	U	Sedation

A = established as effective
B = probably effective
C = possibly effective
U = insufficient evidence

occur in later, more severe stages, and does not exclude the ET diagnosis.[11]

12.2 Pathophysiology and Imaging

12.2.1 Animal Studies

The harmaline-induced tremor animal model of ET suggests pathology within the inferior olivary nucleus, since it induces rhythmic burst-firing in that structure, which contains pathways projecting to Purkinje cells and deep cerebellar nuclei (DCN).[12] The DCN form projections back to the brainstem, eventually engaging the spinal cord as well as the thalamocortical network. Downregulation of this pathway may lead to pathologic tremor.

12.2.2 Post-mortem Studies

ET is associated with multiple pathologies including reduced GABAergic function from the Purkinje cells, cerebellar vermis atrophy, dentate degeneration, and increased brain iron accumulation.[13,14,15] A post-mortem study of 33 ET brains by Louis and colleagues reported 76% had cerebellar changes with Purkinje cell degeneration and cell death associated with marked changes in the dentate nucleus (a component of the DCN) including neuronal loss, microglial clusters and reduction in efferent fibers. These authors also reported pathologic heterogeneity which is consistent with some clinical heterogeneity observed in practice.[14] Others have proposed that a decrease in $GABA_A$ receptors in the dentate nucleus of post-mortem ET brains results in disinhibition of cerebellar pacemaker output activity in the cerebello-thalamo-cortical pathways to generate tremors.[15,16,17]

12.2.3 Imaging Studies

While ET is a clinical diagnosis, fMRI and MRI studies are non-invasive supplements to understand tremor pathophysiology. Involvement of the cerebellum is the most consistent finding with many studies supporting GABAergic dysfunction. Ioflupane I-123 injection scanning (DaTscan™) can distinguish parkinsonian from other tremor types; however, a normal scan does not unequivocally imply an ET diagnosis.[12,18] In practice, most patients do not require imaging unless deep brain stimulation (DBS) is anticipated.[19]

12.3 Treatment

The only FDA approved medication for ET is propranolol, however the most common initial medications for ET are primidone and propranolol.[19] These medications have Level A evidence supporting their efficacy, but 30–50% of patients will not respond to either. Medications that are probably effective with Level B evidence include alprazolam, atenolol, gabapentin, sotalol, and topiramate. Medication selection may depend on their potential side effect profiles (▶ Table 12.2).[20,21,22] Polypharmacy may be required as disability progresses.[23] Botulinum toxin type A injections has Class C evidence for refractory ET. Candidates for surgical therapies including DBS should experience disabling tremor that significantly impairs their ability to carry out daily tasks despite medical therapy.

References

[1] Louis ED. Clinical practice. Essential tremor. N Engl J Med. 2001; 345(12): 887–891

[2] Chopra A, Klassen BT, Stead M. Current clinical application of deep-brain stimulation for essential tremor. Neuropsychiatr Dis Treat. 2013; 9:1859–1865

[3] Louis ED, Dogu O. Does age of onset in essential tremor have a bimodal distribution? Data from a tertiary referral setting and a population-based study. Neuroepidemiology. 2007; 29(3–4):208–212

[4] Deuschl G, Bain P, Brin M, Ad Hoc Scientific Committee. Consensus statement of the Movement Disorder Society on Tremor. Mov Disord. 1998; 13 Suppl 3:2–23

[5] Raethjen J, Deuschl G. The oscillating central network of Essential tremor. Clin Neurophysiol. 2012; 123(1):61–64

[6] Hopfner F, Ahlf A, Lorenz D, et al. Early- and late-onset essential tremor patients represent clinically distinct subgroups. Mov Disord. 2016; 31(10): 1560–1566

[7] Fahn S, Tolosa E, Marin C. Clinical rating Scale for tremor. Parkinson's Disease and Movement disorders. Baltimor-Munich: Urban & Schwarzenberg; 1988:225–34

[8] Elble R. The Essential Tremor Rating Assessment Scale. J Neurol Neuromed. 2016; 1(4):34–38

[9] Putzke JD, Whaley NR, Baba Y, Wszolek ZK, Uitti RJ. Essential tremor: predictors of disease progression in a clinical cohort. J Neurol Neurosurg Psychiatry. 2006; 77(11):1235–1237– Erratum in: J Neurol Neurosurg Psychiatry. 2010;81(1):126. doi:10.1136/jnnp.2006.086579

[10] Louis ED, Gerbin M, Galecki M. Essential tremor 10, 20, 30, 40: clinical snapshots of the disease by decade of duration. Eur J Neurol. 2013; 20(6):949–954

[11] Thenganatt MA, Louis ED. Distinguishing essential tremor from Parkinson's disease: bedside tests and laboratory evaluations. Expert Rev Neurother. 2012; 12(6):687–696

[12] Bhalsing KS, Saini J, Pal PK. Understanding the pathophysiology of essential tremor through advanced neuroimaging: a review. J Neurol Sci. 2013; 335(1–2):9–13

[13] Handforth A. Harmaline tremor: underlying mechanisms in a potential animal model of essential tremor. Tremor Other Hyperkinet Mov (N Y). 2012; 2: 2–92

[14] Louis ED, Faust PL, Vonsattel JP, et al. Neuropathological changes in essential tremor: 33 cases compared with 21 controls. Brain. 2007; 130(Pt 12):3297–3307

[15] Paris-Robidas S, Brochu E, Sintes M, et al. Defective dentate nucleus GABA receptors in essential tremor. Brain. 2012; 135(Pt 1):105–116

[16] Louis ED. Essential tremor: evolving clinicopathological concepts in an era of intensive post-mortem enquiry. Lancet Neurol. 2010; 9(6):613–622

[17] Lorenz D, Deuschl G. Update on pathogenesis and treatment of essential tremor. Curr Opin Neurol. 2007; 20(4):447–452

[18] Sharifi S, Nederveen AJ, Booij J, van Rootselaar AF. Neuroimaging essentials in essential tremor: a systematic review. Neuroimage Clin. 2014; 5:217–231

[19] Zesiewicz TA, Elble RJ, Louis ED, et al. Evidence-based guideline update: treatment of essential tremor: report of the Quality Standards subcommittee of the American Academy of Neurology. Neurology. 2011; 77(19):1752–1755

[20] Pal PK. Guidelines for management of essential tremor. Ann Indian Acad Neurol. 2011; 14 Suppl 1:S25–S28

[21] Gironell A, Kulisevsky J. Diagnosis and management of essential tremor and dystonic tremor. Ther Adv Neurol Disorder. 2009; 2(4):215–222

[22] Loiselle C, Young R.. Gamma knife: a useful tool for treatment of essential tremor. Swedish Radiosurgery. 2014; 3 4. DOI: 10.3978/j.issn.2218-676X.201 4.08.01

[23] Ondo WG. Essential tremor: treatment options. Curr Treat Options Neurol. 2006; 8(3):256–267

13 Surgery for Essential Tremor

Andres l. Maldonado-Naranjo, Joshua Golubovsky, Andre G. Machado

Abstract

Deep brain stimulation of the Ventral Intermedius Nucleus (Vim DBS) is approved by the Food and Drug Administration for the management of essential tremor (ET) or tremor associated with Parkinson's disease. In this chapter we will focus on the treatment of ET and will describe the assessment of candidates for DBS, the operative procedure, post-operative management, risks and complication avoidance strategies. Indications are described, along with our patient selection process. The procedures for surgical planning including target and trajectory planning, the operative approach, intraoperative physiology and macroelectrode implantation are described.

Keywords: essential tremor, thalamus, deep brain stimulation, microeletrode physiology, ventral intermedius nucleus (VIM)

13.1 Patient Selection

Patients considered for surgical treatment of Essential Tremor (ET) are evaluated by an interdisciplinary team with neurological examination, video recording, and brain MRI with gadolinium. Cases are then discussed in a multi-disciplinary conference to determine candidacy and discuss technical choices. Common criteria are listed in ▶ Table 13.1. Prerequisites for surgical treatment include a confirmed diagnosis of ET,[1,2] failure of medical treatment to reduce tremor meaningfully without intolerable side effects, and significant impairment of function and quality of life associated with tremor.

13.2 Preoperative Preparation

Once candidacy is finalized, the patient is scheduled for preoperative assessments aimed at reducing perioperative risks. Internal medicine assessment, cardiology or other medical specialties are requested as needed. Platelet anti-aggregation therapy, anticoagulation, and non-steroidal anti-inflammatory medications are stopped 7 to 10 days before surgery, or a warfarin-to-heparin bridge is initiated in high-risk individuals. A 1.5 or 3 Tesla gadolinium-enhanced volumetric MRI, with T1 -and T2-weighted images is obtained for planning. A high resolution, thin-cut CT scan with contrast is used when MRI is contraindicated. Due to the limited number of MRI sequences

Table 13.1 Inclusion and exclusion criteria for Vim DBS

Indications	Red Flags
Confirmed diagnosis of ET	Cognitive and behavioral issues, unrealistic goals
Failure of medical treatment	Early disease, non-optimized medical therapy
Significant medication intolerance	Abnormal brain imaging, alternative diagnoses
Moderate to severe disability	Significant medical or surgical comorbidities

compatible with deep brain stimulation (DBS) systems, patients requiring frequent MRI imaging post DBS might not be appropriate candidates[3,4] although some DBS systems are now compatible with head as well as body MRIs under specific scanning conditions. It is necessary to consult the labeling of the specific DBS implant for MRI safety instructions.

13.2.1 Targeting

While it is commonplace to utilize both direct and indirect techniques for DBS targeting, commonly available 1.5 T or 3.0 T MRI sequences do not allow for visualization of individual thalamic nuclei parcellations. Therefore, thalamic targeting is dependent primarily on indirect targeting based on the posterior commissure, distance to the wall of the third ventricle and distance to the internal capsule. While it is possible to target the Vim nucleus of the thalamus in the first stereotactic cannulation for placement of the DBS lead, we often prefer to refine stereotactic localization by first targeting the ventrocaudal (Vc) nucleus, the primary sensory relay located posterior to Vim. The Vc is organized with the sensory representation of the face medially and the representation of the lower extremity laterally. The transition between Vc and Vim is typically located 2–4 mm anterior to the posterior commissure (PC) and the upper extremity representation in the Vc located approximately 10–11 mm lateral to the wall of the third ventricle. The bottom of the thalamus is typically at the level of the intercommissural plane. The first microelectrode recording pass can indicate the laterality in relation to the plan. If more tactile units corresponding to the face are identified, this is an indication that the pass was more medial than intended and if more units corresponding to the leg are identified, it suggests a more lateral pass. A second microelectrode recording (MER) pass can be made anteriorly to help define the Vc-Vim transition. The final electrode is typically placed 2–4 mm anterior to the estimated Vc-Vim transition and aimed at the physiological topography of the upper extremity.[5] Although we in general avoid transventricular trajectories[6] some patients require a transventricular approach due to large ventricles or other limitations such as vascular anatomy that narrows the options for trajectory planning.[5,7]

13.3 Operative Procedure

The stereotactic frame is set at the lateral canthus-tragus line to parallel the AC-PC plane. Pins are finger-tightened to avoid frame deformation. Next, a stereo- CT scan is obtained and MRI images are co-registered. Trajectory coordinates are generated with the navigation software. Following scalp prepping, the rings and stereotactic arc are positioned and the coordinates applied. A linear or curvilinear incision is made, burr hole drilled, and remaining internal table removed. The anchoring burr hole device is fixed to the skull and the dura matter is coagulated, opened in a cruciate fashion, and a small corticectomy is performed, with care to avoid any potential injury to superficial vessels. A microdrive is assembled and a premeasured cannula is inserted. The burr hole is packed with Gelfoam and fibrin glue to minimize CSF loss and pneumocephalus.

13.3.1 Microelectrode Recording

We typically start recording 15 mm dorsal to the final target. The microelectrode is advanced along the sagittal angle of a trajectory that parallels the major axis of the Vim, usually 50–60 degrees from the AC-PC line, and with a lateral angle of 15–20 degrees. As it descends, it traverses the Voa/Vop, Vim, VC, ventral border of the thalamus, and the fibers of the medial lemniscus.[8] The anterior thalamic nuclei have low density and slow firing rates, interposed by bursting cells (15 Hz) throughout the Voa/Vop that respond to active movement of contralateral limbs.[8] As the electrode is advanced, Vim kinesthetic units (25 – 30 Hz) and tremor cells may be isolated. Next, proprioceptive fields can be found (responsive to deep muscle palpation), corresponding to the "dorsal shell of the Vc". The Vc contains units that are extremely responsive to light touch. Targeting is adjusted somatotopically, with better outcomes when targeting anterior to the Vc receptive field for the thumb and mouth.[9] An intraoperative O-arm image is combined with the MER track to interpolate electrode location relative to the Vim before final lead implantation. The use of intraoperative O-arm reduces the number of penetrations required for successful localization as demonstrated in a recent study by our team.[10] The final electrode is positioned 3–4 mm anterior to the identified Vim/Vc border.[5] (▶ Fig. 13.1) Microstimulation (10–100 μA) is performed along the trajectory and its effects are observed.

13.3.2 DBS Electrode Implantation and Testing

Once the final target has been selected, the microelectrode and cannula are removed, the frame coordinates are adjusted, and the cannula followed by the DBS lead are inserted and advanced to the target. Contact 0 is positioned at the ventral aspect of the Vim. Using monopolar macrostimulation (pulse width 90 μs, rate 130 Hz), the voltage is increased progressively and the patient is observed for improvements in tremor and for possible side effects. We usually start with the most distal electrode. However, bipolar stimulation might be necessary if adverse effects are elicited, at low thresholds. If electrode repositioning is required, we recommend moving the target by a minimum of 1.5 mm increments to avoid falling into the previous track. Once the Vim DBS electrode is satisfactorily placed, the guide wire and cannula are removed and the electrode is secured with the Stim-Loc device (Medtronic, Minneapolis). Next, the electrode is tunneled under the galea to the parietal region in preparation for stage II surgery. The excess cable is then coiled around the burr hole and the wound is closed. A pulse generator is implanted 7–10 days after the lead is placed.

13.4 Post-Operative Management

A CT scan can be obtained to rule out subclinical intracranial complications, such as an asymptomatic bleed or inadvertent electrode migration. Tremor medications are resumed and perioperative antibiotics are given. The majority of patients are routinely discharged after overnight stay.

13.4.1 Complications

Complications include bleeding, infections, and hardware and stimulation-related complications. Bleeding risk is reported between 1.5 to 3%, with a risk of permanent morbidity of 0.5 and 1%. If bleeding is observed through the cannula, irrigation should continue until it clears. Examination is necessary and surgery can be aborted if signs of progressive deterioration are present. Trajectories that avoid superficial, sulcal or deep vessels may be safer. Infection rates vary from 1 to 15%. Hardware-related complications, such as lead fractures, lead migration,

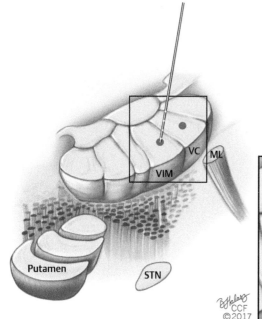
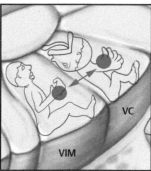

Fig. 13.1 Three dimensional rendering of the left basal ganglia. Primary targeting is aimed at the somatotopic area of the hand/arm in the Vc. Side effects such as capsular (motor) and paresthesias (ML) might be elicited during microstimulation, which will indicate proximity to those structures. Once Vc is confirmed, the microelectrode moved anteriorly to target the hand/arm representation of the Vim. Vim = ventral intermedius nucleus, Vc = ventrocaudal nucleus, ML = medial lemniscus, STN = subthalamic nucleus. Reprinted with permission, Cleveland Clinic Center for Medical Art & Photography © 2019. All Rights Reserved.

lead exposure, disconnection, and pain over the pulse generator site vary significantly from center to center. Vim Stimulation-related complications include paresthesias, muscular contractions, dysarthria, dystonia, gait and balance issues, as well as decreased dexterity.[5,11,12,13] Programming can often minimize such adverse effects while maintaining good benefits.

13.5 Conclusion

Medication-resistant essential tremor is effectively treated with Vim DBS. Alternative options include thalamotomy by radiofrequency, radiosurgery or focus ultrasound, all of which are non-reversible.

References

[1] Jain S, Lo SE, Louis ED. Common misdiagnosis of a common neurological disorder: how are we misdiagnosing essential tremor? Arch Neurol. 2006; 63 (8):1100–1104

[2] Deuschl G, Bain P, Brin M, Ad Hoc Scientific Committee. Consensus statement of the Movement Disorder Society on Tremor. Mov Disord. 1998; 13 Suppl 3: 2–23

[3] Sharan A, Rezai AR, Nyenhuis JA, et al. MR safety in patients with implanted deep brain stimulation systems (DBS). Acta Neurochir Suppl (Wien). 2003; 87:141–145

[4] Rezai AR, Phillips M, Baker KB, et al. Neurostimulation system used for deep brain stimulation (DBS): MR safety issues and implications of failing to follow safety recommendations. Invest Radiol. 2004; 39(5):300–303

[5] Rezai AR, Machado AG, Deogaonkar M, Azmi H, Kubu C, Boulis NM. Surgery for movement disorders. Neurosurgery. 2008; 62 Suppl 2:809–838, discussion 838–839

[6] Gologorsky Y, Ben-Haim S, Moshier EL, et al. Transgressing the ventricular wall during subthalamic deep brain stimulation surgery for Parkinson disease increases the risk of adverse neurological sequelae. Neurosurgery. 2011; 69 (2):294–299, discussion 299–300

[7] Machado A, Rezai AR, Kopell BH, Gross RE, Sharan AD, Benabid AL. Deep brain stimulation for Parkinson's disease: surgical technique and perioperative management. Mov Disord. 2006; 21 Suppl 14:S247–S258

[8] Gross RE, Krack P, Rodriguez-Oroz MC, Rezai AR, Benabid AL. Electrophysiological mapping for the implantation of deep brain stimulators for Parkinson's disease and tremor. Mov Disord. 2006; 21 Suppl 14:S259–S283

[9] Benabid AL, Pollak P, Gao D, et al. Chronic electrical stimulation of the ventralis intermedius nucleus of the thalamus as a treatment of movement disorders. J Neurosurg. 1996; 84(2):203–214

[10] Frizon LA, Shao J, Maldonado-Naranjo AL, Lobel DA, Nagel SJ, Fernandez HH, Machado AG. The Safety and Efficacy of Using the O-Arm Intraoperative Imaging System for Deep Brain Stimulation Lead Implantation. Neuromodulation. 2018 Aug;21(6):588–592

[11] Beric A, Kelly PJ, Rezai A, et al. Complications of deep brain stimulation surgery. Stereotact Funct Neurosurg. 2001; 77(1–4):73–78

[12] Umemura A, Jaggi JL, Hurtig HI, et al. Deep brain stimulation for movement disorders: morbidity and mortality in 109 patients. J Neurosurg. 2003; 98(4): 779–784

[13] Hariz MI. Complications of deep brain stimulation surgery. Mov Disord. 2002; 17 Suppl 3:S162–S166

14 Dystonia: Evaluation, Imaging and Medical Treatment

Travis J. W. Hassell and Fenna T. Phibbs

Abstract

Dystonia is a hyperkinetic movement disorder that involves intermittent or sustained muscle contractions that produce repetitive, patterned, and twisting postures with associated tremor. Accurate recognition of these features and understanding of appropriate pharmacologic therapy, chemodenervation strategies, and surgical interventions will lead to improved patient outcomes. This chapter will provide a concise set of clinical tools to accurately diagnose dystonia review current medical treatment strategies.

Keywords: dystonia, chemodenervation, blepharospasm, spasmodic torticollis, DYTb

14.1 Introduction

Dystonia is a hyperkinetic movement disorder that involves intermittent or sometimes fixed muscle contractions that cause repetitive movements such as tremor or abnormal body postures. While dystonia is represented by a spectrum of clinical features, there are common presentations. Accurate classification begins by identifying the primary phenomenology of the abnormal movement. This chapter provides a concise set of tools to accurately identify and treat the key clinical features of dystonic syndromes.

14.2 Classification and Diagnosis of Dystonia

14.2.1 Clinical Features and Phenomenology

The recognition and diagnosis of dystonia can be difficult given the complex spectrum of clinical features, temporal patterns, wide range of affected ages, and overlap with other associated movements disorders such as essential tremor (ET) and Parkinson's Disease (PD). A growing number of identified genes and genetic dystonic syndromes make it even more important to have a more systematic means to distinguish between dystonic patterns. A consensus statement was published in 2013 that revised the classification of dystonia, which is detailed in ▶ Table 14.1. Accurate classification relies on identification of two main characteristics: clinical features and etiology.[1]

Dystonic contractions are often initiated or worsened by specific tasks or voluntary movements producing abnormal and sometimes painful postures. Dystonic movements are most commonly seen as twisting about a longitudinal axis and often have a characteristic direction or pattern.[2] It is this patterned movement that helps to differentiate dystonia from other hyperkinetic movements. The muscles involved in the presenting posture are usually those affected, but dystonic contractions can occur into a muscle adjacent to the primary movement. This is termed *overflow*. Mirroring is a similar concept however, the dystonic movement is brought on by voluntary movement in the homologous, non-affected body part on the opposite side.[3] For example, dystonic wrist flexion can be brought out in the affected hand by writing with the unaffected hand. Several theories exist for dystonic movements, but a prevailing one is that there is impairment of surround inhibition at multiple levels within the central nervous system. This creates an imbalance of sensorimotor integration and an inappropriate output response that is manifested as abnormal co-contraction of specific muscle groups.[4,5] Electromyography (EMG) has shown that added sensory input changes muscle recruitment patterns. Patients often develop "sensory tricks" that can lessen these dystonic contractions.[4,5,6]

When intermittent, dystonic muscle contractions often produce a tremor especially if there is an antagonist muscle attempting to provide balance. Differentiating dystonic tremor from other movement disorders with tremor as a predominant

Table 14.1 Classification criteria for dystonia. Adapted from Camargos S, Cardoso, F.[2]

Category	Classification	Subgroup
I: Clinical Features	Age at onset	Infancy (birth to 2 yrs.) Childhood (2 to 12 yrs.) Adolescence (13 to 20 yrs.) Early adulthood (21 to 40 yrs.) Late adulthood (40 and older)
	Body distribution	Focal (one body region – blepharospasm, orolingual, laryngeal, cervical, limb) Segmental (2 or more contiguous regions) Multifocal (2 or more non-contiguous) Hemidystonia (hemibody) Generalized (trunk plus 2 other sites)
	Temporal pattern	Course (static vs progressive) Variable (persistent, action-specific, diurnal, paroxysmal)
	Associated features	Isolated (with or without tremor) Combined (with other neuro or systemic disease)
II: Etiology	CNS pathology	Degenerative, structural, or neither
	Heritability	Inherited or Primary (genetic with various inheritance patterns)
	Idiopathic	Acquired or Secondary (metabolic, heavy metal (Wilson's – copper), brain injury, drug induced, vascular, neoplastic, infection, psychogenic) Sporadic vs familial

Table 14.2 Diagnosis of hereditary dystonia. Data from Camargos S, Cardoso, F.[2]

Dystonia Type	Age of Onset	Clinical Hallmark	DYT #
Isolated Dystonia	Childhood or adolescence	Adductor dysphonia	DYT 4
		Generalized with laryngeal sparing	DYT 1
		Focal, multifocal, or generalized	DYT 1, 5, 6
		Cranio-cervical and generalized	DYT 2, 6, 16, 25, 27
	Early adulthood	Isolated cranio-cervical	DYT 23, 24, 27
Dystonia-parkinsonism	Childhood and adult	Dopa-responsive	DYT 5
		X-linked, Filipino	DYT 3
		Rapid onset	DYT 12
Dystonia-myoclonus		Alcohol responsive	DYT 11
		Not alcohol responsive	DYT 26
Paroxysmal dystonia		Non-kinesigenic	DYT 8 – ETOH, benzo resp.
		Kinesigenic (exercise, sudden movement induced)	DYT 18 – Ataxia, epilepsy, hemolytic anemia, low CSF glucose, ketogenic diet resp.
			DYT10 – anticonvulsant resp.

feature can be difficult. However, there are certain features of dystonic tremor that can be helpful. Dystonic tremor can be rhythmic or irregular with a jerky quality and is amplified when there is movement opposite to the direction intended by the dystonic muscle. This is seen in cervical dystonia. Dystonic tremor will generally lessen when the desired dystonic posture is reached. This is called a *null point*.[7] Isolated head tremor, or head tremor that precedes or is more severe than hand tremor is more likely to be a dystonic tremor than ET or PD. Dystonic head tremor often persists in the supine position whereas ET head tremor abates.[8]

> Dystonic tremor lessens when the desired posture or null point is reached.
> Dystonic head tremor persists upon lying down whereas essential head tremor abates

When the diagnosis of dystonia is to be considered, it is important to rule out mimics and secondary causes. These are summarized in ▸ Table 14.1. It is also important to consider the natural history of the symptoms before any testing is initiated. Childhood or early-onset dystonia is more likely to involve lower extremities at onset, have a history of known progression and early generalization, is more likely to be associated with other abnormal movements such as those seen in Parkinson's disease, and be responsive to medical therapy such as dopamine replacement. In contrast, adult-onset (> 26 years of age) is more likely to affect the head or neck instead of a limb such as occurs in early-onset dystonia, remain more focal rather than generalized, have a task-specific nature, and have a short period of progression after onset (average 5 to 7 years).[9]

14.2.2 Genetic Testing

Since the first description of primary generalized or familial dystonia (DYT1) in 1997, many different genes have been identified as associated with dystonic syndromes. A few clinically common syndromes are DYT1 (primary generalized), DYT3 (X-linked dystonia-parkinsonism), DYT4 (dysphonic), DYT5 (dopa-responsive), and DYT11 (dystonia-myoclonus). The likelihood of a dystonic syndrome to be of genetic etiology rather than idiopathic or secondary declines with advancing age.[2] The key genetic dystonic syndromes are summarized in ▸ Table 14.2.

14.2.3 Imaging and Other Diagnostic Tools

Imaging is not used to make the diagnosis of dystonia, but it can be helpful when clinical suspicion is high for a secondary dystonia. To best evaluate for structural, vascular, neoplastic, infectious, or other such causes, MRI is the modality of choice. EMG can provide additional evidence, showing changes in muscle fiber recruitment with sensory tricks. EMG can also show if there is co-contraction of agonist and antagonist muscle groups.[5] EMG rarely leads to a definitive diagnosis, however. Some dystonic syndromes can produce painful muscle spasms. Pain may not occur in all forms of dystonia, but is common for some, such as cervical dystonia, with one study reporting that 75% of patients have neck pain.[10] Pain relief can be helpful diagnostically, and provides a metric for treatment success.

14.3 Treatment of Dystonia

When determining the optimal regimen for the management of dystonic syndromes, a multi-modal approach is used that begins with oral medications and chemodenervation with botulinum toxin, then if needed proceeds to surgical intervention. Dystonia classification often dictates treatment strategy with the focus placed on the level of focality. Chemodenervation is a first-line therapy for focal and segmental dystonias. Botulinum toxin is often preferred over oral medications due to its efficacy and minimal systemic side effects. However, for more generalized dystonia, oral medications provide broader coverage than botulinum therapy allows.[11,12] Surgery is considered for most primary generalized dystonias, and refractory focal and segmental dystonias. ▸ Table 14.3 presents a summary of medical treatment options.

Table 14.3 Treatment of dystonia.[11,12]

Therapeutic Medications[11]	Therapeutic Daily Dose (divided 2 to 4 doses)	Common Side Effects
Trihexyphenidyl (Anticholinergic)	6 – 40 mg	Blurry vision, confusion, constipation, urinary retention, dry mouth
Clonazepam/Diazepam (GABA-A agonist)	1 – 4 mg/10 – 40 mg	Drowsiness, fatigue
Carbidopa-levodopa (Dopamine precursor)	75 mg/300 mg – 500 mg/2000 mg	Nausea
Tetrabenazine (Dopamine depleting)	12.5 mg – 100 mg	Akathisia, anxiety, depression, suicidality, parkinsonism, drowsiness
Baclofen (GABA-B agonist)	40 mg – 120 mg	Drowsiness, fatigue, nausea, weakness
Carbamazepine (VGNaCB, GABA)	800 mg – 1200 mg	For paroxysmal kinesigenic dyskinesia
Botulinum Toxin (Strain)	**Dystonia subtype Indication**	**Level of Evidence/Recommendation** [12]
Abobotulinum (A) (Dysport)	CD, B, L, OM, AD	CD - A; B - B; L - B; OM - C; AD - U
Onabotulinum (A) (BOTOX)	CD, B, L, OM, AD	CD - A; B - A; L - B; OM - C; AD - C
Incobotulinum (A) (Xeomin)	CD, B, L, OM, AD	CD - A; B - A; L - U; OM - U; AD - U
Rimabotulinum (B) (Myobloc)	CD, B, L, OM, AD	CD - A; B - U; L - U; OM - U; AD - U

CD – cervical dystonia, B – blepharospasm, L – limb, OM – Oral mandibular, AD – adductor dysphonia. Recommendation order: A, B, C, U; VGNaCB – voltage-gated Na channel blocker

14.4 Conclusion

The clinical spectrum of dystonic syndromes is broad and can overlap with other neurologic conditions making an accurate diagnosis difficult but important for appropriate treatment. Identifying the predominant phenomenology and applying the appropriate classification improves diagnostic accuracy. Botulinum toxin is effective in treating all forms of dystonia, and is a mainstay of focal dystonia treatment.

References

[1] Albanese A, Bhatia K, Bressman SB, et al. Phenomenology and classification of dystonia: a consensus update. Mov Disord. 2013; 28(7):863–873

[2] Camargos S, Cardoso F. Understanding dystonia: diagnostic issues and how to overcome them. Arq Neuropsiquiatr. 2016; 74(11):921–936

[3] Sitburana O, Wu LJ, Sheffield JK, Davidson A, Jankovic J. Motor overflow and mirror dystonia. Parkinsonism Relat Disord. 2009; 15(10):758–761

[4] Hallett M. Pathophysiology of writer's cramp. Hum Mov Sci. 2006; 25(4–5): 454–463

[5] Sohn YH, Hallett M. Disturbed surround inhibition in focal hand dystonia. Ann Neurol. 2004; 56(4):595–599

[6] Loyola DP, Camargos S, Maia D, Cardoso F. Sensory tricks in focal dystonia and hemifacial spasm. Eur J Neurol. 2013; 20(4):704–707

[7] Erro R, Rubio-Agusti I, Saifee TA, et al. Rest and other types of tremor in adult-onset primary dystonia. J Neurol Neurosurg Psychiatry. 2014; 85(9): 965–968

[8] Agnew A, Frucht SJ, Louis ED. Supine head tremor: a clinical comparison of essential tremor and spasmodic torticollis patients. J Neurol Neurosurg Psychiatry. 2012; 83(2):179–181

[9] O'Riordan S, Raymond D, Lynch T, et al. Age at onset as a factor in determining the phenotype of primary torsion dystonia. Neurology. 2004; 63(8): 1423–1426

[10] Chan J, Brin MF, Fahn S. Idiopathic cervical dystonia: clinical characteristics. Mov Disord. 1991; 6(2):119–126

[11] Jankovic J. Medical treatment of dystonia. Mov Disord. 2013; 28(7):1001–1012

[12] Hallett M, Albanese A, Dressler D, et al. Evidence-based review and assessment of botulinum neurotoxin for the treatment of movement disorders. Toxicon. 2013; 67:94–114

15 Surgical Treatment of Dystonia

John Honeycutt

Abstract

Dystonia was recently defined by the Taskforce on Childhood Movement Disorders as "a movement disorder in which involuntary sustained or intermittent muscle contractions cause twisting and repetitive movements, abnormal postures, or both."[1] It is a difficult disorder to diagnose and treat as the presentation of dystonia, overlaps with that of spasticity, chorea and athetosis. This chapter will discuss intrathecal baclofen therapy (ITB) and deep brain stimulation (DBS) for treatment of medically refractory dystonia.

Keywords: dystonia, baclofen, DBS, infection, intrathecal pumps

15.1 Patient Selection

Medical management begins with intense physical, occupational and speech therapy and a limited range of medications. Surgical management ensues when the movement disorder is refractory to medical management. As with medical treatment, surgical options are limited. The mainstays are ITB and DBS. DBS has replaced pallidotomy and thalamotomy as a surgical option because of the presence of significant side effects from the bilateral and irreversible lesions. Peripheral denervation procedures are also used for focal cervical dystonia, but botulinum toxin injections and DBS therapy and now predominate.

Purely dystonic patients are most often treated by DBS. Most pediatric patients have a mixture of symptomatic spasticity and dystonia. In these cases, a baclofen pump is first considered because families are concerned about the thought of "brain surgery." That said, the complication rate of DBS is similar to that which occurs with ITB. The children become dependent on the medication and pumps require frequent refills. There is always a concern of baclofen withdrawal syndrome after refills and pump changes.[2] Many patients have both a baclofen pump and DBS, which reduces the required baclofen dose.

Before consideration of baclofen pump insertion, a plastic pump is used to assure that there is adequate space between the iliac crest and rib cage for the implanted pump. If there is insufficient room, the child should be given time to grow. Many of these patients have their pump placement delayed because of their low weight. They are often thin and weight gain is difficult for them because of their movement disorder. After pump placement, they are able to gain weight, perhaps because of the lower caloric consumption when the disorder is controlled.

All DBS evaluations involve a multi-disciplinary team comprised of experienced neurologists, therapists and neurosurgeons. Pre operative testing is done to measure and score performance levels. Priority is given to the improvements of speech and upper extremity function. For most patients, progression from a wheelchair to ambulation is not realistic. Patients and their families may have difficulty understanding this.

For primary dystonia, especially for DYT-1 patients, after failure of medical management DBS is considered. Our series shows that DYT-1 dystonia responds quickly and effectively to DBS. Unfortunately, primary dystonia is encountered less frequently than secondary dystonia Other genetic dystonias can also respond to DBS, but usually not to the same extent. Too often, other medical issues associated with their genetic diseases complicate their lives and medical management. Marks et al., summarized our early comparison of primary (DYT1) versus secondary dystonia DBS outcomes: Both groups responded well, but the primary group continued to improve after 18 months to a greater degree than the secondary group.[3] The results of secondary dystonia treatment is variable (▶ Table 15.1).

Enrollment of every DBS patient requires a rigorous consent process approved by the institutional review board in accordance with the current United States FDA Humanitarian Device Exemption status for dystonia. No patient less than seven years old undergoes implantation in our practice. We also encourage participation in PEDiDBS, the international registry of pediatric patients undergoing deep brain stimulation.[2]

> DBS treatment of primary dystonia is more successful in the long term that for secondary dystonia.

15.2 Pre-operative Preparation-ITB

One of the advantages of ITB is that the patient can undergo an intrathecal baclofen trial. A single CSF dose given by lumbar puncture can show efficacy. However, because of the disorder's complexity, we do an extended trial using a lumbar catheter that is placed in the OR. Sedation or general anesthesia is used and the patient is admitted to the rehabilitation unit for several days of extensive physical and occupational therapy evaluation. Besides the small surgical risk, a risk of an extended trial is low

Table 15.1 Summary of demographics and etiology of our 10 year DBS program

Demographics			
Average Age(y)	Age Range (y)		
13.8	7–29.6		
Sex	Male	Female	Total
	57	55	112
Etiology			
Primary Dystonia (DYT1)		17	
Primary Dystonia Other		19	
Secondary Dystonia Cerebral Palsy		38	
Secondary Dystonia Other		30	
Other (non-dystonia)		8	

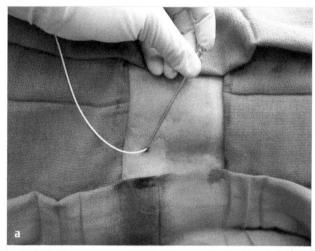

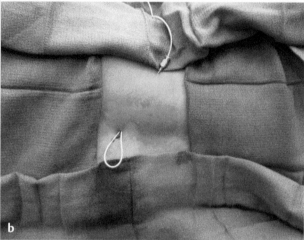

Fig. 15.1 After placement of lumbar drain, the Tuohy needle is measured to maximal tunneling distance **(a)** then used to tunnel the catheter laterally **(b)**

pressure, spinal headache. This can prevent the patient from standing for long, thus limiting trial effectiveness. Fortunately, this is not a common complication and the headaches resolve soon after the catheter is removed .

Lumbar drain placement is a standard procedure. The catheter tip should be threaded to the therapeutic level. The drain is tunneled laterally to the opposite flank from where the baclofen pump would be placed using the same Tuohy needle used to insert the catheter (▶ Fig. 15.1). If the trial is successful, an intrathecal catheter and the baclofen pump are placed one month later.

15.2.1 Operative Technique (ITB)

Baclofen pump placement is done under general anesthesia with the patient in the lateral decubitus position. The legs are flexed as much as possible while allowing access to the abdomen. The patient is secured in position with wide tape (▶ Fig. 15.2). Since many patients have gastrostomy buttons or might need them in the future, the majority of pumps are placed subcutaneously in the right abdominal wall. A midline incision is made in lower lumbar spine for the intrathecal catheter insertion. The incision and dissection needs to be large enough to allow the exiting catheter to curve gently towards the pocket. The catheter is placed using a large Tuohy needle from a paramedian trajectory just off midline. This decreases the incidence of catheter kinking between the spinous processes and decreases the risk of catheter fracture. Intraoperative fluoroscopy with the introducing wire still in place is done to confirms the catheter tip location. We use a two-piece catheter. The connecting piece acts as a scarring source to prevent catheter migration

The baclofen pump is placed submuscular in the abdominal wall. This is because most patients are thin and small. The incision is placed as far away as possible from the pump to help prevent incision breakdown. The pump is placed in the lateral abdominal wall after dissection down to the junction of the external rectus fascia and oblique muscles. The fascia is incised with cautery to expose the deep plane below the rectus and

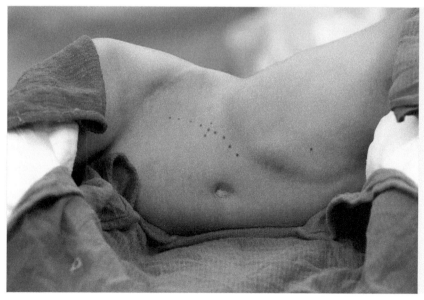

Fig. 15.2 Patient placed in lateral decubitus position with knees flexed as much as possible still allowing appropriate access to abdominal wall. The incision site is marked.

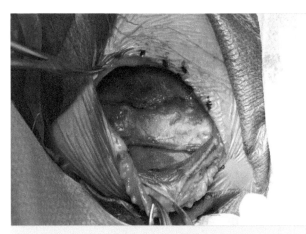

Fig. 15.3 Dissection carried down to internal fascia with overlying intact epigastric vessels showing the lower rectus muscle mobilized to create a pocket for placement of baclofen pump.

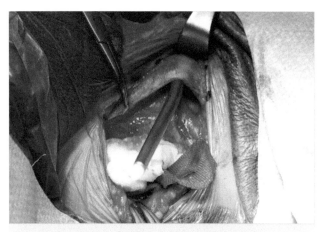

Fig. 15.4 The intrathecal catheter tunneled under the lateral rectus muscle to keep the catheter protected deep to the incision.

oblique muscles (▶ Fig. 15.3). Epigastric arteries and veins are coagulated and a pocket is created in this space above the internal rectus fascia. Since the transversalis fascia is thin below the arcuate line, dissection below it is avoided. By using this submuscular placement, a 40 ml volume pump can be placed in children as young as three years old. The intrathecal catheter is tunneled from the lumbar incision under the lateral rectus muscle to keep the pump and catheter deep to the incision (▶ Fig. 15.4). Finally, the pump and intrathecal catheter are connected, the pump is positioned in the abdominal wall pocket and secured to the internal fascia with non-absorbable sutures (▶ Fig. 15.5). Patients are kept flat for a day after surgery and then mobilized.

The infusion rate is increased during a two-day postoperative hospitalization. Baclofen pump placement for dystonia is not different from placement for spasticity. However, the catheter is usually placed as high as possible, including occasional placement into the lower cisterna magna. Intraventricular placement can also be done.[4] A stim-loc (Medtronic (Minneapolis, MN) skull attachment at the skull may prevent migration.

In thin children, baclofen pumps are placed submuscular to prevent erossion.

15.3 Post-operative Management - ITB

Complications of baclofen pump placement are well described and, unfortunately, frequently seen. Infection is the most serious complication because the pump and catheter must be removed and IV antibiotics given for an extended period. Treating pump infections without removal is rarely effective in our experience. If the pump has been in place for a while, then baclofen withdrawal syndrome must be considered and the

patient closely monitored for it. The patients are admitted to the ICU to watch for this. In our series, for all pump patients treated both for dystonia and spasticity from 1998–2014 195 pumps were placed and 80 replacement surgeries were done. The infection rate was 4.7%. There was no difference in the complication rates for patients that were treated for spasticity or for dystonia. Catheter migration or dislodgement is rare especially after recent catheter modifications that make use of a two-piece catheter. We do see catheter malfunction from wear that requires catheter replacement. True pump malfunction is uncommon, but can occur and requires pump replacement. CSF leak and pseudomeningocele is a difficult challenge. A small lumbar pseudomeningocele often is seen and is initially treated conservatively by keeping the patient flat. Most of these resolve, but the treatment protocol requires frequent clinic visits and reassurance to patient and family. Those that don't resolve require catheter replacement. This usually alleviates the problem. If the leak recurs, then the patient should be evaluated for hydrocephalus. A spine x-ray is needed to make sure that the source of the leak is not catheter migration. The pseudomeningocele can be ignored if it is not bothersome to the patients and they are getting adequate treatment of their movement disorder. Overall, the complication rate is higher than hoped for and patients and families are counseled pre-operatively about the sometimes-difficult management of post-operative complications.

15.3.1 Operative Technique - DBS

Early in our series, we performed awake, frame-based surgery with microelectrode recordings (MER) for placement of leads in an IRB approved fashion. Our pediatric protocol has several notable differences from that used in adult cases. Specifically, before surgery, the patient and family meet with the Team's Child Life specialist (CLS) to select diversion techniques. These include music, videos or movies to calm the child during surgery. The same individual comes to the OR with the child to improve cooperation and communication (▶ Fig. 15.6). The anesthetic used is a combination of iv sedation, dexmedetomidine drip, Lorazepam

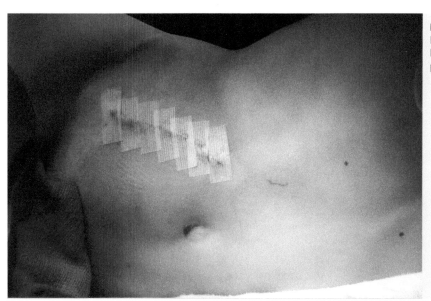

Fig. 15.5 With submuscular placement of 40 ml baclofen pump, the incision is well protected with little tension on closure and the pump with low profile in small thin patient.

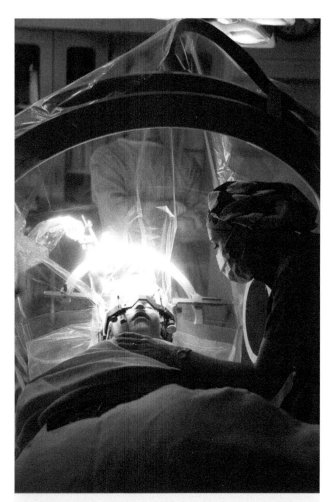

Fig. 15.6 Child life specialist comforting patient while undergoing microelectrode stimulation recording.

bolus, supraorbital, and greater and lesser occipital nerve field blocks. These are delivered before frame application while the child is still in a wheelchair. Hair is not shaved. We use alcohol-based Povidine-iodine prep for those with short hair; otherwise we do Povidine-iodine gel, shampooing and comb the hair parallel to the coronal suture. Hair is parted at the proposed incision site, where intradermal Bupivicaine/Xylocaine buffered with bicarbonate may also be infiltrated. This step may be superfluous when scalp blocks are effective. We use MER off sedation as much as possible with a simultaneous three-pass technique and stimulate intraoperatively to rule out side effects. Relaxation of the dystonia produced by stimulation further confirms accurate lead placement.

Initially, we proceeded to Stage II with extension wire and generator placement at the same time as electrode placement. After placement of electrodes and closure of incisions, the frame was removed, the patient repositioned and intubated and re-prepped. An infection rate of more than 10% in our first 50 patients prompted us to defer Stage II surgery for one week, dropping the infection rate (▶ Fig. 15.7). It is possible these infections were related to surgeon experience, but the change in infection rate was astonishing to us.

We now use intraoperative MRI (iMRI) and the ClearPoint (MRI Interventions, Irvine, CA) stereotactic system.[5] This is more comfortable for our patients. Since using the iMRI-assisted procedure, only two of 30 patients have needed to have more than one pass for electrode placement. The single serious complication in our asleep series was an epidural hematoma. It occurred from laceration of the middle meningeal artery by the frame's pin, and required cessation of the DBS procedure and clot evacuation (▶ Fig. 15.8). Using the hard MRI coil with the 4-in head holder required the pins to be placed below the equator of the calvarium. This provided sufficient room over the vertex to operate. The thin and diminutive skulls of our young patients exacerbate this problem. We now use flexible coils that can be displaced while drilling burr holes, then build the skull-mounted ClearPoint towers (▶ Fig. 15.9a, b). This facilitates a

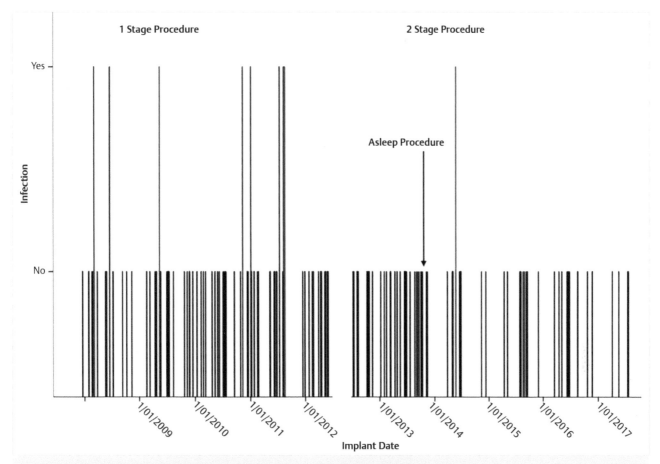

Fig. 15.7 10-year time graph showing infections over the last 10 years in relation to one stage versus two stage DBS placement. Also noted is the start of our asleep DBS protocol. As seen, our infection rate has diminished with the start of the two-stage procedure. No change in infection rate is noted with asleep surgery.

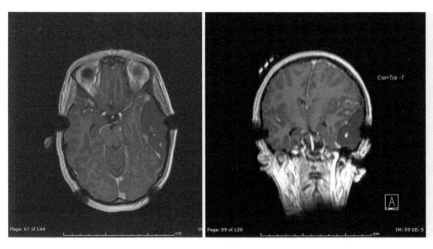

Fig. 15.8 Intraoperative MRI showing acute epidural hematoma from puncture of middle meningeal artery.

more rostral pin placement and reduces the likelihood of skull fracture and arterial laceration.

IPG Selection

Early in our series, we inserted two IPGs after DBS placements. However, since the rechargeable generator has become available (2010), we try to use it exclusively. Most patients and their families can manage generator recharging, though for some the task proves burdensome. For the latter, we have reverted to non-rechargeable generators. Unfortunately, this entails repeated generator replacement. Of 112 patients in our series, there have been 91 generator revisions and 13 generator/extension wire combination revisions. This ratio is decreasing over time with use of rechargeable generators.

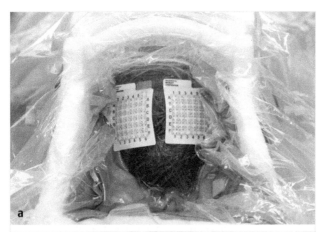

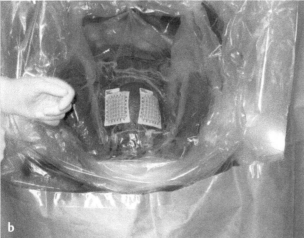

Fig. 15.9 Comparison photographs showing hard coil attachment (a) versus flexible coil attachment (b).

Table 15.2 Summary of DBS electrode target

Implant Site				
	Left Unilateral	Right Unilateral	Bilateral	Total
Globus Pallidus Internus (GPi)	8	6	104	118
Subthalamic Nucleus (STN)	0	1	4	5
Ventral Intermediate Nucleus (VIM)	0	0	5	5
GPi / VIM	0	0	2	2
GPi/STN	0	0	1	1

Target Selection

Our preferred target is the posterior lateral border of the globus pallidus internus (GPi). We have used the subthalamic nucleus (STN) in patients who have sustained too much anatomical damage to the GPi (secondary dystonia series), and this has not decreased efficacy (▶ Table 15.2). Starr's method of targeting the GPi remains our targeting technique.[6] However, we prefer targeting the most lateral border of the nucleus (lateral border

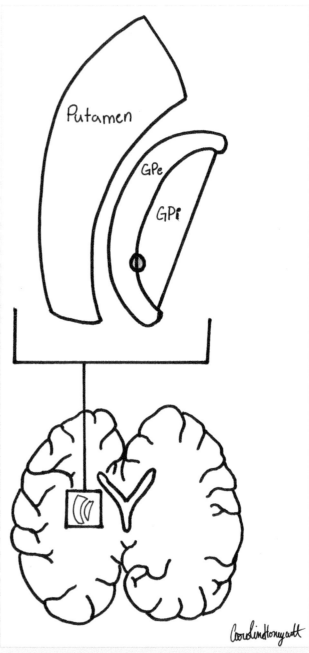

Fig. 15.10 Schematic drawing of our preferred electrode target at lateral border of globus pallidus internus (GPi).

of the GPi at the junction of the globus pallidus externus (GPe) nucleus).[5] This modification positions the electrode slightly further away from the internal capsule, avoiding stimulation side effects (▶ Fig. 15.10). GPi atrophy, often present in patients with secondary dystonia, makes the lamina between the two nuclei more prominent and facilitates localization. The final electrode tip position is 2 mm above the optic tract. We place the leads deep to allow for calvarial growth in younger patients and we have not had to revise leads because of such growth. However, our protocol does not allow surgery until the child is seven years old. Most head growth has already occurred by this age. In younger patients, it could still be an issue. Many of our secondary

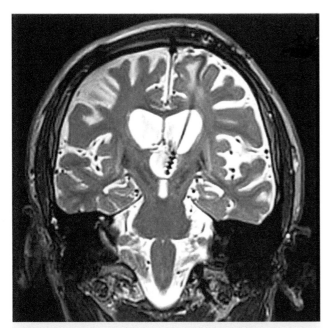

Fig. 15.11 Post-operative coronal MRI showing left DBS lead placement in IIIrd ventricle after awake MER surgery. This illustrates the difficulty with relying on MER on difficult awake patients and the abnormal anatomy commonly seen with our secondary DBS patients (large ventricles, cerebral atrophy, and small target nuclei). By switching to asleep surgery with MRI-assisted placement of electrodes, we have eliminated ineffective lead placement.

dystonia patients have damage to their pallidal structures, which makes targeting difficult and allows less margin for error (▶ Fig. 15.11). Navigation assisted by direct MRI targeting is an improvement over that guided by indirect standard anterior and posterior commissure measurements in this challenging population with smaller head sizes and abnormal anatomy.

15.3.2 Post-Operative Management - DBS

As always, complications can plague surgical management. Of concern is the increased incidence of hardware complications in children. Whether this is related to age or to the hyperkinesis associated with dystonia is not clear. There are also the potential effects of linear growth on indwelling DBS systems. The repetitive torsion movements in neck/trunk and sometimes violent, sudden movements associated with dystonia adds tension and increases the forces placed on indwelling systems. Kaminska et al., summarized his large series of pediatric complications.[7] Our series reflects some of their same issues of worrisome infection rates and frequent hardware malfunctions. We have seen several extension wire fractures or increased lead impedance requiring extension wire revision (6 of 112 patients (5.3%). The new Medtronic (Minneapolis, MN) extension wires (model 37085 /37086), seem to be proving sturdier.

Although the diminutive size and marginal nutritional status of our patients would appear to put them at particular risk for infection, our recent data does not indicate this to be true. Our infection rate since switching to two separated stages (2%) is

close to national adult norms. We avoid making incisions directly over hardware and have not seen tissue breakdown around the DBS system.

> Middle cerebral perforators in children are more sensitive to injury than those in adults and there is a surprising incidence of hemorrhagic and non hemorrhagic stroke along the electrode pathway. Symptoms will resolve.

A surprising complication we have seen is the frequency of both hemorrhagic and non-hemorrhagic stroke. The bleeding seems to be along the electrode track at the level of the caudate. Strokes occur twice as frequently in children younger than ten years old. We postulate that the middle cerebral artery perforators of children are more sensitive to trauma/damage than those of adults. Most strokes are asymptomatic and detected on routine post-operative imaging, but two have had transient hemiparesis. It eventually resolved. In these patients, the electrode path was close to the lateral border of the caudate nucleus and ventricle, so we now use a more lateral pathway. There have been no further such events. Stroke occurrence is not correlated with the number of MER passes. They have not happened when using our asleep protocol but this is more likely because of our switch to a lateral electrode trajectory

15.4 Conclusion

Dystonia is a difficult movement disorder to treat because its presentation overlaps with other hyperkinetic movement disorders, especially that in secondary dystonia. These patients deserve evaluation with a multidisciplinary movement disorder team. Surgical management with ITB and/or DBS is reasonable once medical management has been maximized. Family counseling before surgery helps to manage expectations as results from our clinical series indicates that the outcome from treatment of secondary dystonia is better than that seen with primary dystonia.

References

[1] Sanger TD, Chen D, Fehlings DL, et al. Definition and classification of hyperkinetic movements in childhood. Mov Disord. 2010; 25(11):1538–1549

[2] Varhabhatla NC, Zuo Z. Rising complication rates after intrathecal catheter and pump placement in the pediatric population: analysis of national data between 1997 and 2006. Pain Physician. 2012; 15(1):65–74

[3] Marks W, Bailey L, Reed M, et al. Pallidal stimulation in children: comparison between cerebral palsy and DYT1 dystonia. J Child Neurol. 2013; 28(7):840–848

[4] Rocque BG, Albright AL. Intraventricular versus intrathecal baclofen for secondary dystonia: A comparison of complications. Neurosurgery. 2012; 70(2)(Suppl Operative):321–5

[5] Starr PA, Markun LC, Larson PS, Volz MM, Martin AJ, Ostrem JL. Interventional MRI-guided deep brain stimulation in pediatric dystonia: first experience with the ClearPoint system. J Neurosurg Pediatr. 2014; 14(4):400–408

[6] Marks W, Bailey L, Sanger TD. PEDiDBS: The pediatric international deep brain stimulation registry project. Eur J Paediatr Neurol. 2017; 21(1):218–222

[7] Kaminska M, Perides S, Lumsden DE, et al. Complications of Deep Brain Stimulation (DBS) for dystonia in children - The challenges and 10 year experience in a large paediatric cohort. Eur J Paediatr Neurol. 2017; 21(1):168–175

16 Deep Brain Stimulation for Rare Movement Disorders

Era Hanspal

Abstract

Since it was FDA approved for Essential Tremor (ET), deep brain stimulation (DBS) has been used to treat many other conditions. This chapter reviews off-label and exempted DBS treatment for the hyperkinetic movement disorders of myoclonus, chorea and Tourette's syndrome.

Keywords: myoclonus, chorea, tourette syndrome, hyperkinetic movement disorders

16.1 Introduction

Hyperkinetic movement disorders comprise a heterogeneous group of challenging disorders, either because of lack of medical efficacy or from medication side effects. As such, DBS has been explored as an alternative therapy. This chapter will cover DBS for myoclonus, chorea, and Tourette's syndrome (TS).

16.2 Myoclonus

Myoclonus is defined as a brief, jerking muscle movement. It can be caused by metabolic, post anoxic or degenerative injury. Its medical treatment includes anticholinergics, anti-epileptics and benzodiazepines.

Most of the treatment by DBS in myoclonus has been for myoclonus dystonia, which is a rare, autosomal dominant condition, also known as DYT 11. It is caused by mutations in the epsilon sarcoglycan gene (chromosome 7q). Symptoms of action myoclonus often present in childhood or adolescence; dystonia, either cervical or in the limbs, and psychiatric symptoms, such as obsessive-compulsive disorder (OCD), complete the common phenotype. The myoclonic symptoms be sensitive to alcohol, which along with ET may lead to alcoholism. Pharmacologic agents used include benzodiazepines, anticholinergic, serotonergic and dopaminergic agents. Use of these medications is often limited by their partial benefit and side effects at higher doses.

Given these limitations, DBS has been explored to manage both the myoclonus and dystonia seen in this disorder. Early case studies focused on the ventro-intermedius nucleus of the thalamus (Vim) and Globus pallidus interna (GPi) as stimulation targets based on experience with ET and dystonia treatment, respectively. The literature suggests that GPi may be a preferred target in the treatment of both myoclonus and dystonia.[1]

In the largest case series, published by Gruber et al., ten patients with myoclonus-dystonia were implanted.[2] Eight patients had both GPi and VIM stimulators, one had bilateral Vim electrodes, and one had both GPi and Vim electrodes inserted, but only GPi electrodes connected. Myoclonus symptoms improved when measured on the Unified Myoclonus Rating Scale (UMRS) score. Dystonia did also when assessed by the Burke-Fahn-Marsden Dystonia Rating Scale (BFMDRS) and by measures of quality of life. The UMRS score and BFMDRS disability score improved in all patients, regardless of targets, by

61–66% and 45–48%, respectively on initial evaluation and at 128 months.

Similar findings were supported in a review of 40 cases.[3] Myoclonic symptom improvement was significantly greater than that measured with dystonia. UMRS improved by at least 50% in 94% of cases and BFMDRS improved by at least 50% in 72% of cases.[3]

Youth and a shorter symptom duration before intervention are favorable signs.[3] Single case reports for the treatment of myoclonus of other causes also suggest a favorable outcome with DBS intervention.[4,5] There are fewer reports on the effects of DBS on secondary myoclonus, as may arise from anoxia. In summary, Vim DBS may provide greater improvement in myoclonus, but GPi may be slightly superior overall. It leads to less dysarthria and more effective treatment of dystonia.

16.2.1 Chorea

The term chorea describes the unpredictable, dance-like movements that flow from one body part to another. Neurodegenerative, rheumatogical, and developmental disorders may lead to chorea, as can hyperglycemia, pregnancy, and encephalopathy. Huntington's Disease (HD) is one of the most commonly investigated for possible DBS therapy.

HD is an autosomal dominant neurodegenerative disorder, that derives from an expanded trinucleotide repeat CAG on chromosome 4, encoding for the protein huntingtin. While the abnormal protein is expressed throughout the body, medium spiny neurons in the striatum are affected early and significantly. These changes disrupt the balance between the indirect and direct pathways of movement processing in the basal ganglia causing motor, psychiatric, and cognitive manifestations. The motor signs are diverse, most often of course, including chorea, but also include parkinsonian tremors, dystonia and ataxia. Chorea can involve any voluntary muscle, and as such, can affect, speech, swallowing, balance, and fine motor movements.

Given the benefit of DBS in treatment of levodopa-induced choreic dyskinesias in Parkinson's disease (PD), the GPi has been explored as a target. Moro et al. published the first case report of DBS in a patient with refractory chorea from Huntington's disease. Low frequency stimulation of the dorsal GPi improved the chorea and dystonia without causing further bradykinesia. Higher frequency stimulation correlated with an increase in bradykinesia.

Similar findings were reported in a large, open-label prospective pilot study of seven consecutive patients treated with bilateral GPi DBS for three years.[6] All of the patients had genetically confirmed HD with chorea refractory to tetrabenazine and a combination of a neuroleptic and at least one other drug. They had a United Huntington Disease Rating Scale (UHDRS) independence score of less than or equal to 70, a total functional capacity score of less than or equal to 8, and the absence of severe cognitive or psychiatric impairment.

There was an improvement of 10.91% in the UHDRS total motor score after one year. This worsened over time. The chorea subscore of the UHDRS improved by a mean of 58.34% and the improvement was sustained throughout the study period. In particular, chorea involving the orolingual area and upper limbs improved significantly. In these patients, it was possible to reduce or discontinue drug therapy. Bradykinesia, however, worsened during the study period.

HD presents challenges that arise from the complex origin of the observed movements and multiply affected circuits. Both limbic and cognitive pathways are involved. There is brain atrophy and progressive atrophy in time may alter the implanted lead position relative to the internal capsule. In an autopsy study reported by Vedam-Mai et al. no adverse effects were seen from this migration.[7] The worsening bradykinesia and rigidity leads to postural instability. It may represent stimulation effect or disease progression. The cognitive decline and related apathy is likely to impair assessment of some outcome measures. It may also pose an ethical concern in patient selection for treatment.

16.3 Tourette's Syndrome

Gilles de la Tourette Syndrome (TS) is a childhood onset neuropsychiatric syndrome marked by motor tics, one or more vocal tics associated with OCD and attention deficit hyperactivity disorder (ADHD), anxiety and depression. Symptoms develop in early childhood or adolescence. Tics are defined as sudden, often stereotyped, repetitive movements or sounds. They may be simple, consisting of a single movement or sound, or complex, occurring in an orchestrated pattern. Due to force and repetition, tics can be painful; some can involve self-injury. The majority of TS patients have a favorable prognosis, with either resolution or significant improvement by early adulthood. A small percentage have persistent symptoms or develop severe social and psychological disability despite treatment.

Pharmacologic therapies include dopamine antagonists, benzodiazepines and centrally acting alpha antagonists. Side effects from these agents include sedation, weight gain, and/or tardive movement disorders. Higher doses of benzodiazepines can lead to tolerance or habituation. Treatment failure is defined as no relief with a neuroleptic agent or behavioral therapy and the presence of intolerable side effects. Comorbidities should also be assessed.

While there are proposed guidelines by the Tourette Syndrome Association for DBS patient selection, some criteria are debated. Most agree that DBS should be reserved for treatment refractory tics, and patients 25 or older, as tics often improve in early adulthood.

Since the first DBS case for Tourette syndrome was performed in 1999, at least six targets have been explored in the treatment of TS. This syndrome is thought to disrupt the cortico-striato-thalamo-cortical circuitry. These targets modulate the circuitry at various points: the medial thalamus, Gpi, globus pallidus externus, the nucleus accumbens, anterior limb of the internal capsule, and the subthalamic nucleus.

Outcome is measured by improvements in the Yale Global Tic Severity Scale (YGTSS), Yale-Brown Obsessive Compulsive Score (YBOCS), and direct observation. Overall, using these objective measures DBS in the short term improves tics by 53% regardless of the target selected. Improvement is most robust with thalamic and pallidal targets.[8] Thalamic targets, centromedian, parafascicular, and ventro-oralis internus nuclei, have been associated with improvement in YBOCS, depression, anxiety, and patient-rated impact of symptoms on daily life.

Long-term benefit is less consistent, likely because of a discrepancy between improvement in tic severity and function, and/or patient satisfaction.[8,9] Improvement of tics alone does not address the other aspects of the psychosocial impact of TS. The behavioral manifestations of OCD and ADHD may be more impairing than the tics themselves.

16.4 Conclusion

DBS is an emerging treatment option for an expanding list of neurologic and psychiatric disorders. In this growing field, patient selection criteria, the stimulation targets and the disorders addressed vary widely. Unresolved issues remain with the diverse syndromes discussed in this chapter. Myoclonus-dystonia, while commonly explored in DBS to address the myoclonic aspect, remains an uncommon disorder. The application of DBS for other myoclonic disorders is limited. The progressive neurodegenerative nature of Huntington's disease (HD) makes outcome assessment difficult. Finally, psychosocial issues may limit TS outcome.

References

[1] Smith KM, Spindler MA. Uncommon applications of deep brain stimulation in hyperkinetic movement disorders. Tremor Other Hyperkinet Mov (N Y). 2015; 5:278

[2] Gruber D, Kuhn AA, Schoenecker T, et al. Quadruple deep brain stimulation in Huntington's disease, targeting pallidum and subthalamic nucleus: case report and review of the literature. J Neural Transm (Vienna). 2014; 121(10): 1303–1312

[3] Rughani AI, Lozano AM. Surgical treatment of myoclonus dystonia syndrome. Mov Disord. 2013; 28(3):282–287

[4] Wang JW, Li JP, Wang YP, Zhang XH, Zhang YQ. Deep brain stimulation for myoclonus-dystonia syndrome with double mutations in DYT1 and DYT11. Sci Rep. 2017; 7:41042

[5] Yamada K, Sakurama T, Soyama N, Kuratsu J. Gpi pallidal stimulation for Lance-Adams syndrome. Neurology. 2011; 76(14):1270–1272

[6] Gonzalez V, Cif L, Biolsi B, et al. Deep brain stimulation for Huntington's disease: long-term results of a prospective open-label study. J Neurosurg. 2014; 121(1):114–122

[7] Vedam-Mai V, Martinez-Ramirez D, Hilliard JD, et al. Post-mortem Findings in Huntington's Deep Brain Stimulation: A Moving Target Due to Atrophy. Tremor Other Hyperkinet Mov (N Y). 2016; 6:372

[8] Smeets AY, Duits AA, Leentjens AF, et al. Thalamic Deep Brain Stimulation for Refractory Tourette Syndrome: Clinical Evidence for Increasing Disbalance of Therapeutic Effects and Side Effects at Long-Term Follow-Up. Neuromodulation. 2017. DOI: 10.1111/ner.12556

[9] Servello D, Sassi M, Brambilla A, Defendi S, Porta M. Long-term, post-deep brain stimulation management of a series of 36 patients affected with refractory gilles de la tourette syndrome. Neuromodulation. 2010; 13(3):187–194

17 Lesioning versus Deep Brain Stimulation for Movement Disorders

Tony R. Wang, Robert F. Dallapiazza, Aaron E. Bond, Shayan Moosa, and W. Jeffrey Elias

Abstract

Deep brain stimulation and the creation of stereotactic lesions are both effective means of treating essential tremor (ET) and Parkinson's disease (PD). DBS has largely supplanted lesion generation as the treatment of choice in movement disorders, since it is reversible, adjustable and can be used to safely treat bilateral disease. This chapter highlights differences in efficacy and safety along with the advantages and disadvantages for lesion generation and DBS in the treatment of movement disorders.

Keywords: lesioning, deep brain stimulation, Parkinson's disease, essential tremor

17.1 Historical Considerations

Although lesion generation and deep brain stimulation (DBS) are often viewed as competing procedures, they were at first complementary. In 1947 Spiegel and Wycis designed the first apparatus for accurate human lesion generation in deep brain targets. The device was used for medial thalamotomy for neuropsychiatric disorders as a surgical alternative treatment to lobotomy.[1] Subsequent work in the 1950s, relied on high frequency operative stimulation to identify subcortical targets for lesioning.[2] In the late 1980s, implanted high frequency stimulating electrodes were combined with battery-powered pulse generators as the first DBS devices.[3] DBS has since revolutionized the treatment of movement disorders. This chapter will focus on the use of lesion generation and DBS for treatment of ET and PD.

17.2 Effectiveness

In PD, subthalamic nucleus (STN) DBS may improve Unified Parkinson's Disease Rating Scale, Part III (UPDRSIII) scores 25–89%. Average improvement is 45%. Quality of life measures improve as much as 35%, with an average improvement of 18%.[2] Globus pallidus interna (GPi) DBS leads to comparable improvements in UPDRSIII scores and quality of life measures with average improvements of 35% and 10%, respectively.[4] A recent meta-analysis of ten randomized controlled trials comparing STN-DBS to GPi-DBS for PD showed that STN and GPi were equally effective. STN-DBS, however led to greater decrease in levodopa equivalent daily dose (LEDD).[5] Ventral intermedius nucleus (Vim) DBS and RF Vim thalamotomy for PD improve tremor scores by up to 90%.[4] Both techniques may not address other symptoms of parkinsonism and are generally reserved for tremor dominant PD. STN-DBS, however will treat the other PD symptoms that are known to worsen over time.

For ET, Vim-DBS and RF lesioning have comparable reductions in tremor scores, ranging from 55–90% improvement.[6] A recent prospective trial for Gamma Knife thalamotomy demonstrated average tremor score improvement of 54% at one year

blinded evaluation.[7] MRI-guided focused ultrasound (FUS) has recently been FDA-approved. With this technique, tremor scores improve an average of 40% at 12 months.[8] Long-term clinical data is not yet available. Several studies have compared RF lesioning to DBS at various subcortical targets for PD and ET (▶ Table 17.1).[9,10,11,12,13,14,15] Most of these studies showed no difference in tremors or functional outcome. The majority of the studies compared unilateral lesioning to unilateral or to bilateral DBS.

> Vim DBS and RF Vim thalamotomy are generally reserved for tremor dominant PD.
>
> STN DBS treats other PD symptoms that will likely emerge later.

17.3 Safety/Adverse Events

There is a 0–7% incidence of symptomatic intracerebral hemorrhage (ICH) after DBS.[16] While several groups have reported similar rates in DBS and RF lesioning, others have described a higher hemorrhage incidence during RF lesioning.[16] One hypothesis for this is that during RF coagulation, charred blood vessels may "stick" to the RF probe. A vessel could shear during probe removal and bleed.[12] Transcranial lesioning techniques such as Gamma Knife (GK) and FUS obviate this concern since they do not require an intracerebral probe. The most common adverse events with GK and FUS are sensory changes. The incidence after GK is 8% and 14% after FUS.[17] Regardless of the technique; lesioning avoids the risks of lead migration, fracture and infection, which in large DBS series have a 3%. incidence.[18] While an infrequent occurrence, these complications often require re-operation, potentially further increasing morbidity. Although lesioning avoids hardware-related complications, bilateral lesions of Vim, GPi, and STN all carry higher rates of cognitive, speech, and language dysfunction compared to bilateral DBS.[9,14] Even in unilateral procedures, lesioning may have twice the rate of the aforementioned complications.[9] While these complications are also seen in DBS, they can often be ameliorated by adjustment of stimulation parameters.

Surgery at any of the three most common subcortical locations for PD and ET has adverse risks from injury or involvement of adjacent neural structures. Subthalamotomy risks postoperative hemiballism, contributing to its infrequent use, however the reported incidence is low, ranging from 0.2–10%.[19]

17.4 Recurrence/Tolerance

Symptoms can recur both with lesioning and DBS, but for different reasons. Since these treatments do not address the underlying

Table 17.1 Studies that directly compared lesioning to DBS

Study/year	Study Type	Target	Disease	N	Laterality	Follow-up	Improvement percentages when compared to baseline	
							Tremor score/UPDRSIII	Functional status
Tasker et al., 1998[9]	Retrospective	Vim	ET, PD	26 lesional 19 DBS	4 bilateral lesional, 2 bilateral DBS, otherwise unilateral	At least 3 mo for all	See Below	See below
Merello et al., 1999[10]	Randomized	GPi	PD	7 lesional 6 DBS	Unilateral	3 mo	44 (lesional) 46 (DBS)	46 (lesional) 57.8 (DBS)
Schuurman et al., 2000[11]	Randomized	Vim	ET, PD, MS[#]	34 lesional 34 DBS	Unilateral lesional, unilateral or bilateral DBS*	6 mo	87 (lesional) 91.7 (DBS)	1.5 (lesional) 15.6 (DBS)†
Pahwa et al. 2001[12]	Retrospective matched cohort	Vim	ET	17 lesional 17 DBS	Unilateral	2.2 mo (lesional) 3.1 mo (DBS)	46 (lesional) 49.8 (DBS)	70 (lesional) 64 (DBS)
Esselink et al., 2004[13]	Randomized	GPi (lesional) STN (DBS)	PD	14 lesional 20 DBS	Unilateral pallidotomy Bilateral STN-DBS	6 mo	20.4 (lesional) 48.5 (DBS)†	34.5 (lesional) 46.3 (DBS)
Merello et al., 2008[14]	Randomized	STN	PD	6 lesional 6 DBS 6 DBS + lesional	Bilateral DBS, bilateral lesioning, or unilateral lesion + contralateral DBS	12 mo	52.2 (lesional) 60.9 (DBS) 61.8 (lesional + DBS)	45.5 (lesional) 70.5 (DBS) 69.1 (lesional + DBS)
Anderson et al., 2009[15]	Randomized	Vim	ET	10 lesional 10 DBS	Unilateral	6 mo	40 (lesional) 40 (DBS)	N/A

Tasker et al. do not report average (per patient) percentage improvements in tremor or functional status. They do report that 69% of lesional patients and 79% of DBS patients experienced "near abolition" of tremor. Regarding functional outcome, 48% of lesional paients and 49% of DBS patients had suppression of rigidity; 68% of lesional patients and 38% of DBS patients had improved dexterity. Little improvement in writing, speech, or gait was seen with either group.
#55 PD patients, 13 ET patients, 10 MS patients
*For patients assigned to the lesional group if unilateral tremor was present, unilateral thalamotomy was performed; if bilateral tremor was present, thalamotomy was performed to treat the more symptomatic side, the contralateral side would receive thalamic DBS. All patients assigned to DBS group either underwent unilateral or bilateral thalamic stimulation based on symptoms.
†denotes statistically significant improvement over lesioning

Table 17.2 Advantages/disadvantages of surgical procedures in the treatment of movement disorders

	Bilateral treatments	Adjustability	High cost/ maintenance	Transcranial	Infectious risk	Neurologic complications
DBS	✓	✓	✓	×	✓	Lowest
RF lesioning	×	×	×	×	×	Low
Gamma Knife	✓	×	×	✓	×	Low
Focused ultrasound	Unknown	×	×	✓	×	Low

cause of PD or ET, benefit may diminish when the disease progresses. Patients with DBS may also become tolerant to their stimulation. This issue may be under recognized. In a series of 45 patients with ET who were followed for an average of 56 months, 73% of patients reported waning benefit and/or needed reprogramming.[20] For this reason, patients with ET should turn off their stimulation at night, not only to preserve battery life but also to prevent tolerance from emerging. For PD, waning clinical benefit from DBS may be harder to determine. While both STN and GPi-DBS may improve UPDRSIII scores for 5–10 years, less levodopa responsive axial symptoms often progress. This may lead to overall worsening. Tolerance has also been seen in DBS for PD. Patients frequently must increase stimulation parameters 5–8 years after STN-DBS.[21] While waning of clinical effect is also observed in GPi-DBS, STN-DBS may be used as a salvage therapy in select cases.[22]

Repeat lesion generation, or salvage therapy, may also be done after RF lesioning when clinical benefit diminishes. This may occur in up to 23% of Vim thalamotomies and 38% of pallidotomies[9,23] Long-term outcomes for GK thalamotomy is durable, with minimal tremor recurrence, even up to 4 years.[17] Long-term data for FUS thalamotomy is not yet available. Recurrent tremor scores increased 23% at one year after surgery.[8]

17.5 Advantages/Disadvantages

DBS can be done bilaterally since no lesion is made and the stimulation settings can be adjusted to limit side effects or to treat disease progression. Programming requires multiple clinic visits and may not be ideal for patients who live in remote areas or have limited means of traveling to and from the clinic. Moreover, DBS incurs increased costs compared to lesioning because of the need to manage and replace the hardware. Such costs may be prohibitive, especially in developing nations.[24] As previously noted, hardware-related complications such as lead fracture, migration, and infection all are disadvantages of DBS.

ET patients may be averse to surgery and device implantation.[25] Lesion creation by GK and FUS is perceived as less invasive than RF lesioning and DBS. They may provide ET patients an option they might otherwise have avoided. GK has a latent clinical effect but has been used successfully for bilateral symptoms.[15] Finally, DBS may be contraindicated in patients with comorbidities that require frequent MRI studies. ▶ Table 17.2 summarizes the advantages and disadvantages of lesioning and DBS in the treatment of movement disorders.

17.6 Conclusion

DBS is currently the primary surgical treatment for PD and ET, but lesioning procedures can be effective in properly selected cases, particularly those in which symptoms are asymmetrical. Both have low morbidity, but the type of complication is different and will need to be considered when patients, families, and neurosurgeons make interventional choices.

References

[1] Spiegel EA, Wycis HT, Marks M, Lee AJ. Stereotaxic Apparatus for Operations on the Human Brain. Science. 1947; 106(2754):349–350

[2] Hariz MI, Blomstedt P, Zrinzo L. Deep brain stimulation between 1947 and 1987: the untold story. Neurosurg Focus. 2010; 29(2):E1

[3] Benabid AL, Pollak P, Louveau A, Henry S, de Rougemont J. Combined (thalamotomy and stimulation) stereotactic surgery of the VIM thalamic nucleus for bilateral Parkinson disease. Appl Neurophysiol. 1987; 50(1–6):344–346

[4] Krack P, Martinez-Fernandez R, Del Alamo M, Obeso JA. Current applications and limitations of surgical treatments for movement disorders. Mov Disord. 2017; 32(1):36–52

[5] Tan ZG, Zhou Q, Huang T, Jiang Y. Efficacies of globus pallidus stimulation and subthalamic nucleus stimulation for advanced Parkinson's disease: a meta-analysis of randomized controlled trials. Clin Interv Aging. 2016; 11:777–786

[6] Zesiewicz TA, Elble R, Louis ED, et al. Quality Standards Subcommittee of the American Academy of Neurology. Practice parameter: therapies for essential tremor: report of the Quality Standards Subcommittee of the American Academy of Neurology. Neurology. 2005; 64(12):2008–2020

[7] Witjas T, Carron R, Krack P, et al. A prospective single-blind study of Gamma Knife thalamotomy for tremor. Neurology. 2015; 85(18):1562–1568

[8] Elias WJ, Lipsman N, Ondo WG, et al. A Randomized Trial of Focused Ultrasound Thalamotomy for Essential Tremor. N Engl J Med. 2016; 375(8):730–739

[9] Tasker RR. Deep brain stimulation is preferable to thalamotomy for tremor suppression. Surg Neurol. 1998; 49(2):145–153, discussion 153–154

[10] Merello M, Nouzeilles MI, Kuzis G, et al. Unilateral radiofrequency lesion versus electrostimulation of posteroventral pallidum: a prospective randomized comparison. Mov Disord. 1999; 14(1):50–56

[11] Schuurman PR, Bosch DA, Bossuyt PM, et al. A comparison of continuous thalamic stimulation and thalamotomy for suppression of severe tremor. N Engl J Med. 2000; 342(7):461–468

[12] Pahwa R, Lyons KE, Wilkinson SB, et al. Comparison of thalamotomy to deep brain stimulation of the thalamus in essential tremor. Mov Disord. 2001; 16 (1):140–143

[13] Esselink RA, de Bie RM, de Haan RJ, et al. Unilateral pallidotomy versus bilateral subthalamic nucleus stimulation in PD: a randomized trial. Neurology. 2004; 62(2):201–207

[14] Merello M, Tenca E, Pérez Lloret S, et al. Prospective randomized 1-year follow-up comparison of bilateral subthalamotomy versus bilateral subthalamic stimulation and the combination of both in Parkinson's disease patients: a pilot study. Br J Neurosurg. 2008; 22(3):415–422

[15] Anderson VC, Burchiel KJ, Hart MJ, Berk C, Lou JS. A randomized comparison of thalamic stimulation and lesion on self-paced finger movement in essential tremor. Neurosci Lett. 2009; 462(2):166–170

[16] Zrinzo L, Foltynie T, Limousin P, Hariz MI. Reducing hemorrhagic complications in functional neurosurgery: a large case series and systematic literature review. J Neurosurg. 2012; 116(1):84–94

[17] Young RF, Li F, Vermeulen S, Meier R. Gamma Knife thalamotomy for treatment of essential tremor: long-term results. J Neurosurg. 2010; 112(6):1311–1317

[18] Falowski SM, Ooi YC, Bakay RA. Long-Term Evaluation of Changes in Operative Technique and Hardware-Related Complications With Deep Brain Stimulation. Neuromodulation. 2015; 18(8):670–677

[19] Alvarez L, Macias R, Lopez G, et al. Bilateral subthalamotomy in Parkinson's disease: initial and long-term response. Brain. 2005; 128(Pt 3):570–583

[20] Shih LC, LaFaver K, Lim C, Papavassiliou E, Tarsy D. Loss of benefit in VIM thalamic deep brain stimulation (DBS) for essential tremor (ET): how prevalent is it? Parkinsonism Relat Disord. 2013; 19(7):676–679

[21] Fasano A, Romito LM, Daniele A, et al. Motor and cognitive outcome in patients with Parkinson's disease 8 years after subthalamic implants. Brain. 2010; 133(9):2664–2676

[22] Volkmann J, Allert N, Voges J, Sturm V, Schnitzler A, Freund HJ. Long-term results of bilateral pallidal stimulation in Parkinson's disease. Ann Neurol. 2004; 55(6):871–875

[23] Hariz MI, Bergenheim AT. A 10-year follow-up review of patients who underwent Leksell's posteroventral pallidotomy for Parkinson disease. J Neurosurg. 2001; 94(4):552–558

[24] Benabid AL, Chabardes S, Mitrofanis J, Pollak P. Deep brain stimulation of the subthalamic nucleus for the treatment of Parkinson's disease. Lancet Neurol. 2009; 8(1):67–81

[25] Thenganatt MA, Louis ED. Personality profile in essential tremor: a case-control study. Parkinsonism Relat Disord. 2012; 18(9):1042–1044

18 Spasticity: Evaluation, Medical and Preoperative Considerations

Pouya Entezami, Roy S. Hwang, and Vishad Sukul

Abstract

Spasticity is described as velocity-dependent resistance to passive joint motion. The characteristic muscle stiffness is both from hyper-excitability of the stretch reflex and loss of inhibition from ascending efferent pathways. Spasticity as a symptom is often a result of a variety of disease processes that involve some degree of neurologic injury. While this may seem to be a painful and debilitating concern, spasticity can be helpful as a functional aid for a patient given their degree of neurologic compromise. Some spasticity can be helpful with gait or transfer. Thus, careful pre-operative evaluation and observation are often necessary so as to ensure appropriate treatment response. Several modalities exist for therapy, all aimed at improving a patient's functional status. Because of complexity associated with the diagnosis and management of spasticity, a multi-modality approach to treatment that involves physical therapists, movement-disorder specialists, and neurosurgeons is recommended.

Keywords: spasticity, functional

18.1 Introduction

Spasticity is described as velocity-dependent resistance to passive movement of a joint, due to hyper-excitability of the stretch reflex and loss of inhibition from ascending efferent pathways. It can be a compensatory tool for loss of motor function, and may be useful in certain instances. Thus, the presence of spasticity itself should not be a trigger for surgical intervention unless it is causing significant pain, functional loss, or significant decrease in quality of life.[1]

In patients with functional losses attributable to the patient's spastic musculature, surgical approaches may be an effective adjunct to medical or physical therapy treatment modalities. The goal of intervention in these scenarios is to re-calibrate a balance between paretic and spastic muscles, providing relief from debilitation due to excess tone.[1] Appropriate treatment should leave the patient with enough motility and tone to be useful during the activities of daily living. For patients with poor baseline functionality, surgery may also help to correct progressive orthopedic deformities and appearance.[2]

Spasticity treatments range from minimally invasive to open surgical interventions. Options include botulinum toxin injection, selective peripheral neurotomy intrathecal baclofen, dorsal rhizotomy, and various orthopedic surgeries designed to correct deformities that result from increased tone.[3] In all cases, a multi-modality and disciplinary approach should be adopted.[1,4]

18.2 Evaluation

There are two core components to spasticity, or muscle "stiffness" as patients often describe it. First, velocity-dependent or dynamic muscle shortening due to increased tone may manifest as hyperreflexia, clonus, and resistance to movement. Second, fixed muscle shortening can occur and cause contractures that persist even under anesthesia or nerve block. Contractures must be approached differently than the former category. From a surgical perspective, should medical management fail, orthopedic and neurosurgical procedures may need to be done in tandem to achieve success.[5]

When evaluating the spastic patient for intervention, the first steps are to obtain a thorough history and do a physical exam. It is essential to take time for a period of observation, to assess the patient's range of motion and degree of contracture at individual joints. Next is a qualitative clinical evaluation in which response to deep tendon reflex testing and resistance to passive stretch is measured. The response strength is not as important as whether there is symmetry to the responses. The patient's position during the examination is important. Resistance may be more pronounced when the patient is upright or in a wheelchair.[1] Also, spasticity changes after stress and muscle fatigue.

A number of manual and electrophysiological testing options are available to measure passive quantifiable motion. These efforts measure the gradual increase in resistance present during movement. That resistance may subside when limits to the motion are reached. The change is proportional to the velocity and position-dependent resistance. The measurement of spasms with electrophysiology may also be useful in planning.[1,6]

To best document clinical status and progression and compare pre and post-operative function, spasticity should be graded using the Ashworth scale (▶ Table 18.1). Numerous other outcomes measures have also been reported. Treatment can have a placebo effect and has been reported in up to 50% of patients, so an objective measurement tool is crucial.

Lastly, it is important to develop a good understanding of whether a patient's spasticity is causing pain or discomfort and thus affecting their quality of life. These determinations will help in the choice of intervention.

18.3 Medical and Pre-Operative Considerations

The non-surgical management of spasticity should involve a multidisciplinary approach that uses multiple treatment

Table 18.1 Modified ashworth scale for assessment of spasticity

Score	Characteristic
1	No increase in tone
2	Slight increase in tone A "catch" occurs when affected part is moved in flexion and extension
3	More marked increase in tone Affected parts are easily flexed
4	Considerable increase in tone Passive movement is difficult
5	Affected parts rigid in flexion or extension

modalities. The categories of non-surgical management include: therapeutic interventions such as physical occupational therapy, orthotics, oral medications, and injectables. Physical and occupational therapy are critical in the management of focal and generalized spasticity, especially by stretching, static positioning, strengthening orthotics and splints.

Pharmacological management makes use of anti-spastic medications that work directly on the muscle tone, These medications include dantrolene, baclofen, and other medications that are CNS modulating such as tizanidine, benzodiazepines, gabapentin, and nabiximols. Dantrolene is an antagonist to the ryanodine receptor and inhibits calcium release thus depressing excitation-contraction coupling and reducing muscle contraction. Baclofen affects GABA B activity in the spinal cord thus modulating spinal motor reflexes and reducing spasticity from reflex input. Tizanidine works on adrenoreceptors and increases pre-synaptic inhibition of motor neurons. Gabapentin works centrally by increasing GABA activity in the brain. Nabiximols are often used as adjunctive therapy. Is mechanism of action is not entirely clear though they appear to work on canniboid receptors. Botox modifies synergic movements when it is injected into key muscles..

Other non-surgical, non-pharmacologic treatments include: transcutaneous electric nerve stimulation (TENS), transcranial magnetic stimulation (TMS), cryotherapy, thermotherapy, ultrasound therapy, vibration therapy, and continuous passive motion robotic therapy. These therapies are thought to act on the motor pathways to decrease spasticity. TMS is believed to improve plasticity of motor circuits by modulating corticospinal output through long-term potentiation. TENS may decrease spasticity by local effects on reflex pathways and inhibitory Renshaw cells. Vibration therapy modulates the muscle spindle and Golgi tendon reflexes to modify their reflex input. Ultrasound improves the viscoelastic properties of local muscles. Thermal and cryotherapy modulate reflex organ pathways. Robotic therapies may decrease afferent input to reduce hyper-reflexic activity.

When any interventional technique is considered for treating spasticity, the specific aims and goals of therapy must be well defined by the physician and discussed with the patient, relatives, and caregivers. As always, there are differences in indications for the various surgical modalities available and appropriate patient selection will help deliver a favorable outcome.

The approach to lower extremity spasticity may vary from that used for the upper extremities. Lower extremity spasticity may be treated with selective dorsal rhizotomies or intrathecal baclofen.[7] Focal spasticity can be treated with botulinum toxin injections as an adjunct. Upper limb spasticity can often be treated with botulinum toxin injections as a primary treatment. Injections can be repeated annually or bi-annually assuming the patient does not develop immune-resistance to the drug.[1]

Intrathecal baclofen requires preoperative testing. Side effects of medications must be considered. Neither drugs nor surgical interventions have simple physiologic effects. An intrathecal baclofen trial is done by lumbar puncture to assess benefit and titrate an appropriate dosage prior to permanent implantation of a drug-delivery system.[4,8,9]

Intrathecal baclofen targets the dorsal gray matter of the spinal cord to decrease the hyper-excitability of motor pathways.

The treatment is essentially empirical, and response to treatment must be carefully interpreted. While systemic delivery could produce the same concentration of drug in the spinal cord at a high dosage, the result would be altered cognition. In addition, the infusion rate can be titrated for treatment effectiveness and physiological effects.

18.4 Special Considerations for Spasticity in Children

Spasticity in children is often a consequence of cerebral palsy Grouped in this broad category are various disorders of movement and/or posture. Much like adults, spasticity in children can be useful. The same treatment modalities that exist for adults exist for children. However, there are a few additional considerations for clinical evaluation of a pediatric patient.[8]

Children retain the potential for improvement. Surgical planning must consider its effect in conjunction with the child's extrapolated psychomotor development.

As in adults, the first steps are to obtain a thorough history and physical examination followed by a period of observation. Range of motion and functional need assessments will guide the decision making process. The Gross Motor Function Measure assessment can characterize the evolution of gross motor function throughout the child's development and growth. The assessment should be repeated every 6 to 12 months to help predict the prognosis for motor functionality. Surgical intervention may be delayed if motor function is improving, or may be indicated if the progression of function stagnates or declines.[10]

Upper extremity spasticity in children may be approached differently from lower extremity spasticity. The smaller muscle bulk of the pediatric patient can allow for greater benefit from botulinum toxin local injections. They may be used in combination with physical therapy, bracing and casting before considering extensive neurosurgical treatment.[7]

The use of intrathecal baclofen therapy is often more complex in children than in adults. Because of the smaller size of the child compared to the fixed size of the implanted pumps, dorsal rhizotomy may be preferred in children younger than six years old. Specialized dosing may also be necessary, and as with adults, these dosages can be roughly defined before proceeding to surgery.[11]

18.5 Final Thoughts

Because of the complexities involved in diagnosing and managing spasticity, a multi-modality approach to treatment is demanded. A variety of medical, interventional, and surgical options are available, can be used in tandem and yield varying degrees of effectiveness. Interventions must be tailored to the patient so as to reduce the symptoms of spasticity that cause functional disability while preserving those that are helpful.

References

[1] Alterman RL, Lozano AM. Functional Neurosurgery. In: Winn HR, ed. Youman's Neurological Surgery. Philadelphia, PA: Elsevier-Saunders; 2011
[2] Farmer SE, James M. Contractures in orthopaedic and neurological conditions: a review of causes and treatment. Disabil Rehabil. 2001; 23(13):549–558

[3] Naro A, Leo A, Russo M, et al. Breakthroughs in the spasticity management: Are non-pharmacological treatments the future? J Clin Neurosci. 2017; 39:16–27

[4] Sindou M, Mertens P. Surgery for Intractable Epilepsy. In: Quinones-Hinojosa A, ed. Schmidek & Sweet Operative Neurosurgical Techniques. Vol. 2. 6th ed. Philadelphia, PA: Elsevier-Saunders; 2012

[5] Boyd RN, Morris ME, Graham HK. Management of upper limb dysfunction in children with cerebral palsy: a systematic review. Eur J Neurol. 2001; 8(Suppl 5):150–66

[6] Pizzi A, Carlucci G, Falsini C, Verdesca S, Grippo A. Evaluation of upper-limb spasticity after stroke: A clinical and neurophysiologic study. Arch Phys Med Rehabil. 2005; 86(3):410–415

[7] Steinbok P. Selective dorsal rhizotomy for spastic cerebral palsy: a review. Childs Nerv Syst. 2007; 23(9):981–990

[8] Boster AL, Bennett SE, Bilsky GS, et al. Best Practices for Intrathecal Baclofen Therapy: Screening Test. Neuromodulation. 2016; 19(6):616–622

[9] Nair KP, Marsden J. The management of spasticity in adults. BMJ. 2014; 349: g4737

[10] Farmer JP, Sabbagh AJ. Selective dorsal rhizotomies in the treatment of spasticity related to cerebral palsy. Childs Nerv Syst. 2007; 23(9):991–1002

[11] Kan P, Gooch J, Amini A, et al. Surgical treatment of spasticity in children: comparison of selective dorsal rhizotomy and intrathecal baclofen pump implantation. Childs Nerv Syst. 2008; 24(2):239–243

19 Surgery for Spasticity: Rhizotomy and Intrathecal Therapy

Carolina Gesteira Benjamin, Jugal Shah, Alon Mogilner, and David Harter

Abstract

In cases of spasticity refractory to medical management, the most common neurosurgical procedures that can ameliorate symptoms and prevent complications of persistently increased tone include dorsal rhizotomy and intrathecal baclofen pump placement. Common indications for surgical intervention include cerebral palsy, traumatic brain injury, spinal cord injury, and multiple sclerosis. Dorsal rhizotomy involves transecting sensory lumbar and sacral nerve roots to reduce excitatory input to the spinal cord, thereby decreasing spasticity and improving motor function in the lower limbs. Unlike rhizotomy, an ablative procedure, intrathecal baclofen therapy is a procedure with reversible therapeutic effects. It requires permanent implantation of a lumbar-subarachnoid catheter and a subcutaneous pump apparatus that can deliver baclofen, a GABA-B agonist that increases the inhibitory effect interneurons on motor neurons, thus decreasing tone. Both procedures can have serious adverse effects that can either be severely debilitating or even fatal. Therefore, meticulous patient selection involving a thorough pre-operative evaluation by experienced clinicians is crucial, ideally utilizing a multidisciplinary approach to maximize the success of these surgical procedures and minimize complications.

Keywords: baclofen, intrathecal therapy, intrathecal baclofen pump, rhizotomy, selective dorsal rhizotomy, spasticity, hypertonicity

19.1 Introduction

When spinal spasticity is refractory to medical management, the neurosurgical procedures currently most performed are dorsal rhizotomy and intrathecal baclofen pump placement. Conditions requiring such intervention include cerebral palsy, traumatic brain injury, spinal cord injury, and multiple sclerosis.[1,2,3,4] In dorsal rhizotomy, the sensory lumbar and sacral nerve roots are transected to reduce excitatory input to the spinal cord. This decreases spasticity and improves lower limb function.[5] Unlike rhizotomy, which is an ablative procedure, intrathecal baclofen therapy is therapeutically reversible. It requires an implanted lumbar-subarachnoid catheter and a subcutaneous pump for infusion of baclofen, a GABA-B agonist that increases the inhibitory effect of interneurons on motor neurons.[6]

19.2 Rhizotomy

19.2.1 Patient Selection

The most common condition to require selective dorsal rhizotomy (SDR) is spastic diplegia associated with cerebral palsy), a consequence of non-progressive injury to the fetal or infantile brain. This injury leads to insufficient inhibitory interneuron input, excessive alpha motor neuron excitatory activity, and thus spasticity.[5,7] The resultant hypertonicity makes ambulation difficult. It may also cause orthopedic deformities of the lower extremities.[8] Patients that benefit from SDR are those with disabling hypertonicity secondary to spasticity. The presence of significant dystonia is, however, a contraindication to SDR because the dystonia can be unmasked or exacerbated by rhizotomy.[7] Before considering SDR, patients should have undergone a trial of physical and occupational therapy, oral medication, intramuscular botulinum toxin injections, and tendon release. Candidates should be between the 3–10 years of age. Most procedures are done before the age of 15 years.[9,10]

19.2.2 Preoperative Preparation

For both procedures, the degree of spasticity and extent of motor function must be quantified before surgery. Hypertonicity in upper and lower extremity muscle groups is measured using the Modified Ashworth Scale (MAS). Motor function is quantified using the Gross Motor Function Classification System Score (GMGMS). Gait is assessed using the Visual Gait Assessment Scale (VGAS). Patients should have some motor strength and control so as to prevent deterioration in crouching, lateral trunk sway, and knee hyperextension post operatively.[11] A magnetic resonance imaging scan should be done before surgery to identify the level of the conus medullaris and any possible structural abnormality.

19.2.3 Operative Procedure

Before 1991, SDR was done with L2-S2 laminectomies but the technique has been modified to a selective, single level (L1) or two level (L1–2) osteoplastic laminotomy to avoid delayed spinal deformity.[8,12,13] A short acting, non-depolarizing neuromuscular blocking agent is used during intubation for general anesthesia so as to not interfere with neurophysiologic monitoring. Direct stimulation and electromyography (EMG) are used to guide the surgery along with sensory and motor evoked potentials. After the monitoring leads are placed and initial levels obtained, the patient is positioned prone on the operating room table over gel rolls. The L1 spinous process is identified for the skin incision and a high-speed drill is used to create a laminotomy, which is plated to the spine after completion of the rhizotomy. Ultrasound can be used to identify the conus location, but this can be confirmed grossly when the dura is opened.

A midline durotomy is made and, once the dura is opened, saline irrigation is no longer used so as to not interfere with the EMG responses. Under the operating microscope, the spinal roots between L2 and S2 bilaterally are dissected so as to separate the dorsal roots and ventral roots both anatomically and electrophysiologically. After the rootlets are anatomically identified, a single 0.1 msec square-wave pulse is applied to each dorsal rootlet at a rate of 0.5 Hz. The intensity of the stimulus is

Table 19.1 Criteria used for assigning rootlet grades. CMAP = Compound muscle action potential

Grade	Interpretation
0	Unsustained CMAP in any muscle ('normal')
1 +	Sustained CMAP from muscles innervated by the segmen tal level of the stimulated dorsal rootlet
2 +	Same as grade 1 + with CMAP in muscles innervated by an adjacent segmental level
3 +	Same as grade 2 + with CMAP in muscles innervated by multiple ipsilateral segmental levels
4 +	Same as grade 3 + with motor response in the contralateral leg

Adapted from: Warf BC, Nelson KR. (1996) The electromyographic responses to dorsal rootlet stimulation during partial dorsal rhizotomy are inconsistent. Pediatric Neurosurgery 25: 13–19.

increased until a reflex response is obtained from the ipsilateral corresponding muscle. Once the reflex is established, a 50-Hz train of tetanic stimulation is applied for 1 second and the response is graded on a scale of 1 + to 4 + (▶ Table 19.1). Rootlets that produce 1 + and 2 + responses are spared and those that produce 3 + and 4 + responses are sectioned. The decision to transect a given rootlet depends on the intensity of the response and on the number of rootlets that produce that response at a given level. Abnormal roots are identified in this manner, coagulated using bipolar electrocautery and cut sharply with micro-scissors. To achieve maximal clinical benefit, 50–70% of motor roots are transected.[5,11] Stimulation of the penis or clitoris and perianal area while monitoring the activity in the S2 rootlets is done to identify those rootlets to preserve in order to avoid bowel and bladder dysfunction.[5,9,11] The portion of the dorsal S2 root that is sectioned is limited to less than 35% to limit such morbidity.[5]

The subdural space is copiously irrigated, and the dura is closed with a running suture in a water-tight fashion. The bone is secured in placed either using sutures absorbable or titanium miniplates. The wound is then closed in multiple layers including muscle, fascia, and skin.

19.2.4 Postoperative Management

Patients are observed in a monitored setting for the first day post operatively and slowly mobilized. Comprehensive physical and occupational therapy is started in the hospital and most patients require transfer to an acute rehabilitation facility for the first 2–3 weeks. After patients are able to ambulate independently, they may be discharged home but aggressive outpatient physical and occupational therapy should continue.

While lower extremity weakness and bowel and bladder dysfunction are the two most disabling complications that can occur, they can be largely prevented with meticulous intraoperative neurophysiologic monitoring.[9,11] Transient parasthesias and dysesthesias can also occur and can be treated with agents that mitigate neuropathic pain.[11] Common complications of the laminectomies or osteoplastic laminotomies done for SDR are the development of progressive deformities such as scoliosis, kyphosis, hyperlordosis, or hip subluxation requiring orthopedic intervention.[7,8,9] If cerebrospinal fluid leak occurs, it should be aggressively treated to reduce the risk of meningitis.

19.3 Intrathecal Therapy

19.3.1 History of Baclofen Treatment

Baclofen (B-[4-chlorophenyl]-g-aminobutryic acid) is a muscle relaxant and antispasmodic agent that works as an agonist to GABA-B receptors. There is a high density of GABA-B receptors in the dorsal horn of the spinal cord. Activation of pre-synaptic receptors causes inhibition of Ca2 + influx into presynaptic terminals resulting in inhibition of release of excitatory neurotransmitters such as aspartate and glutamate into the polysynaptic pathways of the dorsal horn.[6] Oral baclofen was first described in 1976 and showed clinical benefits for some patients with spasticity, but many patients failed to respond or had intolerable systemic adverse effects at doses required to penetrate the blood-brain barrier.[6] Subsequently, intrathecal delivery of baclofen was used to maximize therapeutic effects while diminishing systemic adverse effects.[6,14,15] Single dose intrathecal administration for human spinal spasticity was first reported by Penn in 1984. Continuous administration via an implantable pump was performed for patients with spinal spasticity after clinical trials carried out in Europe and the United States. The United States Food and Drug Administration granted approval for intrathecal use in 1992. With continuous spinal intrathecal baclofen (ITB) infusions, the concentration achieved in CSF is 10 to 80 times greater than oral administration.[6,16]

19.3.2 Patient Selection

The most common indications for intrathecal baclofen therapy are anoxic or traumatic brain injury (including cerebral palsy), spinal cord injury, and multiple sclerosis. Rare hereditary conditions can also cause spasticity requiring intrathecal therapy. There is a consensus that, in the appropriate patient population, ITB therapy can reduce tone thus facilitating the management and care of these patients. This ultimately leads to a decrease in complications such as ulcerations secondary to positioning and also leads to a decrease in the need for corrective orthopedic procedures.[8] For patients who are ambulatory, ITB can help maintain independent ambulation.[4,14]

The determination of which patients will benefit from an ITB pump is made preoperatively. The degree of spasticity prior to surgery is again measured using the Modified Ashworth scale score. Most patients will undergo a lumbar puncture trial for intrathecal baclofen trial injection. The dose injected is determined by the degree of pre-operative spasticity, the patient's weight, and the etiology of the spasticity (00mcg for traumatic brain injury patients, 50mcg for patients with cerebral palsy, and 75mcg for patients with cerebral palsy with a component of dystonia). Following the lumbar puncture trial, serial assessments by a physical therapist, nurse, or physician are made at two and six hours after injection. Improvement in tone compared to preoperative spasticity using the Modified Ashworth Scale indicates a positive result.

19.4 Operative Procedure

Intrathecal pump placement is usually done under general anesthesia, although select cases can be done under intravenous sedation/monitored anesthesia care. The patient is positioned in the lateral decubitus position with appropriate padding of all bony prominences. An important consideration that may determine the side of pump placement is the presence of a gastrostomy tube, suprapubic catheter, scoliotic deformity or any other previous scar. Fluoroscopic guidance may facilitate identification of the midline and trajectory. A 14-gauge Tuohy needle is used to enter the intrathecal space either percutaneously, or following a cutdown to the lumbodorsal fascia, depending on the surgeon's preference. An oblique paramedian approach has been recommended to minimize the possibility of catheter fracture. Ideally, the dura is only punctured once with the Tuohy needle to prevent the risk of persistent cerebrospinal fluid (CSF) leak from multiple punctures.[17] Once clear CSF is obtained, the stylet is removed and the implantable catheter is advanced cephalad to the desired level. The catheter is advanced to approximately T8–12 for spastic diplegia, to C5-T2 for spastic quadriparesis, or to C1–4 for generalized secondary dystonia.[4]

Catheter tip position may be confirmed with fluoroscopy. If the percutaneous approach is taken, a 2 cm skin incision is made sharply around the Tuohy needle in the rostral caudal direction and the soft tissues are dissected using electrocautery down to the fascia. A 2–0 silk purse string suture is then placed around the needle entry point in the fascia and the needle is removed. After the catheter is anchored with its tip buried in the fascia, the purse string suture is tied down. The anchor is again secured to the fascia with additional 2–0 silk sutures.

For placement of the pump, a 6–8 cm incision is made at least 2–3 cm below the costal margin on the desired side. Electrocautery is used to dissect through the soft tissue down to the rectus sheath. A subfascial technique may be used in thin patients to allow for improved healing and cosmesis, as well as to lower the risk of skin erosion.[18,19,20] When the subfascial technique is done, the rectus sheath is incised horizontally, and blunt dissection with Kittner "peanut" dissectors is used to develop a plane between the muscle and fascia. Once an adequate pocket is made and hemostasis is obtained, a passer is used to tunnel the catheter from the lumbar incision to the abdomen. The catheters are trimmed and fixed appropriately and the pump is placed in the previously made pocket with any excess catheter placed posterior to the pump to avoid damage when the pump is accessed for refilling. The most commonly used pump is the programmable Synchromed II device that can either be 20cc or 40cc in volume (Medtronic, Inc., Minneapolis, MN). The wounds are both copiously irrigated either with bacitracin or vancomycin irrigation. The wounds are then closed in multiple layers.

19.5 Post Operative Management and Complications

The battery-powered pump can be adjusted using an RF-controlled external probe and computer to adjust flow rates, continuous or bolus infusions, or total dose. For complication due to overdose, the pump can be emergently shut off, and information regarding the remaining dose and battery life can be queried.

Complications from ITB therapy may occur because of the side effects of baclofen, the surgery, or hardware. Baclofen toxicity can present as over sedation, dizziness, blurred vision, and slurred speech. Overdose may result in respiratory depression, coma, hypotension, and bradycardia, in addition to weakness and flaccidity.[1,4,14] Withdrawal, a potentially life threatening complication, can occur from pump malfunction or blockage of the catheter and results in confusion, hyperthermia, seizures, psychiatric manifestation, and rebound spasticity.[21,22,23,24] Withdrawal can be treated with oral baclofen, benzodiazepenes, periactin, and oral dantrolene.[25] For significant withdrawal, emergent intrathecal bolus dosing, either via pump or lumbar puncture, may be indicated.

Other surgical complications include seromas or skin breakdown over the device in addition to disconnection, kinking, or breaking of the catheter. Leakage of CSF at the catheter insertion site has also been reported.[4,25] Issues related to the size of the pump and local problems tend to be more pronounced in thin patients and younger children and can be mitigated with subfascial placement (▶ Fig. 19.1).[18,19,20] Infection may be treated with systemic antibiotics, but often the pump removal is necessary. If complicated by leakage of CSF, meningitis becomes a concern.

If system malfunction is suspected, it is important to understand that infection, alcohol withdrawal, benzodiazepine withdrawal, or serotonin syndrome may present with similar symptoms and should also be ruled out. The initial tests of choice are AP and lateral abdominal radiographs to evaluate the integrity of the pump and catheter.[26] The newer catheters (Ascenda®, Medtronic), cannot always be visualized on plain x-rays and a CT scan may be necessary. If plain films are non-diagnostic and

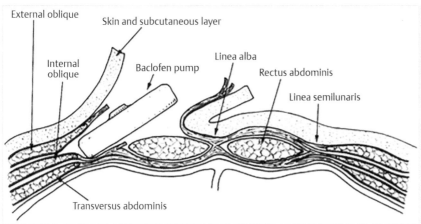

External oblique
Skin and subcutaneous layer
Internal oblique
Baclofen pump
Linea alba
Rectus abdominis
Linea semilunaris
Transversus abdominis

Fig. 19.1 Schematic illustration of a cross section of the subfascial pocket for baclofen pump placement in thin individuals.
From: Kopell BH, Sala D, Doyle WK, Feldman DS, Wisoff JH, Weiner HL: Subfascial implantation of intrathecal baclofen pumps in children: Technical note. Neurosurgery 2001; 49:753–6

pump and catheter malfunction remains a concern, more invasive testing may be done. A needle can be inserted percutaneously into the pump side port and 2–3 mL of fluid should be withdrawn, both to establish catheter patency and to clear residual baclofen to avoid overdose during subsequent contrast injection. If CSF is successfully aspirated and the patient's symptoms are relatively mild, programming an intrathecal medication bolus through the system as a therapeutic trial may be done. If the symptoms are severe or there is no response to a therapeutic bolus, fluoroscopy during contrast injection through the accessory port is indicated, which may visualize disconnection of the catheter from the pump, leaks, catheter tip migration, or macroscopic perforations.[27] When CSF is successfully aspirated, one should remember that the pump should be reprogrammed for a single bolus to deliver back the medication aspirated from the port so as to prevent withdrawal.

The intrinsic battery life of an intrathecal baclofen pump is 4–7 years depending on the infusion rate.[4] The pump should be replaced prior to final expiration to prevent withdrawal.

References

[1] Steinbok P. Selection of treatment modalities in children with spastic cerebral palsy. Neurosurg Focus. 2006;21(2):e4.

[2] Grunt S, Fieggen AG, Vermeulen RJ, Becher JG, Langerak NG. Selection criteria for selective dorsal rhizotomy in children with spastic cerebral palsy: a systematic review of the literature. Dev Med Child Neurol. 2014;56(4):302-312.

[3] Dudley RW, Parolin M, Gagnon B, et al. Long-term functional benefits of selective dorsal rhizotomy for spastic cerebral palsy. J Neurosurg Pediatr. 2013;12(2):142-150.

[4] Albright AL, Turner M, Pattisapu JV. Best-practice surgical techniques for intrathecal baclofen therapy. Journal of neurosurgery. 2006;104(4 Suppl):233-239.

[5] Steinbok P. Selective dorsal rhizotomy for spastic cerebral palsy: a review. Child's nervous system : ChNS : official journal of the International Society for Pediatric Neurosurgery. 2007;23(9):981-990.

[6] Penn RD, Kroin JS. Intrathecal baclofen alleviates spinal cord spasticity. Lancet. 1984;1(8385):1078.

[7] van Schie PE, Schothorst M, Dallmeijer AJ, et al. Short- and long-term effects of selective dorsal rhizotomy on gross motor function in ambulatory children with spastic diplegia. J Neurosurg Pediatr. 2011;7(5):557-562.

[8] Steinbok P, Hicdonmez T, Sawatzky B, Beauchamp R, Wickenheiser D. Spinal deformities after selective dorsal rhizotomy for spastic cerebral palsy. Journal of neurosurgery. 2005;102(4 Suppl):363-373.

[9] Graham D, Aquilina K, Cawker S, Paget S, Wimalasundera N. Single-level selective dorsal rhizotomy for spastic cerebral palsy. J Spine Surg. 2016;2(3):195-201.

[10] Peter JC, Arens LJ. Selective posterior lumbosacral rhizotomy in teenagers and young adults with spastic cerebral palsy. British journal of neurosurgery. 1994;8(2):135-139.

[11] Oki A, Oberg W, Siebert B, Plante D, Walker ML, Gooch JL. Selective dorsal rhizotomy in children with spastic hemiparesis. J Neurosurg Pediatr. 2010;6(4):353-358.

[12] Peacock WJ, Arens LJ, Berman B. Cerebral palsy spasticity. Selective posterior rhizotomy. Pediatr Neurosci. 1987;13(2):61-66.

[13] Peacock WJ, Arens LJ. Selective posterior rhizotomy for the relief of spasticity in cerebral palsy. S Afr Med J. 1982;62(4):119-124.

[14] Penn RD. Intrathecal baclofen for spasticity of spinal origin: seven years of experience. Journal of neurosurgery. 1992;77(2):236-240.

[15] Penn RD. Medical and surgical treatment of spasticity. Neurosurg Clin N Am. 1990;1(3):719-727.

[16] Knutsson E, Lindblom U, Martensson A. Plasma and cerebrospinal fluid levels of baclofen (Lioresal) at optimal therapeutic responses in spastic paresis. Journal of the neurological sciences. 1974;23(3):473-484.

[17] Seeberger MD, Kaufmann M, Staender S, Schneider M, Scheidegger D. Repeated dural punctures increase the incidence of postdural puncture headache. Anesth Analg. 1996;82(2):302-305.

[18] Thakur SK, Rubin BA, Harter DH. Long-term follow-up for lumbar intrathecal baclofen catheters placed using the paraspinal subfascial technique. J Neurosurg Pediatr. 2016;17(3):357-360.

[19] Kopell BH, Sala D, Doyle WK, Feldman DS, Wisoff JH, Weiner HL. Subfascial implantation of intrathecal baclofen pumps in children: technical note. Neurosurgery. 2001;49(3):753-756; discussion 756-757.

[20] Bassani L, Harter DH. Paraspinal subfascial placement of lumbar intrathecal baclofen catheters: short-term outcomes of a novel technique. J Neurosurg Pediatr. 2012;9(1):93-98.

[21] Siegfried RN, Jacobson L, Chabal C. Development of an acute withdrawal syndrome following the cessation of intrathecal baclofen in a patient with spasticity. Anesthesiology. 1992;77(5):1048-1050.

[22] Reeves RK, Stolp-Smith KA, Christopherson MW. Hyperthermia, rhabdomyolysis, and disseminated intravascular coagulation associated with baclofen pump catheter failure. Arch Phys Med Rehabil. 1998;79(3):353-356.

[23] Mandac BR, Hurvitz EA, Nelson VS. Hyperthermia associated with baclofen withdrawal and increased spasticity. Arch Phys Med Rehabil. 1993;74(1):96-97.

[24] Kofler M, Arturo Leis A. Prolonged seizure activity after baclofen withdrawal. Neurology. 1992;42(3 Pt 1):697-698.

[25] Ghosh D, Mainali G, Khera J, Luciano M. Complications of intrathecal baclofen pumps in children: experience from a tertiary care center. Pediatric neurosurgery. 2013;49(3):138-144.

[26] Miracle AC, Fox MA, Ayyangar RN, Vyas A, Mukherji SK, Quint DJ. Imaging evaluation of intrathecal baclofen pump-catheter systems. AJNR Am J Neuroradiol. 2011;32(7):1158-1164.

[27] Woolf SM, Baum CR. Baclofen Pumps: Uses and Complications. Pediatr Emerg Care. 2017;33(4):271-275.

20 Epilepsy: Preoperative Evaluation, EEG and Imaging

Ika Noviawaty and Oguz Cataltepe

Abstract

Surgical management of epilepsy is a well-established treatment option for drug resistant epilepsy. Preoperative assessment of epilepsy patients aims to select the surgical candidates and most appropriate surgical approaches for the patients. Patients undergo extensive work up for preoperative evaluation that includes long term video-EEG monitoring, imaging studies, neuropsychological tests as well as invasive electrophysiological monitoring in many cases. The collected data is reviewed by a multidisciplinary team to determine the patient's surgical candidacy and best surgical approach.

Keywords: seizure, epilepsy surgery, EEG, video-EEG monitoring, MRI

20.1 Introduction

Epilepsy is one of the most common neurological disorders in both adults and children. Reported annual incidence of epilepsy is around 60/100,000 person-years and point prevalence of active epilepsy is about 6/1000 persons.[1] Epilepsy is defined by the International League Against Epilepsy (ILAE) as "enduring predisposition to generate epileptic seizures."[2,3,4] Epileptic seizures might be focal or generalized and significantly affect the patient's quality of life. Medical management with anti-epileptic drugs (AED) is the first line of treatment in epilepsy patients. However, approximately one third of epilepsy patients fail to respond to medical management and they are considered candidates for surgical treatment.[2,5,6]

20.2 Selection of Surgical Candidates

Drug resistant epilepsy can be defined as failure of seizure freedom despite adequate trials of two appropriately chosen AED therapies, whether as monotherapy or in combination.[2,5,6,7] Epilepsy surgery is a well-established management option for this patient group not only to control the seizures but also to prevent and/or control associated co-morbiditiy, cognitive and developmental decline, especially in young children. The goal of epilepsy surgery is to excise the epileptogenic zone without causing any functional deficit. The selections of the proper surgical candidate and most appropriate surgical approach is the most critical first step to reach this goal.

20.3 Preoperative Assessment

The main goal of preoperative assessment of epilepsy patients is to define the epileptogenic zone. The ideal candidate for epilepsy surgery is a patient with a well-defined epileptogenic zone without involvement of eloquent cortex. This should be demonstrated by a fully congruent data base obtained from electrophysiological, imaging and semiological investigations.

Epileptogenic zone is a conceptual term and can be described as those cortical areas or networks responsible for the generation of seizures. An extensive work-up that includes assessment of clinical semiology, various electrophysiological and radiological tests is needed to define the epileptogenic zone and to determine its anatomo-electro-clinical correlations.[7,8,9]

20.3.1 Seizure Semiology

Seizure semiology is the clinical manifestations of habitual seizures of the patient and it has an important lateralizing and localizing value. For example, temporal lobe and temporal plus epilepsy are typically seen with auras, vegetative or visceral symptoms such as behavioral arrest, staring spells, vague epigastric sensation, nausea, auditory or visual hallucinations, dream states, and/or language dysfunction. On the other hand, seizure semiology in extratemporal epilepsy is less stereotypical and much more variable. It changes widely based on the location of seizure onset and its propagation pathways. Typical frontal lobe seizures are seen with motor automatisms, dystonic posturing, head and eye deviation, tonic, clonic, or atonic activity, drop attacks, olfactory manifestations, vocalization and complex behaviors. Parietal lobe seizures are frequently associated with somatosensory, abdominal symptoms (nausea or choking), and gustatory sensations and they spread to frontal or temporal regions easily. Occipital lobe seizure symptoms are mostly present as visual phenomena, hallucinations, flashes, scotomas, hemianopia, contraversive and ipsiversive eye and head movements. All these semiological characteristics of the seizures help to locate the epileptogenic zone and accurate description of clinical semiology can be most reliably obtained through long-term video EEG monitoring.[8,10,11,12]

20.3.2 Electroencephalography

Electroencephalography (EEG) remains the cornerstone of preoperative workup in determining the epileptogenic zone. Electrophysiological data may be obtained with non-invasive techniques such as routine EEG, long-term scalp video EEG monitoring (LTM), and magnetoencephalography (MEG). However, routine EEG may be normal in about 30–50% of the patients with epilepsy.[8,9,10,11,12,13] Therefore, although abnormal interictal EEG findings are helpful, a normal EEG does not rule out presence or location of epilepsy. The value of ictal EEG is much higher and documenting the abnormal electroencephalographic activity during the onset of habitual seizures constitutes the single most significant information. LTM plays the most critical role in obtaining both ictal and interictal EEG recordings and also documenting the clinical characteristics of habitual seizures. Correlation of clinical semiology and abnormal EEG findings are essential to lateralize and localize the epileptogenic zone. LTM with scalp EEG is a routine part of the preoperative assessment of surgical candidates in Phase I and might be sufficient to select surgical candidates in many cases. However, if the non-invasive electrophysiological techniques fail to define the epileptogenic zone or the results from diagnostic work up are discordant, then invasive monitoring techniques are used to locate the epileptogenic zone. Invasive LTM is performed by using surgically placed intracranial electrodes such as subdural strip, grid and intraparenchymal depth electrodes. These electrodes can also be used to map cortical functions by stimulating cortical and subcortical areas.[8,9,10]

Invasive monitoring is indicated if:

- surface EEG data is inconclusive to lateralize and/or localize the epileptogenic zone,
- clinical, electrophysiological, and radiological data is non-congruent,
- multiple epileptogenic areas or structural abnormalities are present,
- there is a single structural lesion with ill-defined borders,
- MRI is negative despite electrographically well-documented epileptogenic activity in a certain cortical region,
- epileptogenic zone extends in or abuts the eloquent cortex,
- suspicious epileptogenic zone is in a deep-seated location.

The goal of invasive monitoring is precise determination of the epileptogenic zone, seizure propagation pathways and mapping of the eloquent cortex. It provides a reliable electrophysiological recording directly from cortical surface or deep structures. However, the goal can be achieved only after determining the appropriate coverage area to place intracranial electrodes. Coverage area is defined based on a hypothesis about possible location or network of the epileptogenic zone. Non-invasive electrophysiological data, imaging studies, Positron emission tomography (PET), Single-photon emission computed tomography (SPECT), and clinical semiology are used to develop a reasonable hypothesis regarding the possible location of the epileptogenic zone and propagation paths before proceeding to invasive LTM.

The most commonly used intracranial electrodes are subdural strip, grid and depth electrodes. They have different indications, advantages and disadvantages. Strip electrodes are single row of electrode arrays imbedded in thin silastic sheets and can be placed easily through a simple burr hole. They are ideal to lateralize the seizures. Grid electrodes are rectangular arrays with several parallel rows of contacts. They cover a larger area and are ideal to localize and map the borders of epileptogenic zone and adjacent eloquent cortex. However, relatively large craniotomies are needed for subdural grid placement. Depth electrodes are multi-contact electrode arrays embedded in a very thin, tubular silastic material. They provide excellent recordings from deep structures such as the amygdala, hippocampus, cingulum, and orbitofrontal cortex. They are placed through small drill holes using stereotactic technique. The most common application of depth electrode is hippocampal placement and stereo-electroencephalography (SEEG).[9,10]

Placement of subdural electrodes has a higher risk for CSF leak, infection, hemorrhage, cortical injury and cerebral edema. Although these risks are much less with depth electrodes, there are some disadvantages of depth electrodes. The main disadvantages are it provides minimal cortical coverage, limited functional stimulation capability and limited cortical sampling (tunnel vision). Selection of the electrodes should be determined by coverage strategy. If the purpose is covering an electrographically well-defined epileptogenic lesion and adjacent eloquent cortex, then subdural grid electrode might be the best option for cortical EEG recording as well as stimulation and mapping of the cortex. If the epileptogenic zone is not well defined and multiple potential epileptogenic areas are present or the epileptogenic zone is deep seated, then stereotactically placed depth electrodes are more appropriate to explore the epileptogenic network.[9,10]

20.3.3 Neuroimaging

MRI is the main imaging modality in epilepsy patients' preoperative assessment. It provides critical information on diagnosis of any structural abnormality and also helps for surgical planning. High resolution MRI with appropriate sequences provides detailed information regarding both well-defined lesions and also radiological characteristics of the brain tissue such as signal intensity and structural changes in hippocampus, abnormalities in gray-white matter differentiation, cortical thickness, and architecture. Most common epileptogenic substrates for focal epilepsy are mesial temporal sclerosis, low-grade tumors, vascular lesions and focal cortical dysplasia (▶ Fig. 20.1). Most common neoplasms associated with epilepsy are low-grade astrocytoma, dysembryoplastic neuroepithelial tumors (DNET), ganglioglioma and oligodendroglioma (▶ Fig. 20.2). All these lesions can be diagnosed on high-field MRI studies within a reasonable degree of certainty.[8,14]

Advanced MRI techniques such as functional MRI and diffusion tensor imaging also contribute in the preoperative assessment. Other functional imaging techniques such as PET and SPECT provide valuable information by measuring the local changes in brain metabolism during interictal and ictal activities. PET study might be very helpful diagnostically in temporal lobe epilepsy if it shows unilaterally decreased metabolism in temporal lobe during interictal period. Ictal SPECT is also useful to localize the epileptogenic zone, It will document increased blood flow to certain brain regions during the seizure.[14]

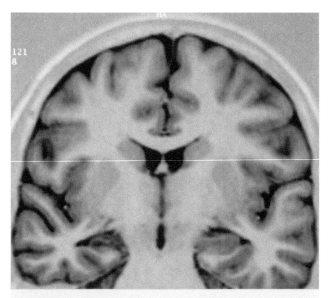

Fig. 20.1 Hippocampal atrophy has been seen on the right side in coronal cuts of the MRI study.

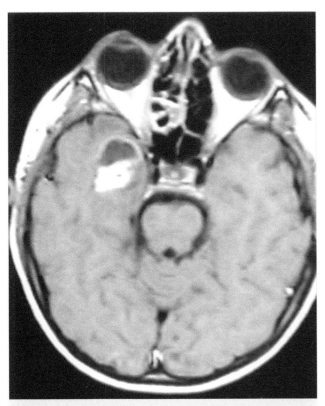

Fig. 20.2 A mesial temporal lobe tumor has been seen in axial cuts of the MRI study. The pathology was ganglioglioma.

20.3.4 Neuropsychological Tests

Neuropsychological tests help to define functional deficit zone, determine language, memory and visuospatial functions, and predict the risk of postoperative deficits. Localizing the functional deficit zone helps to identify location of the "lesion" and determine whether the dysfunction is focal or multifocal. The epileptogenic focus might be within this dysfunctional cortex. For example, language or verbal memory deficits suggests dominant hemisphere dysfunction. Visualspatial memory deficits suggest non-dominant temporal dysfunction. Deficits in both areas suggest bitemporal disease. Neuropsychological test results are also beneficial to counsel the patient regarding postoperative potential risks.[8]

The intracarotid amobarbital procedure (WADA test) helps to determine cerebral dominance for language, memory and visuospatial functions. This is an invasive procedure that is performed in the angiography suit. It is valuable in predicting postoperative risk for language and memory function. Functional MRI is also very helpful to lateralize and localize speech area non-invasively and it has been replacing WADA test in many centers.

20.3.5 Surgical Decision

After completing the preoperative assessment, the multidisciplinary team discusses the findings and decides whether or not the patient is a good surgical candidate and which surgical approach is the most appropriate option. This may not be a straightforward decision in many cases. Although the presence of a structural lesion has a high association with the epileptogenic zone, it may not contain the complete epileptogenic zone. Therefore, even if the imaging studies show a lesion in the brain, documenting the relationship between lesion and epileptogenic zone is still needed to determine the best surgical approach for seizure control. Again, in some other cases, the patient may have focal seizures without any well-defined electrographic focus and any visible abnormality in a high-resolution MRI study. These cases are the most challenging in epilepsy surgery. Extensive investigation with PET, SPECT, MEG and invasive monitoring techniques such as SEEG might be helpful to identify the epileptogenic zone in these cases.

20.4 Conclusion

Surgical management of epilepsy is a well-established, safe and efficacious treatment modality, but needs an extensive diagnostic work up with a multidisciplinary approach and collaborative effort between medical and surgical teams that have experience and expertise in the management of these patients. Selection of surgical candidates and determination of the most appropriate surgical technique constitute the main challenge in this patient population. Determining the right candidate and most appropriate surgical technique for each patient in a multi-disciplinary fashion is a pre-requisite for success in epilepsy surgery.

References

[1] Fiest KM, Sauro KM, Wiebe S, et al. Prevalence and incidence of epilepsy: A systematic review and meta-analysis of international studies. Neurology. 2017; 88(3):296–303

[2] Kwan P, Schachter SC, Brodie MJ. Drug-resistant epilepsy. N Engl J Med. 2011; 365(10):919–926

[3] Fisher RS, Acevedo C, Arzimanoglou A, et al. ILAE official report: a practical clinical definition of epilepsy. Epilepsia. 2014; 55(4):475–482

[4] Berg AT, Berkovic SF, Brodie MJ, et al. Revised terminology and concepts for organization of seizures and epilepsies: report of the ILAE Commission on Classification and Terminology, 2005–2009. Epilepsia. 2010; 51 (4):676–685

[5] Devinsky O. Patients with refractory seizures. N Engl J Med. 1999; 340(20): 1565–1570

[6] Berg AT, Kelly MM. Defining intractability: comparisons among published definitions. Epilepsia. 2006; 47(2):431–436

[7] Elger CE, Schmidt D. Modern management of epilepsy: a practical approach. Epilepsy Behav. 2008; 12(4):501–539

[8] Rosenow F, Lüders H. Presurgical evaluation of epilepsy. Brain. 2001; 124(Pt 9):1683–1700

[9] Kovac S, Vakharia VN, Scott C, Diehl B. Invasive epilepsy surgery evaluation. Seizure. 2017; 44:125–136

[10] Noachtar S, Rémi J. The role of EEG in epilepsy: a critical review. Epilepsy Behav. 2009; 15(1):22–33

[11] Beniczky S, Neufeld M, Diehl B, et al. Testing patients during seizures: A European consensus procedure developed by a joint taskforce of the ILAE - Commission on European Affairs and the European Epilepsy Monitoring Unit Association. Epilepsia. 2016; 57(9):1363–1368

[12] Tufenkjian K, Lüders HO. Seizure semiology: its value and limitations in localizing the epileptogenic zone. J Clin Neurol. 2012; 8(4):243–250

[13] Salinsky M, Kanter R, Dasheiff RM. Effectiveness of multiple EEGs in supporting the diagnosis of epilepsy: an operational curve. Epilepsia. 1987; 28(4): 331–334

[14] Nagae LM, Lall N, Dahmoush H, et al. Diagnostic, treatment, and surgical imaging in epilepsy. Clin Imaging. 2016; 40(4):624–636

21 Epilepsy: Temporal Lobectomy with Invasive Monitoring

Ashwin G. Ramayya, Gordon H. Baltuch

Abstract

Over the past half century, temporal lobectomy has emerged as a well-established surgical therapy for temporal lobe epilepsy. In this chapter, we review basic concepts involving temporal lobectomy surgery, including recent developments in patient selection, preoperative evaluation, surgical technique, and postoperative outcomes. We describe in detail the surgical technique we use at our institution and briefly discuss emerging future developments.

Keywords: temporal lobectomy, temporal lobe epilepsy, anteromedial temporal lobectomy, medial temporal lobe sclerosis, standard temporal lobectomy, epilepsy

21.1 Patient Selection

Temporal lobectomy emerged in the 1950s as a surgical procedure used to treat seizures arising from the temporal lobe.[1,2] The primary indication is medically-refractory temporal lobe epilepsy, however, it can also be useful to treat lesions in the anterior temporal lobe such as cavernomas or low-grade gliomas. Classically, patients were identified as candidates for temporal lobectomy if they had partial seizures that were medically refractory, and they did not have diffuse or progressive brain disease.[3] However, these requirements have been substantially revised over the past several decades.[4,5,6] When selecting patients for this procedure, three basic questions must be answered.

21.1.1 Have the Patients Failed Medical Treatment?

The patient must have failed medical treatment with two anti-epileptic medications either in terms of seizure control or tolerance of these medications.

21.1.2 Are Seizures Arising from the Temporal Lobe?

Temporal lobectomy is only successful if there is a seizure focus in the temporal lobe. To assess whether this is the case, it is important to integrate data from several diagnostic modalities. These include clinical semiology, neuropsychological testing, neuroimaging, non-invasive electrocroticography (EEG), and in select cases, invasive electrocorticography (EEG). The ideal candidate for temporal lobectomy will have converging evidence to suggest that seizures arise from the temporal lobe. However, in many cases the data is mixed and requires collaborative decision-making from a multi-disciplinary team to make a surgical decision.

21.1.3 Is There a High Risk of Post-operative Functional Deficits?

Temporal lobectomy can result in damage to structures that are important to language (lateral dominant temporal lobe), vision (optic radiations, Meyer's loop), and memory (hippocampus). Preoperative studies to assess the baseline status of these cognitive functions and their anatomical localization relative to the temporal lobe are important to assess the risk of further injury during surgery. Additionally, as with all major surgical procedures, the patient's cardiovascular status, nutritional status and overall health should be assessed to as to estimate a perioperative risk of cardiovascular and infectious complications.

21.2 Preoperative Evaluation

We briefly discuss several diagnostic modalities that are useful for pre-operative assessment of patients (see Chapter 19 for a further discussion of these modalities, including specific indications for surgery).

21.2.1 Semiology

Seizures arising from the temporal lobe are classically complex partial seizures with hand and face automatisms such as lip smacking. With involvement of the amygdala, they are often preceded by aura involving fear ("feeling of impending doom"), or a difficult to describe epigastric sensation. Involvement of the ipsilateral basal ganglia can lead to contralateral hemiplegia or dystonia. When these signs are observed in the setting of persistent ipsilateral automatisms, they may be falsely localized to the contralateral motor cortex.

21.2.2 Non-invasive Scalp Electroencephalograpy (EEG)

Scalp EEG can be used to assess for interictal spikes, markers of pathological neural activity arising from epileptogenic tissue in between seizures. The observation of unilateral interictal spikes arising from the temporal lobe provides a strong indication for temporal lobectomy.[7] Additionally, scalp EEG recordings can be used in conjunction with video recordings to capture clinical and subclinical seizures. Here, one can assess intra ictal electrophysiological patterns of activity to anatomically localize a seizure focus.

21.2.3 Neuropsychological Testing

Specific patterns of cognitive deficits as identified by neuropsychological testing may provide clues to the site of the epileptogenic focus. For example, a selective reduction in verbal memory performance may suggest that the epileptogenic focus involves the patient's dominant medial temporal lobe.

21.2.4 Language Localization: The WADA Test and Functional Magnetic Imaging (fMRI)

The main goal of these tests is to determine which cerebral hemisphere is dominant for language function, which of course has major implications for surgical planning. The WADA test is an invasive procedure and involves injecting a barbiturate into each of the carotid arteries and testing the subsequent effects on language. Functional MRI (fMRI) is a non-invasive neuroimaging method to study patterns of blood oxygenation during various cognitive tasks. Recent data suggests that fMRI provides concordant results to the WADA test in most cases of temporal lobe epilepsy.[8]

21.2.5 MRI Evaluation

MRI scans can reveal evidence of sclerosis in the medial temporal lobe, suggesting ischemic injury and gliosis, and a potential substrate for seizure generation. Unilateral mesial temporal sclerosis (MTS) on MRI is a strong indication that the epileptogenic focus is within the temporal lobe; as such, these cases are associated with favorable postsurgical outcomes (n = 161, 71% seizure freedom at 2 years).[9] However, favorable post-surgical outcomes have been observed in "MRI-normal" patients with other indicators of temporal lobe epilepsy, albeit in a smaller study (n = 40; 60% seizure freedom with at least 1 year of follow-up).[10] See the outcomes section below for further discussion.

21.2.6 Other Imaging Modalities (PET, SPECT, MEG)

Other imaging modalities can provide important evidence in preoperative evaluation but vary in their utility across institutions.[11] Positron emission tomography (PET) can be used to study metabolic activity in the medial temporal lobe. Relative hypometabolism in one hemisphere is an indicator of epileptic activity. Subtraction ictal single photon emission computed tomography (SPECT) imaging can be used in with EEG activity to assess whether the mesial temporal lobe shows increased activity during seizure generation. Magnetoencephalography (MEG) can be used with source-localization algorithms to spatially localize the onset of ictal activity with greater detail than scalp EEG.

21.2.7 Intracranial Invasive EEG Monitoring with Depth and Subdural Electrodes

When the above studies fail to identity a seizure focus, patients can undergo invasive monitoring with intracranial EEG subdural and depth electrodes. Intracranial EEG offers the temporal resolution of scalp EEG recordings with greater spatial resolution. However, because of the limited coverage offered by these electrodes, they are most useful when preoperative studies yield specific hypotheses about particular locations where the seizure focus may be located. Subdural electrodes can be "grids" or "strip" electrodes that can be used to cover cortical surface, and can also be used to map motor and language function. Depth electrodes are inserted into the parenchyma and can sample from deeper subcortical tissue, such as the mesial temporal lobe.

21.2.8 Operative Procedure

Before discussing the specific operative technique for temporal lobectomy, it is important to briefly discuss two major concepts related to this procedure.

21.2.9 Standard Temporal Lobectomy vs. Selective Amygdalohippocampectomy

There are two major surgical procedures to treat temporal lobe epilepsy - the "standard" temporal lobectomy (STL) and the more selective amygdalohippocampectomy (SAH).[5,12,13,14] The STL involves removal of the lateral temporal cortex in addition to the medial temporal lobe. In contrast, SAH selectively removes medial temporal lobe structures that are thought to contain the epileptic focus while largely sparing the presumably functional lateral temporal cortex. However, recent data has shown largely similar outcomes, both in terms of seizure freedom and functional deficits.[15,16,17,18] These data suggest that the lateral temporal cortex removed during STL may largely be non-functional, or alternatively, that the SAH results in damage to the anterio-lateral temporal lobe by removing the surrounding medial temporal structures.[6]

21.2.10 Standardized Approach vs. Tailored Approach

There are two general approaches to temporal lobectomy surgery. In the standardized approach the extent of lateral and medial resection are pre-determined for each patient so as to maximize post-operative seizure freedom and minimize functional deficits. A prominent randomized control trial demonstrated improved post-surgical outcomes compared to medical management with temporal lobectomy when resecting a "maximum of 6.0 to 6.5 cm of the anterior lateral non dominant temporal lobe or 4.0 to 4.5 cm of the dominant temporal lobe."[19] In keeping with this data, surgeons resect 4–5 cm of the temporal tip in the non-dominant hemisphere and 3–4 cm in the dominant hemisphere. This excludes resection of the superior temporal gyrus, which frequently has language representation.[1] Early evidence suggested that a maximal medial resection improves post-surgical seizure freedom. Recent data now suggests that outcome is also favorable when 2.5 cm instead of 3.5 cm of the hippocampus is resected.[20]

In the tailored approach, the extent of resection is individually determined for each patient based on pre-operative and intra-operative mapping studies.[21] These studies attempt to identify the seizure focus in each patient by recording interictal spikes, intra ictal electrophysiological patterns, and by identifying eloquent language and motor with simulation studies.

There has been no high quality clinical data showing improved outcomes with such a fully tailored approach. As such, the degree to which the temporal lobectomy is tailored to the individual patient is institution-dependent.

21.3 Operative Technique

Here, we describe our technique for performing a standardized temporal lobectomy on the right side.

21.3.1 Positioning and Extradural Surgery

Place the patient in the supine position, and secure him in the Mayfield headrest (Integra LifeSciences Corp., Plainsboro, NJ). The head is positioned so as to bring the Sylvian fissure parallel to the table and the floor. This requires rotation of at least 45 degrees to the left, head extension, and tilting of the vertex towards the floor. The incision is planned in the form of a question mark. In addition to providing adequate anatomical exposure, this incision has the following advantages: (1) it is behind the hairline (2) preserves blood supply to scalp and temporalis; (3) avoids the facial nerve; and (4) avoids the ear canal. The scalp may be reflected in one or two layers.

Next, perform a pterional craniotomy. Opened mastoid air cells along the floor must be thoroughly waxed. It is helpful to drill off some of the sphenoid wing, but not to extend into the superior orbital fissure.

21.3.2 Durotomy

The dural flap should be anteriorly based. We measure 4 cm from the temporal tip to ensure that the craniotomy is satisfactory and to plan the lateral temporal lobectomy. Intra-operative electrocorticography can be performed at this time if indicated by pre-operative testing or institutional practice (see Chapter 19 for further discussion).

21.3.3 Lateral Temporal Resection

This resection may begin while using the operating microscope, or it may first be used for the medial temporal resection. Use a #7 Frazier suction and bipolar cautery to make the initial pial incision approximately 4 cm posterior to the temporal tip, preserving large surface veins. The vein of Labbé has variable anatomy and is usually located over the posterior temporal lobe. We extend the resection 4 cm from the temporal tip regardless of the side of surgery. Make a coronal cut through the middle temporal gyrus, working deep to identify the ventricle. This will mark the medial extent of the lobectomy. Close the ventricular opening with a cottonoid patty. For the inferior limb, extend this coronal cortisectomy inferiorly towards the floor of the middle fossa, and then anteriorly towards the temporal tip. For the superior limb, work along the inferior edge of the superior temporal gyrus towards the anterior temporal tip. Next, connect the superior and inferior limbs for the lateral temporal cortisectomy. Elevate the lateral temporal cortex, along with the uncus and the anterolateral part of the amygdala. During this step it is important to maintain the depth of the resection at the lateral edge of the ventricle wall, which is in the same

sagittal plane as the collateral sulcus. Be careful not to resect any tissue posterosuperior to the tip of the temporal horn. This tissue may contain fibers of Meyer's loop and damaging them causes a contralateral superior temporal quadrantanopsia. In general, excessive posterolateral resection or retraction can damage the optic radiations.

21.3.4 Microsurgical Retraction of Medial Temporal Lobe

After completing the lateral temporal resection, you should see a resection cavity that extends to the depth of the lateral wall of the temporal horn and the collateral sulcus. Deep (medial) to these structures, we find medial temporal lobe structures, the basal ganglia and brain stem. Begin your microsurgical dissection by unroofing the lateral ventricle and identifying the inferior choroidal point as the anterior most extent of the choroid in the temporal horn. An imaginary line between this point and the lesser wing of the sphenoid (or the site of the MCA bifurcation) will guide your resection of deep structures and keep you out of the basal ganglia.[22] Next, remove the parahippocampal gyrus, uncus, and remaining amygdala. To do this, follow the pia from the collateral sulcus along the tentorial incisura to the medial pial surface. At the medial extent of the resection, deep to the medial pial surface, one should identify the posterior cerebral artery, and the oculomotor nerve in the ambient cistern. It is critical not to violate this medial pial border and cause damage to these structures. During this antero-medial dissection, avoid removing the hippocampal head (which lies anterior to the inferior choroidal point). The head of the hippocampus can also be removed during this dissection, but we prefer to remove it en bloc with the remainder of the hippocampus in a subsequent step.

To remove the hippocampus, place a 3/8' retractor lateral to the ventricle and another where needed, usually superiorly. The choroidal point marks the beginning of the choroidal fissure and also marks the division between the hippocampal head anteriorly and body posteriorly. Open the choroidal fissure and coagulate the small hippocampal feeders along the pial surface along the medial surface of the fimbria. Once the hippocampal body is mobilized from these vascular feeders, work anteriorly to posteriorly to remove the hippocampus en bloc. The posterior extent of the hippocampal resection should be carried out to at least 2.5 cm posteriorly. A complete hippocampal resection enables you to see the contents of the ambient and crural cisterns as well as the cerebral peduncle, colliculi, and the pulvinar of the thalamus.

21.4 Closure

Obtain hemostasis. Because the ventricle is open, a watertight dural closure is needed. Backfill the resection cavity with irrigation before placing the final stitch, as pneumocephalus will often cause a severe headache. Complete the closure in standard fashion.

21.5 Postoperative Management

Postoperative management is similar to that with a standard craniotomy. The patient is admitted to the intensive care unit overnight and continues on preoperative anti-seizure medication. We obtain a head CT scan within 24 hours of surgery to assess for immediate post-operative complications such as hemorrhage. The patient is transferred to the floor and out of the hospital within 3 to 5 days. A follow-up MRI scan can be obtained at 3 months once the resection cavity has settled into its final position.[5,6] Repeat neuropsychological testing and EEG testing can be done at 6 months and one year to assess for post-operative cognitive deficits and persistent inter ictal activity.

21.5.1 Outcomes and Complications

Several studies have shown that temporal lobectomy improves seizure freedom more than medical management alone.[19] A recent systematic review estimated that surgery results in seizure freedom in approximately 60% of patients, with reports in the literature ranging from 34 to 74%.[17] They also reported the best seizure-free outcomes for patients with lesions in the temporal lobe, such as hippocampal sclerosis or low grade tumors compared to non-lesional temporal lobe epilepsy, or extratemporal lesional epilepsy.

Temporal lobectomies have a low perioperative mortality rate (0.1 – 0.5%,).[17] Overall morbidity (including cerebrospinal fluid leaks, infection, hemorrhage) is approximately 8%.[23] Permanent neurologic complications occur in about 5% of patients and are most commonly visual field defects that are well tolerated.[24] Common neurocognitive deficits after surgery include a decline in verbal naming and memory. Verbal memory is more often affected after left (approximately 44%) as compared to right (approximately 20% temporal lobectomy.[25] Overall IQ is spared.

21.6 Conclusions

Temporal lobectomy remains a core neurosurgical procedure for the treatment of medically refractory temporal lobe epilepsy. It has undergone significant evolution since its conception in the 1950s, particularly in terms of patient selection, preoperative work up, and the emergence of variations in surgical technique. It remains an effective and safe procedure and has been shown to be reliably better than medical management in carefully selected patients. Exciting future directions include the further development of minimally invasive surgical approaches and more detailed preoperative workup to identify "subtypes" of medically refractory temporal lobe epilepsy that may respond differently to the various emerging surgical treatments.[26,27]

References

[1] Falconer MA, Meyer A, Hill D, Mitchell W, Pond DA. Treatment of temporal-lobe epilepsy by temporal lobectomy; a survey of findings and results. Lancet. 1955; 268(6869):827–835

[2] Penfield W, Flanigin H. Surgical therapy of temporal lobe seizures. AMA Arch Neurol Psychiatry. 1950; 64(4):491–500

[3] Cahan LD, Engel J , Jr. Surgery for epilepsy: a review. Acta Neurol Scand. 1986; 73(6):551–560

[4] Kwon CS, Neal J, Telléz-Zenteno J, et al. CASES Investigators. Resective focal epilepsy surgery - Has selection of candidates changed? A systematic review. Epilepsy Res. 2016; 122:37–43

[5] Spencer DD, Spencer SS, Mattson RH, Williamson PD, Novelly RA.. 1984

[6] Torres-Reveron and Spencer. Standard Temporal Lobectomy. Youmann's Neurological Surgery

[7] Holmes MD, Dodrill CB, Wilensky AJ, Ojemann LM, Ojemann GA. Unilateral focal preponderance of interictal epileptiform discharges as a predictor of seizure origin. Arch Neurol. 1996; 53(3):228–232

[8] Janecek JK, Swanson SJ, Sabsevitz DS, et al. Language lateralization by fMRI and Wada testing in 229 patients with epilepsy: rates and predictors of discordance. Epilepsia. 2013; 54(2):314–322

[9] Janszky J, Janszky I, Schulz R, et al. Temporal lobe epilepsy with hippocampal sclerosis: predictors for long-term surgical outcome. Brain. 2005; 128(Pt 2): 395–404

[10] Bell ML, Rao S, So EL, et al. Epilepsy surgery outcomes in temporal lobe epilepsy with a normal MRI. Epilepsia. 2009; 50(9):2053–2060

[11] Knowlton RC. The role of FDG-PET, ictal SPECT, and MEG in the epilepsy surgery evaluation. Epilepsy Behav. 2006; 8(1):91–101

[12] Çataltepe O, Weaver J. Anteromesial temporal lobectomy. Pediatric epilepsy surgery: preoperative assessment and surgical treatment. New York: Thieme; 2010

[13] Conolly P, Baltuch GH. Temporal Lobectomy and Amygdalohippocampectomy. 2009. Operative Techniques in Epilespy Surgery. New York: Thieme; 2009

[14] Wieser HG, Yaşargil MG. Selective amygdalohippocampectomy as a surgical treatment of mesiobasal limbic epilepsy. Surg Neurol. 1982; 17(6): 445–457

[15] Helmstaedter C. Cognitive outcomes of different surgical approaches in temporal lobe epilepsy. Epileptic Disord. 2013; 15(3):221–239

[16] Hu WH, Zhang C, Zhang K, Meng FG, Chen N, Zhang JG. Selective amygdalohippocampectomy versus anterior temporal lobectomy in the management of mesial temporal lobe epilepsy: a meta-analysis of comparative studies. J Neurosurg. 2013; 119(5):1089–1097

[17] Jobst BC, Cascino GD. Resective epilepsy surgery for drug-resistant focal epilepsy: a review. JAMA. 2015; 313(3):285–293

[18] Sagher O, Thawani JP, Etame AB, Gomez-Hassan DM. Seizure outcomes and mesial resection volumes following selective amygdalohippocampectomy and temporal lobectomy. Neurosurg Focus. 2012; 32(3):E8

[19] Wiebe S, Blume WT, Girvin JP, Eliasziw M, Effectiveness and Efficiency of Surgery for Temporal Lobe Epilepsy Study Group. A randomized, controlled trial of surgery for temporal-lobe epilepsy. N Engl J Med. 2001; 345(5):311–318

[20] Schramm J, Lehmann TN, Zentner J, et al. Randomized controlled trial of 2.5-cm versus 3.5-cm mesial temporal resection in temporal lobe epilepsy–Part 1: intent-to-treat analysis. Acta Neurochir (Wien). 2011; 153(2):209–219

[21] Silbergeld DL, Ojemann GA. The tailored temporal lobectomy. Neurosurg Clin N Am. 1993; 4(2):273–281

[22] Tubbs RS, Miller JH, Cohen-Gadol AA, Spencer DD. Intraoperative anatomic landmarks for resection of the amygdala during medial temporal lobe surgery. Neurosurgery. 2010; 66(5):974–977

[23] McClelland S , III, Guo H, Okuyemi KS. Population-based analysis of morbidity and mortality following surgery for intractable temporal lobe epilepsy in the United States. Arch Neurol. 2011; 68(6):725–729

[24] Hader WJ, Tellez-Zenteno J, Metcalfe A, et al. Complications of epilepsy surgery: a systematic review of focal surgical resections and invasive EEG monitoring. Epilepsia. 2013; 54(5):840–847

[25] Sherman EM, Wiebe S, Fay-McClymont TB, et al. Neuropsychological outcomes after epilepsy surgery: systematic review and pooled estimates. Epilepsia. 2011; 52(5):857–869

[26] Bonilha L, Martz GU, Glazier SS, Edwards JC. Subtypes of medial temporal lobe epilepsy: influence on temporal lobectomy outcomes? Epilepsia. 2012; 53(1):1–6

[27] Chang EF, Englot DJ, Vadera S. Minimally invasive surgical approaches for temporal lobe epilepsy. Epilepsy Behav. 2015; 47:24–33

22 Epilepsy: Extra-Temporal Surgery with Invasive Monitoring

Andres I. Maldonado-Naranjo, Zachary Fitzgerald, Jorge Gonzalez-Martinez

Abstract

The goal of epilepsy surgery is the complete resection or disconnection of the cortical and subcortical areas that are responsible for the generation and early spread of seizures. This is known as the epileptogenic zone (EZ). The EZ may overlap with eloquent cortex, which must be preserved. Standard, non-invasive monitoring provides a rather broad overview of the anatomical location of epileptogenic areas and respective cortical functioning. The goal of invasive monitoring is to better understand the anatomical boundaries of the EZ as well as cortical and subcortical function. This chapter discusses the indications, advantages, disadvantages, and the role of invasive monitoring in medically refractory extra-temporal focal epilepsy, focusing primarily on subdural grid and strip and stereo-electroencephalography (SEEG) methodologies.

Keywords: extra-temporal epilepsy, stereo-electroencephalography, stereotaxy, invasive monitoring

22.1 Patient Selection

To best define the anatomical location of the epileptogenic zone (EZ) and its proximity to cortical and subcortical eloquent areas, a range of non-invasive tools can be used. Such tools include the analysis of patient semiology, magnetocencephalography (MEG), Magnetic resonance imaging (MRI), ictal single-photon emission computed tomography (SPECT), functional MRI (fMRI), magnetic resonance spectroscopy (MRS) and positron emission tomography (PET). These methods are complementary to one another and may define cortical zones of interest as symptomatic, irritative, ictal, and functionally deficient in addition to the EZ, which is defined as the minimal amount of brain tissue that needs to be removed or disconnected to achieve seizure freedom.[1] However, under circumstances in which: (1) the non-invasive data is insufficient to precisely define the location of the hypothetical EZ, (2) there is suspicion for early involvement of eloquent cortical and subcortical areas or, (3) there is the possibility for multi-focal seizures, invasive monitoring may be indicated.[2,3,4]

22.2 Preoperative Preparation

22.2.1 Localizing the Epileptogenic Zone

Prolonged video-EEG monitoring with analysis of clinical semiology is the standard for diagnosis and localization of the EZ.[1] This noninvasive sampling technique gives an excellent overview of the epileptogenic areas but often only approximates the boundaries of both the irritative zone and the EZ. Scalp EEG detects only epileptiform activity that results from EEG synchronization of large areas of cortex, while recordings are disturbed by the effect of high-resistance structures.[1,5] MEG may provide better identification of the epileptic activity localized in a tangential orientation such as the inter-hemispheric fissure or opercular areas, but with limited information regarding the interictal epileptic activity.[6] In malformations of cortical development (MCD), 85%-100% of patients exhibit epileptiform discharges on inter ictal scalp EEG recordings. These discharges can range from lobar to lateralized, and from non-localizing to diffuse. In some cases of subependymal heterotopia, they can include generalized spike-wave patterns.[7] The spatial distribution of interictal spikes is usually more extensive than the structural abnormality when assessed by intraoperative inspection or visual MRI analysis.[7,8] For these reasons, when subtle forms of cortical dysplasia are suspected as the pathological substrate of medically intractable epilepsy, mainly in patients with extra-temporal epilepsy and non-lesional imaging, extra-operative invasive monitoring is recommended to provide a more accurate and effective localization of the EZ.[2,9,10,11]

22.2.2 Localization of the Functional/Eloquent Zone

Localization of functional areas in the brain, and the anatomical boundaries of these areas with the EZ, is an essential part in the process of developing an adequate and individualized surgical strategy.[1,12,13] An understanding of the functional status of the involved region(s) and its anatomical or pathological correlation is essential.[1,12,14] For example, some focal MCD-related lesions that are characterized by significant FLAIR signal increase on MRI and are located in anatomically functional areas such as Broca's area, are not functional on direct electrical stimulation.[15] Additionally, the same lesions may show no evidence of intrinsic epileptogenicity when assessed by mapping of the ictal onset zones (▶ Fig. 22.1).[16] On the other hand, MCD lesions with mild or no FLAIR signal increase may be functional and at times epileptogenic with persistent eloquent function in MCD devoid of balloon cells.[9,17] Similar electrocorticogram (EcoG) patterns have been reported in patients with low-grade glial tumors (DNET and ganglioglioma), whereas dysplastic and epileptic cortical areas were found immediately surrounding these lesions.[18] Functional cortex may be displaced. Of course, the precise location of eloquent cortex that may be in the vicinity or within the limits of the hypothetical EZ is essential information that will guide the completion of a safe operation.

22.3 Operative Procedure

22.3.1 Indications, Advantages, and Disadvantages of the Subdural Method in Evaluating Medically Refractory Extra-temporal Lobe Epilepsy

Intracranial electrodes are used to identify the EZ and functional or eloquent cortex. Subdural grids have an advantage,

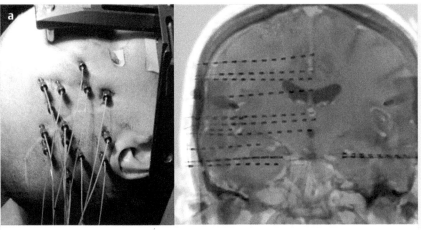

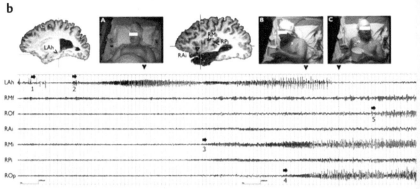

Fig. 22.1 Mapping using the SEEG method. **(a)** shows images of the final implantation aspect of a bilateral frontal-temporal SEEG exploration, demonstrating the position of 14 depth electrodes (right). Note the precise parallel placement, with electrodes covering extensive bilateral brain areas. **(b)** shows the SEEG anatomo-electro-clinical analysis of seizures, demonstrating the 3D temporal-spatial pattern of the epileptic network activation that correlates with seizure semiology, with identification of the EZ in the left hippocampus and insula.

however. They can be left in place long enough to record both spontaneous seizures and inter ictal activity during various stages of arousal. They can be used for continuous preoperative mapping and surveying of adjacent cortex.[9,15,19,20] However, subdural grids also have disadvantages. These are: increased risks of wound infection, flap osteomyelitis, acute meningitis, cerebral edema, increased intracranial pressure, and hemorrhage, greater financial costs, and limited access to deep cortical regions. Two such regions are the mesial orbitofrontal cortex and the anterior cingulate gyrus.[21,22,23,24] While implanted depth electrodes that use a non or semi-stereotactic technique can compensate for these deficiencies, high precision and clear localization of the EZ may be lacking.[25]

22.3.2 The Subdural Operative Technique in Evaluating Medically Refractory Extra-temporal Lobe Epilepsy

Pre-operative, non-invasive studies are used to determine areas of coverage. Perioperative antibiotics, dexamethasone and 0.25 g/kg mannitol are given. The craniotomy should allow room for electrode insertion in addition to lesion resection. Stereotactic guidance might be necessary if depth electrodes are needed, as well as a sizable craniotomy if extensive cortical surface area is to be covered. Orbitofrontal access can be obtained if the craniotomy includes the neurosurgical keyhole. Inter-hemispheric access requires an incision to the midline. Planned depth electrodes are inserted first, using stereotactic guidance. Cortical draining veins can impede basal and medial surface electrode placement. These surfaces should be carefully inspected before a grid is positioned

beyond the craniotomy edge. Any resistance to placement likely indicates the presence of a draining vein and the trajectory of the array should be adjusted. The lateral cortical surface is covered as the final step. Once in place, each electrode wire is secured to the nearest dural edge with a stitch. The closure is done using standard technique.

22.4 The Stereo-electroencephalography Method

22.4.1 Indications, Advantages, and Disadvantages of the SEEG Method in Evaluating Medically Refractory Extra-temporal Lobe Epilepsy

The modern principle of SEEG is still similar to that described by Bancaud and Talairach in 1973. It is based on anatomo-electro-clinical correlations (AEC) designed to conceptualize the spatial-temporal organization of the epileptic discharge within the brain.[11,26,27]

Specific indications for SEEG include: (1) the possibility of a deep-seated or difficult to cover EZ location; (2) failure of a previous subdural invasive study to clearly outline the exact location of the seizure onset zone; (3) the need for extensive bi-hemispheric explorations; (4) pre-surgical evaluation that is suggestive of a functional network involvement, such as the limbic system, with a normal MRI. The main disadvantage of SEEG is its restricted ability to complete functional mapping. Because the number of contacts in the superficial cortex is limited, a contiguous mapping of eloquent brain areas cannot be obtained as in the subdural method of mapping. To overcome this relative disadvantage, SEEG can be complemented with DTI imaging or awake craniotomies.[11]

22.4.2 Planning SEEG Implantation for Extra-Temporal Lobe Coverage

An adequate implantation plan requires the formulation of precise AEC hypotheses. These are determined during multidisciplinary patient management conferences and based on the results of all non-invasive tests. Depth electrodes should sample the anatomic lesion if it has been identified, the most likely structures of ictal onset, the early and late spread regions, and the interactions with the functional networks. By analyzing the available non-invasive data and the temporal evolution of the ictal and clinical manifestations, a hypothesis of the EZ's anatomical location is then formulated.[28] Adequate knowledge of the functional networks involved in the primary organization of the epileptic activity is mandatory. In addition, surgeons and epileptologists will have to account for the three dimensional aspects of depth electrode recordings. Despite its limited coverage of the cortical surface, they accurately sample the structures along its trajectory. A full investigation must also include the lateral and mesial lobar surfaces, deep-seated cortex at sulcal depths, the insula, and the posterior inter-hemispheric cortical surface. The focus of the implantation strategy is to map epileptogenic networks, which usually involves multiple lobes, rather than individual lobes or lobules. The strategy should consider alternative hypotheses of localization.[29,30,31] Note that it is rare to implant more than 15 depth electrodes. Yet, when eloquent regions may be in the ictal discharge area, judicious coverage is needed. The strategy is: (1) to assess the role of the eloquent cortex in the seizure organization and; (2) to define the boundaries of a safe surgical resection.

22.4.3 SEEG Implantation Technique in Evaluating Medically Refractory Extratemporal Lobe Epilepsy

Once SEEG planning is finalized, the desired targets are reached using commercially available depth electrodes in various lengths and number of contacts, depending on the specific brain regions to be explored. The depth electrodes are implanted using conventional stereotactic technique or by the assistance of stereotactic robotic devices. Depth electrodes are inserted through 2.5 mm diameter drill holes, using orthogonal or oblique orientation, allowing intracranial recording from lateral, intermediate, or deep cortical and subcortical structures in a three-dimensional arrangement, thus accounting for the dynamic, multidirectional, spatiotemporal organization of the epileptogenic pathways.

Frame-based implantation has been described in detail elsewhere.[11] More recently, robotically assisted devices have been applied. Similar to the conventional approach, volumetric preoperative MRIs are obtained and DICOM format images are digitally transferred to the robot's native planning software. Individual trajectories are planned within the 3D imaging reconstruction according to predetermined target locations and intended trajectories. Trajectories are selected to maximize

sampling from superficial and deep cortical and subcortical areas within the pre-selected zones of interest and are oriented orthogonally in the majority of cases to avoid possible trajectory shifts due to excessively angled entry points.

All trajectories are evaluated for safety and target accuracy. Any trajectory that appears to compromise vascular structures is adjusted appropriately without affecting the sampling from areas of interest. External trajectory positions are examined for any entry sites that would be prohibitively close (less than 1.5 cm distance).

Patients are then placed under general anesthesia and the head is placed into a three-point fixation head holder. The robot is locked into position and the head holder device is secured to the robot. Next, image registrations are performed using a semi-automatic laser based facial recognition followed by manual selection of preset landmarks. The areas defined by the manually entered anatomic landmarks subsequently undergo automatic registration using laser based facial surface scanning. Accuracy is then confirmed. After successful registration, the accessibility of planned trajectories is automatically verified by the robot's software. A drilling platform, with a 2.5 mm diameter working cannula is secured to the robotic arm. After trajectory confirmation, the arm movement is initiated. The robotic arm automatically locks the drilling platform into a stable position. A 2 mm diameter handheld drill is introduced through the platform and used to create a pinhole. The dura is then opened with an insulated dural perforator using monopolar cautery at low settings. A guiding bolt is screwed firmly into each pinhole. The distance from the drilling platform to the retaining bolt is measured and this value is subtracted from the standardized 150 mm platform-to-target distance. The resulting difference is recorded for later use as the final length of the electrode to be implanted. This process is repeated for each trajectory. A 2 mm diameter stylet is set to the previously recorded electrode distance and passed gently into the parenchyma, guided by the implantation bolt, followed immediately by the insertion of the pre-measured electrode.

22.5 SEEG Guided Resections

Our center reported on 200 patients who underwent a total of 2,663 SEEG electrode implantations for the purposes of invasive intracranial EEG monitoring. They were inserted to investigate and anatomically characterize the extension of the EZ in accordance with a tailored pre-implantation hypothesis. This group was a challenging one because of the paucity of non-invasive data and/or the possibility of a more diffuse pathology than was suggested by previous failed invasive explorations. Nearly one-third (29.0%) of the studied patients had undergone prior surgical intervention for medically refractory epilepsy and had seizure recurrence. SEEG was able to confirm the EZ in 154 patients (77%). Of these, 134 patients (87%) underwent subsequent craniotomy for SEEG guided resection. Within this cohort, 90 patients had a minimum post-operative follow-up of at least 12 months; 61 patients (68%) no longer had disabling epileptic activity. The most common pathological diagnosis in this group was focal cortical dysplasia type I (55 patients, 61%). These results of seizure treatment outcome and complications are compatible with published results from other groups.[32,33,34]

22.6 Postoperative Management and Complications

CT is obtained shortly after surgery to rule out hemorrhagic complications and to confirm the adequacy of electrode trajectories. All patients are admitted to the epilepsy-monitoring unit and routine prophylactic antibiotics are given. In the Cleveland Clinic SEEG series, the complication rate was 3%. Other groups have reported similar results. Cossu et al., reported a 5.6%, morbidity. One percent of these had permanent deficits.[35] All three complications were hemorrhagic, which has been reported in several studies to be the most common complication in depth electrodes placement.[11] Other published series reporting complications for subdural grids and depth electrodes reported rates ranging from 0% to 26%.[23,36,37] Although, it is difficult to compare morbidity rates between subdural grids and SEEG due to the variability in patient selection and variable numbers of implanted electrodes, it is our preliminary impression that SEEG provides at least a similar degree of safety to that of with subdural grids or strips. This impression is also shared by others.[38,39,40,41]

22.7 Conclusions

The goals of invasive monitoring in extra-temporal refractory focal epilepsy may include: (1) the need for better anatomical delineation of the hypothetical epileptogenic zone and; (2) the need for a thorough definition of cortical and subcortical functional brain areas. Extra-operative mapping with the subdural method using subdural grids and strips has the advantage of allowing an optimal coverage of the subdural space adjacent cortex with adequate and continuous superficial functional mapping capabilities. Subdural implantations are open procedures making management of intracranial hemorrhagic simpler. The disadvantages of the subdural method are related to the inability to record and stimulate from deep cortical and subcortical areas such as the insula, posterior orbito-frontal, cingulate gyrus, and the depths of sulci. In these scenarios, SEEG may be a more efficient and safer option. Finally, SEEG has the advantages of allowing extensive and precise deep brain recordings and stimulations while maintaining minimal associated morbidity.

References

[1] Luders H, Comair Y. Epilepsy Surgery. 2nd ed. LWW; 2001

[2] Adelson PD, O'Rourke DK, Albright AL. Chronic invasive monitoring for identifying seizure foci in children. Neurosurg Clin N Am. 1995; 6(3):491–504

[3] Jayakar P. Invasive EEG monitoring in children: when, where, and what? J Clin Neurophysiol. 1999; 16(5):408–418

[4] Winkler PA, Herzog C, Henkel A, et al. [Noninvasive protocol for surgical treatment of focal epilepsies]. Nervenarzt. 1999; 70(12):1088–1093

[5] Engel JJ, Henry TR, Risinger MW, et al. Presurgical evaluation for partial epilepsy: Relative contributions of chronic depth-electrode recordings. Relative contributions of chronic depth-electrode recordings versus FDG-PET and scalp-sphenoidal ictal EEG. Neurology. 1990; 40:1670–1677

[6] Kakisaka Y, Kubota Y, Wang ZI, et al. Use of simultaneous depth and MEG recording may provide complementary information regarding the epileptogenic region. Epileptic Disord. 2012; 14(3):298–303

[7] Marnet D, Devaux B, Chassoux F, et al. [Surgical resection of focal cortical dysplasias in the central region]. Neurochirurgie. 2008; 54(3):399–408

[8] Kellinghaus C, Möddel G, Shigeto H, et al. Dissociation between in vitro and in vivo epileptogenicity in a rat model of cortical dysplasia. Epileptic Disord. 2007; 9(1):11–19

[9] Marusic P, Najm IM, Ying Z, et al. Focal cortical dysplasias in eloquent cortex: functional characteristics and correlation with MRI and histopathologic changes. Epilepsia. 2002; 43(1):27–32

[10] Francione S, Nobili L, Cardinale F, Citterio A, Galli C, Tassi L. Intra-lesional stereo-EEG activity in Taylor 's focal cortical dysplasia. Epileptic Disord. 2003; 5(September) Suppl 2:S105–S114

[11] Gonzalez-Martinez J, Bulacio J, Alexopoulos A, Jehi L, Bingaman W, Najm I. Stereoelectroencephalography in the "difficult to localize" refractory focal epilepsy: early experience from a North American epilepsy center. Epilepsia. 2013; 54(2):323–330

[12] Wieser HG. Epilepsy surgery. Baillieres Clin Neurol. 1996; 5(4):849–875

[13] Bancaud J. [Epilepsy after 60 years of age. Experience in a functional neurosurgical department]. Sem Hop/La Sem des hôpitaux organe fondé par l"Association d"enseignement médical des hôpitaux Paris. 1970; 46 (48):3138–3140

[14] Jeha LE, Najm I, Bingaman W, Dinner D, Widdess-Walsh P, Lüders H. Surgical outcome and prognostic factors of frontal lobe epilepsy surgery. Brain. 2007; 130(Pt 2):574–584

[15] Najm IM, Bingaman WE, Lüders HO. The use of subdural grids in the management of focal malformations due to abnormal cortical development. Neurosurg Clin N Am. 2002; 13(1):87–92, viii–ix

[16] Widdess-Walsh P, Jeha L, Nair D, Kotagal P, Bingaman W, Najm I. Subdural electrode analysis in focal cortical dysplasia: predictors of surgical outcome. Neurology. 2007; 69(7):660–667

[17] Ying Z, Najm IM. Mechanisms of epileptogenicity in focal malformations caused by abnormal cortical development. Neurosurg Clin N Am. 2002; 13 (1):27–33, vii

[18] Battaglia G, Chiapparini L, Franceschetti S, et al. Periventricular nodular heterotopia: classification, epileptic history, and genesis of epileptic discharges. Epilepsia. 2006; 47(1):86–97

[19] Jayakar P, Duchowny M, Resnick TJ. Subdural monitoring in the evaluation of children for epilepsy surgery. J Child Neurol. 1994; 9 Suppl 2:61–66

[20] Nair DR, Burgess R, McIntyre CC, Lüders H. Chronic subdural electrodes in the management of epilepsy. Clin Neurophysiol. 2008; 119(1):11–28

[21] Lee WS, Lee JK, Lee SA, Kang JK, Ko TS. Complications and results of subdural grid electrode implantation in epilepsy surgery. Surg Neurol. 2000; 54(5): 346–351

[22] Simon SL, Telfeian A, Duhaime AC. Complications of invasive monitoring used in intractable pediatric epilepsy. Pediatr Neurosurg. 2003; 38(1): 47–52

[23] Önal C, Otsubo H, Araki T, et al. Complications of invasive subdural grid monitoring in children with epilepsy. J Neurosurg. 2003; 98(5):1017–1026

[24] Vadera S, Mullin J, Bulacio J, Najm I, Bingaman W, Gonzalez-Martinez J. Stereoelectroencephalography following subdural grid placement for difficult to localize epilepsy. Neurosurgery. 2013; 72(5):723–729, discussion 729

[25] Bulacio JC, Jehi L, Wong C, et al. Long-term seizure outcome after resective surgery in patients evaluated with intracranial electrodes. Epilepsia. 2012; 53 (10):1722–1730

[26] Bancaud J, Angelergues R, Bernouilli C, et al. Functional stereotaxic exploration (SEEG) of epilepsy. Electroencephalogr Clin Neurophysiol. 1970; 28(1): 85–86

[27] Bancaud J, Favel P, Bonis A, Bordas-Ferrer M, Miravet J, Talairach J. [Paroxysmal sexual manifestations and temporal lobe epilepsy. Clinical, EEG and SEEG study of a case of epilepsy of tumoral origin]. Rev Neurol (Paris). 1970; 123 (4):217–230

[28] Chauvel P, McGonigal A. Emergence of semiology in epileptic seizures. Epilepsy Behav. 2014; 38:94–103

[29] Cardinale F, Cossu M, Castana L, et al. Stereoelectroencephalography: surgical methodology, safety, and stereotactic application accuracy in 500 procedures. Neurosurgery. 2013; 72(3):353–366, discussion 366

[30] Cardinale F, Lo Russo G. Stereo-electroencephalography safety and effectiveness: Some more reasons in favor of epilepsy surgery. Epilepsia. 2013; 54(8): 1505–1506

[31] Gonzalez-Martinez J, Mullin J, Vadera S, et al. Stereotactic placement of depth electrodes in medically intractable epilepsy. J Neurosurg. 2014; 120(3):639–644

[32] Munari C, Hoffmann D, Francione S, et al. Stereo-electroencephalography methodology: advantages and limits. Acta Neurol Scand Suppl. 1994; 152: 56–67, discussion 68–69

[33] Guenot M, Isnard J, Ryvlin P, et al. Neurophysiological monitoring for epilepsy surgery: the Talairach SEEG method. StereoElectroEncephaloGraphy. Indications, results, complications and therapeutic applications in a series of 100 consecutive cases. Stereotact Funct Neurosurg. 2001; 77(1–4):29–32

[34] Tanriverdi T, Ajlan A, Poulin N, Olivier A. Morbidity in epilepsy surgery: an experience based on 2449 epilepsy surgery procedures from a single institution. J Neurosurg. 2009; 110(6):1111–1123

[35] Cossu M, Schiariti M, Francione S, et al. Stereoelectroencephalography in the presurgical evaluation of focal epilepsy in infancy and early childhood. J Neurosurg Pediatr. 2012; 9(3):290–300

[36] Wyler AR, Walker G, Somes G. The morbidity of long-term seizure monitoring using subdural strip electrodes. J Neurosurg. 1991; 74(5):734–737

[37] Rydenhag B, Silander HC. Complications of epilepsy surgery after 654 procedures in Sweden, September 1990–1995: a multicenter study based on the Swedish National Epilepsy Surgery Register. Neurosurgery. 2001; 49(1):51–56, discussion 56–57

[38] Cossu M, Chabardès S, Hoffmann D, Lo Russo G. [Presurgical evaluation of intractable epilepsy using stereo-electro-encephalography methodology: principles, technique and morbidity]. Neurochirurgie. 2008; 54(3):367–373

[39] Guenot M, Isnard J. [Epilepsy and insula]. Neurochirurgie. 2008; 54(3):374–381

[40] Devaux B, Chassoux F, Guenot M, et al. [Epilepsy surgery in France]. Neurochirurgie. 2008; 54(3):453–465

[41] Chabardès S, Minotti L, Hamelin S, et al. [Temporal disconnection as an alternative treatment for intractable temporal lobe epilepsy: techniques, complications and results]. Neurochirurgie. 2008; 54(3):297–302

23 Neuromodulation in Epilepsy

Kevin Mansfield, Joseph S. Neimat

Abstract

Targeted neuromodulation can be used to reduce seizure frequency in patients with medically intractable epilepsy who are not candidates for surgical resection. Vagus Nerve Stimulation (VNS), Deep Brain Stimulation (DBS), and Responsive Neurostimulation (RNS) can be used for different types of epilepsy and in varied patient populations. The indications differ slightly, and each requires unique surgical approaches. All require the placement of a pulse generator in an accessible location, and precise placement of electrodes at a target point in the nervous system. The procedures are well tolerated, and have risks comparable to other similar operations. In this chapter, we review the indications and anticipated benefit for each mode of neuromodulation.

Keywords: neuromodulation, vagus nerve stimulation, deep brain stimulation, responsive neurostimulation, epilepsy, seizures

23.1 Patient Selection

Epilepsy affects an estimated 1% of the world's population.[1,2] In 20–30% of those individuals medication is not effective.[1,3,4] Whereas resection or ablation of a seizure focus can produce great improvements in seizure control in well-selected patients, a substantial population of refractory patients is not appropriate for surgical resection. Those not eligible for resection or ablation may be considered for targeted neuromodulation.

Current stimulation works by using electrical waveforms to inhibit pathologic signal transmission through the central nervous system. Vagus Nerve Stimulation (VNS) and Deep Brain Stimulation (DBS) decrease the excitability of seizure circuitry. Both are open-looped systems. Responsive Neuromodulation (RNS) detects a seizure and instantaneously blocks propagation with a high frequency stimulus burst. This is a closed loop system. Both types can reduce seizure frequency, but will rarely produce seizure freedom.[5,6,7] Partial, focal and multifocal and generalized epilepsy syndromes have been studied, with variable results (▶ Table 23.1).[8,9,10,11]

An algorithm for selecting the appropriate neuromodulation therapy is provided (▶ Fig. 23.1). Patients with a clear seizure focus in a non-eloquent area that can be safely resected or ablated should undergo surgical resection. Resection can provide a 50–70% chance of seizure free outcome. If the focus or foci can be identified but cannot be resected, then RNS may be better than the less specific VNS and DBS therapies. The inability to resect may be because either the focus is in eloquent cortex or arises from both hippocampi. If greater than two foci are present or if the foci cannot be identified, then VNS and DBS are the best options. Although slight differences in VNS and DBS therapeutic efficacy exist, they are comparable. The merits and challenges of each mode should be discussed with each patient and family in the selection process. Table 23.2 compares the practical requirements of each form of neuromodulation.

23.1.1 Preoperative Preparation

Patients with medically-refractory epilepsy should be evaluated for the option of surgical resection. The elements of the workup depend upon the patient's seizure pattern, and their tolerance for the testing. The goal is to identify the seizure foci, characterize the epilepsy type and clarify the risks of neurologic injury from the surgery. Neuropsychiatric evaluation should be included, to aid in localization and surgical risk assessment, and because depression and other psychiatric disorders may be exacerbated by the intervention. Even if a patient is not a candidate for resection or ablation, this data can guide the selection of the appropriate neuromodulation therapy.

23.1.2 Operative Procedure

Neuromodulation involves two components: an electrode to deliver the signal, and a pulse generator containing the energy source and controlling circuitry. The operative planning, positioning and scheduling must accommodate for the placement of both elements.

23.1.3 Electrode Placement

Vagus Nerve Stimulation

A carotid dissection is done to expose the left vagus nerve in the carotid sheath. Placement is always on the left vagus to avoid the risk of cardiac arrhythmias, since the right vagus nerve innervates the cardiac atria. A flexible, helical electrode is coiled around the vagus nerve. At least 3 cm of isolated nerve is

Table 23.1 Epilepsy studies and results

Therapy	% Seizure Reduction (during blinded phase)	% Responders (Achieving > 50% reduction by 1 year)	Notable Side Effects
VNS[12,13]	28	27	66.3% experienced voice alteration
DBS[6]	40.4	43	Incidence of depression (14%) and memory impairment (11%) in active group.
RNS[14]	37.9	46	2.1% experienced significant hemorrhage without permanent deficit. Death from SUDEP in 3 subjects with stimulation enabled

Note: Cohorts in the DBS and RNS studies included some patients that had failed VNS.

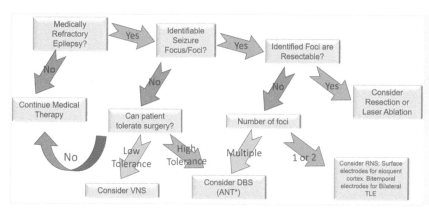

Fig. 23.1 Algorithm for determining surgical therapy for epilepsy:
*ANT = Anterior Nucleus of thalamus. Other targets may be suitable depending on the seizure type/ onset; TLE = Temporal Lobe Epilepsy

Table 23.2 Patient selection

Modality	Preoperative Planning	Surgical Stress	Inpatient Required	Time to Initiation
VNS	Standard workup only	Minimal	No	Same-day
DBS	Additional imaging, surgical planning*	Moderate; awake surgery sometimes required. Often staged over 1–2 weeks	Cranial portion only; generator placement is outpatient	2–4 weeks after generator placement
RNS	Possible additional imaging, surgical planning*	High, must tolerate craniotomy; performed asleep	Yes	1–2 months after placement

*Image acquisition for frame targeting and trajectory planning; some platforms require planning 1 week prior to implantation.

required for proper placement. A serpentine loop of redundant wire is secured to the overlying muscle to prevent tension on the nerve with neck movement, and the lead is tunneled, superficial to the clavicle, to the upper chest, where it connects to the generator in its pocket.

Deep Brain Stimulation

Some variation in the logistical requirements of scheduling and anesthetic technique exist, depending on the type of stereotactic platform used for lead placement and whether intraoperative microelectrode recording (MER) will be used. Target selection and trajectory planning are completed preoperatively using high-resolution imaging. Standard stereotactic technique is used intraoperatively by inserting a straight, multi-contact electrode through a burr hole to the target deep in the brain. In some cases, MER and/ or test stimulation can be done in awake patients to evaluate for correct placement or unwanted side effects. The extracranial ends of the electrodes are tunneled toward the side where the generator will reside.

Responsive Neurostimulation

Cortical surface or depth electrodes (or both) can be used for RNS. For depth electrodes, electrode placement is similar to the process for DBS. Pre-operative target selection and electrode trajectory planning are critical. Targets are selected based on presumed or documented seizure foci and placement may follow phase II monitoring of a patient's seizures with depth or subdural grid electrodes. Depth electrodes, if required, are placed using the standard stereotactic technique. Cortical surface electrodes that usually are in a 4-contact 4X5 cm strip are placed after craniotomy. Intraoperative ECoG will confirm proper electrode positioning.

23.1.4 Generator Placement

Vagus Nerve Stimulation & Deep Brain Stimulation

A pocket is created in the upper chest wall, several centimeters below the clavicle. It can be subcutaneous or submuscular. Care should be taken to avoid excessive tissue depth, since it could interfere with the wireless interface between the programming device and the generator. VNS leads usually connect directly to the generator, as the working end of the electrode is nearby. DBS leads usually require extension leads. Many surgeons will create a partial-thickness channel in the parietal skull to reduce tension on the working end of the electrode, and prevent creep of the connections down into the neck.

Responsive Neurostimulation

The sensor/generator for the RNS system is placed into a customized craniotomy defect in the skull. Once the electrodes are positioned and tested, a craniotomy shaped to match the device is made on the same side of the skull, usually centered on the parietal boss. A securing-tray (or 'ferrule') is secured into the craniotomy with screws, and the device is locked into the ferrule after the electrodes are connected. The scalp is then closed over the device. This location reduces motion artifact and other sources of interference in the sensing loop of the circuit.

23.1.5 Postoperative Management

After implantation of the complete system, programming and activation of a targeted neuromodulation system is done using a wireless interface device. System diagnostics can also be completed. Stimulation current, pulse frequency and pulse width are the parameters adjusted. More sophisticated paradigms are under investigation. Initial programming can occur on the day of implantation for VNS, but DBS and RNS generally require a separate visit. The effect of stimulation seems to increase over time. Within the first 3–12 months, decreases in seizure frequency of around 30%-40% are seen with all three systems. After two or more years DBS can decrease seizure frequency by more than 50%, and the percentage of patients reporting more than 50% reduction (responder rate) over the same period can range between 54% and 67%.[6] RNS benefits also improve with time, ranging from 44% after one year to as much as 66%, with a 60% responder rate.[7]

Complications are uncommon but will occur, and are a possibility each time the generator requires replacing (usually every 3–6 years). Infection, bleeding, skin erosion and mechanical/electrical failure of the system can occur, and potentially require explantation. Hoarseness can occur with VNS, but is usually well tolerated and improves with time. DBS carries various neuropsychiatric risks depending on the target. Stimulation to the anterior nucleus of the thalamus may cause subjective worsening of memory or depression, or possible worsening of seizures.[6,15,16] RNS may be associated with an increased risk of sudden death in epilepsy (SUDEP), but this has not been demonstrated with statistical significance to-date.[7]

23.2 Conclusion

Targeted neuromodulation can be an effective treatment for patients with medically refractory epilepsy who are not candidates for resection or ablation. Vagus Nerve Stimulation (VNS), tonic or scheduled Deep Brain Stimulation (DBS) and Responsive Neurostimulation systems (RNS) are effective in reducing the seizure frequency in these patients, and can improve the quality of life for patients and their families. Selection of an appropriate system depends on many factors, including the type of epilepsy and the patient's tolerance of various diagnostic and therapeutic procedures. All modalities are well tolerated with few common side effects. VNS has a long history of use, both in partial epilepsy (for which it is FDA approved), and in other kinds of epilepsy. DBS and RNS both show promise in achieving greater reduction in seizures in long-term observational studies; however, more data is required to optimize target selection. The greater potential efficacy of the intracranial therapies is balanced by a more significant surgical risk and the increased preparation, hospital time, operative time, and possibly stress on the patient. Further study of DBS and RNS is needed to identify risks of neuropsychiatric complications, and whether changes in rates of SUDEP are true risks.

References

[1] Thomas GP, Jobst BC. Critical review of the responsive neurostimulator system for epilepsy. Med Devices (Auckl). 2015; 8:405–411

[2] Schachter SC, Saper CB. Vagus nerve stimulation. Epilepsia. 1998; 39(7):677–686

[3] Panebianco M, Rigby A, Weston J, Marson AG. Vagus nerve stimulation for partial seizures. Cochrane Database Syst Rev. 2015(4):CD002896

[4] Kwan P, Brodie MJ. Early identification of refractory epilepsy. N Engl J Med. 2000; 342(5):314–319

[5] Rolston JD, Englot DJ, Wang DD, Shih T, Chang EF. Comparison of seizure control outcomes and the safety of vagus nerve, thalamic deep brain, and responsive neurostimulation: evidence from randomized controlled trials. Neurosurg Focus. 2012; 32(3):E14

[6] Fisher R, Salanova V, Witt T, et al. SANTE Study Group. Electrical stimulation of the anterior nucleus of thalamus for treatment of refractory epilepsy. Epilepsia. 2010; 51(5):899–908

[7] Bergey GK, Morrell MJ, Mizrahi EM, et al. Long-term treatment with responsive brain stimulation in adults with refractory partial seizures. Neurology. 2015; 84(8):810–817

[8] Sprengers M, Vonck K, Carrette E, Marson AG, Boon P. Deep brain and cortical stimulation for epilepsy. Cochrane Database Syst Rev. 2014(6): CD008497

[9] Fridley J, Thomas JG, Navarro JC, Yoshor D. Brain stimulation for the treatment of epilepsy. Neurosurg Focus. 2012; 32(3):E13

[10] Lega BC, Halpern CH, Jaggi JL, Baltuch GH. Deep brain stimulation in the treatment of refractory epilepsy: update on current data and future directions. Neurobiol Dis. 2010; 38(3):354–360

[11] Velasco AL, Velasco F, Jiménez F, et al. Neuromodulation of the centromedian thalamic nuclei in the treatment of generalized seizures and the improvement of the quality of life in patients with Lennox-Gastaut syndrome. Epilepsia. 2006; 47(7):1203–1212

[12] Salinsky MC, Uthman BM, Ristanovic RK, Wernicke JF, Tarver WB, Vagus Nerve Stimulation Study Group. Vagus nerve stimulation for the treatment of medically intractable seizures. Results of a 1-year open-extension trial. Arch Neurol. 1996; 53(11):1176–1180

[13] Handforth A, DeGiorgio CM, Schachter SC, et al. Vagus nerve stimulation therapy for partial-onset seizures: a randomized active-control trial. Neurology. 1998; 51(1):48–55

[14] Morrell MJ, MD on behalf of the RNS System in Epilepsy Study Group. Responsive cortical stimulation for the treatment of medically intractable partial epilepsy. Neurology. 2011; 77(13):1295–1304

[15] Salanova V, Witt T, Worth R, et al. SANTE Study Group. Long-term efficacy and safety of thalamic stimulation for drug-resistant partial epilepsy. Neurology. 2015; 84(10):1017–1025

[16] Loring DW, Kapur R, Meador KJ, Morrell MJ. Differential neuropsychological outcomes following targeted responsive neurostimulation for partial-onset epilepsy. Epilepsia. 2015; 56(11):1836–1844

24 Laser Interstitial Thermal Therapy for Epilepsy

Dario J. Englot, Hamid M. Shah and Peter E. Konrad

Abstract

Laser interstitial thermal therapy (LITT) guided by magnetic resonance imaging (MRI) is a minimally invasive treatment option to ablate epileptogenic tissue or focal lesions in drug-resistant epilepsy patients. LITT induces less tissue injury and reduces perioperative pain and length of hospital stay when compared to open surgery. Laser energy is delivered using a long, flexible optical fiber stereotactically placed into the parenchymal region or lesion. Once MRI verifies the probe position, ablation induces thermal coagulation and tissue destruction at the probe tip. Injury extent can then be tracked using MRI thermography. Thermal ablation of the amygdalohippocampal complex in mesial temporal lobe epilepsy (MTLE) is the most common use of LITT in epilepsy patients. Published studies suggest seizure free rates of approximately 50% after LITT for MTLE, which is less favorable than open resection. Some authors have noted improved outcomes in certain neuropsychological parameters after LITT compared to resection in MTLE, although these results are preliminary. Other potential uses of LITT in epilepsy surgery include the ablation of an epileptogenic tumor, tuber, cavernoma, focal cortical dysplasic lesion or hypothalamic hamartoma. It can also be used to complete a corpus callosotomy. Long-term seizure and neuropsychological outcomes must be investigated in future prospective studies, and a better understanding of complication rates and strategies for avoidance is needed. In the future, LITT is likely to be a prominent procedure for the treatment of drug-resistant epilepsy.

Keywords: ablation, epilepsy, laser, MRI-guided, stereotactic

24.1 Overview and Technique

With the introduction of new technology, the surgical treatment of epilepsy continues to evolve. Laser interstitial thermal therapy (LITT) guided by magnetic resonance imaging (MRI) is a minimally invasive treatment for stereotactic ablation of epileptogenic tissue or focal lesions. It has the advantages of producing less tissue damage, reduced perioperative pain and a shorter hospital stay when compared to open surgery. It has a high level of precision, and provides for real-time imaging feedback.

In LITT, laser energy is delivered using a long, flexible optical fiber stereotactically placed into the parenchymal region or lesion intended for ablation. Several software solutions already available to functional neurosurgeons for planning stereotactic procedures may also be used to plan targets and trajectories for LITT. A stab incision in the skin and small burr hole are required at the entry site, and an anchor bolt is used to fix the laser probe. Precise probe placement is essential and can be achieved with a traditional stereotactic frame, a patient-specific 3D-printed platform and an adjustable navigated micropositioner system, or using frameless stereotaxy with neuronavigation. MRI-guided surgical platforms are also available with which a

probe is inserted while the patient is inside the MRI scanner. This gives near immediate confirmation of placement accuracy.

Once MRI verifies probe position, laser energy creates thermal coagulation of tissue at the probe tip. Serial ablations may be done after partial withdrawal of the laser probe. During the ablation, MRI thermography imaging using the water proton resonance frequency shift is done to monitor tissue temperature.[1] A recent FDA letter sent to physicians however has warned that magnetic resonance thermometry may be inaccurate in certain conditions and lead to overheating.[2] A cooling cannula controls thermal spread within tissue and protects the probe tip from damage caused by overheating. If a pre selected temperature threshold is reached adjacent to critical structures, ablation can be aborted.[3] The FDA recommends setting the low temperature targets on nearby critical structures to 43 degrees Celsius or less. After probe removal, the incision can be closed with a single stitch. Hospital discharge the next morning is feasible.

24.2 Treatment of Mesial Temporal Lobe Epilepsy

Thermal ablation of the amygdalohippocampal complex in mesial temporal lobe epilepsy (MTLE) is the most common use of LITT for epilepsy treatment. The hippocampus is approached from an occipital or posterolateral trajectory. By reaching it along its longitudinal axis a large portion of the structure can be engaged while the medial basal cisterns and the inferior horn of the lateral ventricle lateral to the target create a "heat sink" to avert thermal injury to nearby structures and vessels.[4] Example MRI images from a LITT case for MTLE are depicted in ▶ Fig. 24.1.

In one early series, Willie and others described 13 adult patients who underwent LITT for MTLE with or without mesial temporal sclerosis.[6] The investigators observed a 60% mean ablation volume for the amygdalohippocampal complex with a median length of stay of one day. After a median of 14 months follow-up, 54% of patients were seizure free, including 67% (6 of 9) of individuals with mesial temporal sclerosis. All seizure recurrences occurred within the first six months. Neither the ablation volume nor length correlated with the clinical outcome. There was one adverse event. An aberrant insertion of a stereotactic aligning rod caused a visual defect. The probe trajectory was corrected before ablation. A follow-up investigation using a prospective, non-randomized, parallel-group designed protocol compared neuropsychological outcome in 19 patients undergoing LITT for MTLE with 39 patients who underwent standard resection.[7] Naming in patients with dominant hemisphere MTLE with LITT was improved compared to open surgical resection. There was better object recognition in individuals with MTLE of the non-dominant hemisphere. Overall, no patient had a decline in object recognition and naming tasks after LITT.

Another group evaluated LITT outcomes in 20 MTLE patients and measured ablation volumes.[8] After six months 53% of 15

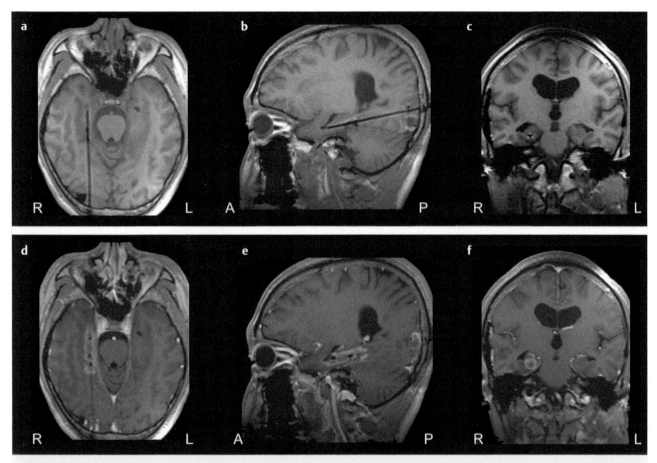

Fig. 24.1 Laser interstitial thermal therapy (LITT) for mesial temporal lobe epilepsy. (A-C) Shown are T1-weighted MRI axial **(a)**, sagittal **(b)**, and coronal **(c)** images showing during laser probe placement along the axis of the left hippocampus, prior to SLA in a patient with mesial temporal lobe epilepsy. **(d-f)** Contrast-enhanced T1-weighted MRI axial **(ad)**, sagittal **(be)**, and coronal **(fc)** images obtained approximately 5–10 minutes after thermal ablation of mesial temporal lobe structures, with contrast enhancement seen in the region of ablation. Lesioning is performed with real-time MRI thermal measurements. A: anterior; L: left; P: posterior; R: right. Adapted with permission from Englot et al., 2016.[5]

patients were seizure free; 36% of 11 patients were free after one year, and 60% of 5 individuals were free after two years (median follow-up was 13 months). No differences were found in the ablated volumes of the hippocampus, amygdala, parahippocampal gyrus, entorhinal cortex, or fusiform gyrus in patients with favorable versus unfavorable seizure outcomes. Contextual verbal memory performance was preserved, although declines in non-contextual memory task scores occurred, and no major complications were observed. Finally, a recent review of all published LITT series for MTLE estimated an overall seizure free rate of 53% (follow-up range 6 to 39 months). Morbidity was reported in 16% of 74 procedures on 68 patients.[9] Adverse events included visual field deficits (6), cranial nerve III or IV injury (2), and intracranial hemorrhage (3). There were no deaths.

Overall, published results to date suggest favorable seizure outcomes after LITT for MTLE, although seizure free rates remain below those published for open resection with either anterior temporal lobectomy or selective amygdalohippocampectomy.[10] Advantages of LITT over resection for MTLE are: the minimally invasive nature of the procedure, and potentially improved neuropsychological outcomes, although the latter will require further study in larger cohorts.

24.3 Treatment of Other Epilepsy Syndromes

LITT has been used for ablation of other epileptogenic lesions in both children and adults. In one series of 19 pediatric patients undergoing LITT for intractable epilepsy, seizure freedom was reported in 41% of individuals after a mean follow-up of 16 months (range 4–36).[11] Nearly all of these individuals suffered from focal neocortical epilepsy, with 11 patients harboring focal cortical dysplasia. Four patients with tuberous sclerosis complex underwent ablation of epileptogenic tubers. Ten patients in the series had failed a previous resection, suggesting a potential role for LITT in repeat epilepsy surgery. Seizure outcome after LITT for focal neocortical epilepsy is inferior to that in MTLI similar to results with resection,

Another small series reported the use of LITT to treat cavernous malformations associated with medically-refractory epilepsy in 5 patients, achieving seizure freedom in 4 (80%) individuals 12 to 28 months after treatment.[12] In addition, some practitioners have successfully used LITT to ablate hypothalamic harmartomas associated with epilepsy. Hamartomas are a challenge to safely access with open surgery.[13] LITT has

Table 24.1 Selected potential indications for LITT in focal epilepsy treatment

Amygdalohippocampectomy	Insular epilepsy
Cavernous malformation	Hypothalamic hamartoma
Completion corpus callosotomy	Periventricular lesions
Epileptogenic tumor	Residual lesion after resection/ablation
Focal cortical dysplasia	Tuberous sclerosis complex

also been used to ablate other deep seated lesions, including subependymal giant cell astrocytoma, ganglioglioma, pleomorphic xanthoastrocytoma, and optic glioma.[14] Finally, LITT is used to complete minimally-invasive anterior corpus callosotomy.[15] Overall, these studies suggest that LITT may offer a minimally invasive alternative to craniotomy in individuals with extra-temporal epilepsy who harbor a discrete radiographic lesion. However, given the small size of studies reported to date, these results remain quite preliminary.

24.4 Conclusions and Future Directions

LITT is a new and important treatment option for the surgical treatment of epilepsy. It has the advantages of reduced perioperative pain and a shorter hospital stay compared to craniotomy for resection. Planning and probe placement can be done using a variety of techniques, and MRI thermography offers a unique opportunity to track ablation in real-time while protecting critical structures. The accumulated data regarding the results of amygdalohippocampal ablation is becoming robust, and suggests favorable seizure outcomes. Seizure free rates however are lower than is obtained with lesion resection. Early reports suggesting better neurocognitive outcomes with LITT in MTLE surgery are encouraging, but preliminary, and larger prospective cohorts are needed. Fewer studies have examined LITT for extra-temporal epileptogenic lesions, but the technology is well positioned for the treatment of deep, well-circumscribed, radiographically apparent lesions, particularly those that may be challenging to access with open surgery. When tissue diagnosis is required, stereotactic biopsy can often be performed immediately preceding laser probe placement, during the same procedure. ▶ Table 24.1 summarizes the potential uses for LITT in surgical epilepsy treatment.

Patients less well suited for LITT include those with a large or complex epileptogenic zone that requires extensive or tailored resection, and individuals with non-lesional epilepsy in whom invasive electrographic recordings may be beneficial. Long-term seizure and neuropsychological outcomes will be required in future prospective studies, and a better understanding of complication rates and strategies for avoidance is needed. Furthermore, the role of resection versus LITT in patients with residual epileptogenic lesion after prior surgical treatment requires further investigation. Going forward, it is apparent that LITT and other minimally-invasive surgical technologies will serve a prominent role in the treatment of drug-resistant epilepsy.

References

[1] Patel NV, Mian M, Stafford RJ, et al. Laser Interstitial Thermal Therapy Technology, Physics of Magnetic Resonance Imaging Thermometry, and Technical Considerations for Proper Catheter Placement During Magnetic Resonance Imaging-Guided Laser Interstitial Thermal Therapy. Neurosurgery. 2016; 79 Suppl 1:S8–S16

[2] Maisel W. Magnetic Resonance-guided laser Interstitital Thermal Therapy (MRgLITT) Devices: Letter to Health Care Providers-Risk of Tissue Overheating Due to Inaccurate magnetic Resonance Thermometry. In: Health CfDaR, ed. Silver Spring, MD: CDRH Division of Industry Communication and Education; 2018

[3] Sun XR, Patel NV, Danish SF. Tissue Ablation Dynamics During Magnetic Resonance-Guided, Laser-Induced Thermal Therapy. Neurosurgery. 2015; 77(1): 51–58, discussion 58

[4] Wu C, Boorman DW, Gorniak RJ, Farrell CJ, Evans JJ, Sharan AD. The effects of anatomic variations on stereotactic laser amygdalohippocampectomy and a proposed protocol for trajectory planning. Neurosurgery. 2015; 11 Suppl 2: 345–356, discussion 356–357

[5] Englot DJ, Birk H, Chang EF. Seizure outcomes in nonresective epilepsy surgery: an update. Neurosurg Rev. 2016

[6] Willie JT, Laxpati NG, Drane DL, et al. Real-time magnetic resonance-guided stereotactic laser amygdalohippocampotomy for mesial temporal lobe epilepsy. Neurosurgery. 2014; 74(6):569–584, discussion 584–585

[7] Drane DL, Loring DW, Voets NL, et al. Better object recognition and naming outcome with MRI-guided stereotactic laser amygdalohippocampotomy for temporal lobe epilepsy. Epilepsia. 2015; 56(1):101–113

[8] Kang JY, Wu C, Tracy J, et al. Laser interstitial thermal therapy for medically intractable mesial temporal lobe epilepsy. Epilepsia. 2016; 57(2): 325–334

[9] Waseem H, Vivas AC, Vale FL. MRI-guided laser interstitial thermal therapy for treatment of medically refractory non-lesional mesial temporal lobe epilepsy: Outcomes, complications, and current limitations: A review. J Clin Neurosci. 2016

[10] Englot DJ, Chang EF. Rates and predictors of seizure freedom in resective epilepsy surgery: an update. Neurosurg Rev. 2014; 37(3):389–404, discussion 404–405

[11] Lewis EC, Weil AG, Duchowny M, Bhatia S, Ragheb J, Miller I. MR-guided laser interstitial thermal therapy for pediatric drug-resistant lesional epilepsy. Epilepsia. 2015; 56(10):1590–1598

[12] McCracken DJ, Willie JT, Fernald BA, et al. Magnetic Resonance Thermometry-Guided Stereotactic Laser Ablation of Cavernous Malformations in Drug-Resistant Epilepsy: Imaging and Clinical Results. Oper Neurosurg (Hagerstown). 2016; 12(1):39–48

[13] Wilfong AA, Curry DJ. Hypothalamic hamartomas: optimal approach to clinical evaluation and diagnosis. Epilepsia. 2013; 54 Suppl 9:109–114

[14] Buckley R, Estronza-Ojeda S, Ojemann JG. Laser Ablation in Pediatric Epilepsy. Neurosurg Clin N Am. 2016; 27(1):69–78

[15] Ho AL, Miller KJ, Cartmell S, Inoyama K, Fisher RS, Halpern CH. Stereotactic laser ablation of the splenium for intractable epilepsy. Epilepsy Behav Case Rep. 2016; 5:23–26

25 Vagus Nerve Stimulation for Epilepsy

Ryan B. Kochanski and Sepehr Sani

Abstract

Vagus nerve stimulation (VNS) is a well-established treatment option for patients suffering from partial and generalized epilepsy. Although it is rarely curative, it is still an effective palliative treatment option aimed at reducing seizures and antiepileptic medications in a select group of patients. In this chapter, key considerations prior to the operation along with the surgical technique and postoperative management are discussed in detail.

Keywords: vagal nerve, stimulation, epilepsy, neuromodulation, seizures

25.1 Patient Selection

The concept of VNS originated in the work of Zabara in 1992. He found that repetitive vagal stimulation stopped chemically induced seizures in dogs. Ensuing studies led, in 1997, to approval by the United States Federal Drug Agency for the treatment of medically refractory partial seizures in adults and adolescents over 12 years of age by VNS. There is Class I evidence for the safety and effectiveness of VNS therapy for epilepsy, but VNS is considered a palliative adjunct to pharmacotherapy with only rare instances of complete seizure remission. It is generally reserved for pharmacoresistant patients with partial or secondarily generalized epilepsy who are poor candidates for resection. These patients lack a localizable focus, have bilateral foci, or foci in eloquent cortex. VNS can significantly reduce medication needs. There have been several randomized controlled trials of high frequency VNS stimulation that showed statistically significant reductions in seizure frequency in 20–30% patients and at least a 50% decrease in seizure frequency in 31% of patients with either complex partial or secondarily generalized seizures. Because VNS is an extracranial procedure, it has a side effect profile that is safer than, for example, than corpus callostomy for disabling drop attack seizures. VNS can improve the quality of life by reducing anti epileptic drug burden and seizure frequency.

25.2 Preoperative Preparation

Pre-operative assessment for patients with medication refractory epilepsy includes inpatient video EEG monitoring, neuropsychological testing, and structural and functional neuroimaging including brain MRI and subtraction ictal SPECT co-registered to MRI. A multidisciplinary review of these results should eliminate candidacy for seizure focus resection.

Candidates must have an intact and functional vagus nerve. The nerve on the left side is the preferred site of treatment. Animal studies show that the right vagus nerve preferentially innervates the sinoatrial node of the heart. Stimulation of this side can produce bradycardia or even asystole; however, there are clinical reports of safe implantation and stimulation of the right vagus nerve. Pre-existing recurrent laryngeal nerve injury on the side opposite to the planned left side implant may preclude implantation. Patients who have had previous neck surgery or recurrent laryngeal nerve injury should have their vocal cord function evaluated preoperatively by video laryngoscopy.

25.3 Operative Procedure

The surgery is done under general endotracheal anesthesia with the head positioned in neutral position with slight extension. The head of the operating table is elevated by 15 degrees to facilitate venous return. The midline of the thyroid cartilage and the medial border of the middle portion of the sternocleidomastoid (SCM) are marked. A horizontal skin incision is made from the midline to the medial border of SCM at the level of the thyroid cartilage within a skin crease. The platysma muscle is divided and the medial border of the SCM is identified. The plane of fascia at the medial border of the SCM and lateral border of the pharyngeal strap muscles is bluntly dissected until the carotid sheath is visible. The omohyoid muscle can be divided if necessary and re-approximated at closure.

The carotid sheath is opened and a plane is developed between the more medial common carotid artery and lateral internal jugular vein. The vagus nerve is found within this plane, either medial or deep to the internal jugular vein. A 3–4 cm segment of nerve is mobilized with sharp dissection and by removing all fibrous adhesions and a vascular loop is placed around it. The helical coils of the stimulating electrode (LivaNova, Houston, TX) are then wrapped around the nerve starting superiorly and proceeding inferiorly using two microsurgical forceps, one preferably with a curved tip. A strain loop beneath the underside of a strap muscle and the inner belly of the SCM secures the electrode wire.

The subcutaneous pocket for the generator can be created in several different locations. These include: the lateral portion of the pectoralis muscle through an axial incision; above the superior medial pectoralis major through a subclavicular incision; or intrascapular through a posterior midline incision. Lead impedance is checked before completing generator implantation. When the Aspire 106 generator (LivaNova, Houston, TX) is implanted, accurate heart rate sensing should also be confirmed. The initial programming is delayed until two weeks after implantation.

The helical coils can become adherent to the nerve. When lead removal without re-implantation is required, they can be left in situ by cutting the lead before it enters the carotid sheath. This does not prevent MRI studies from being done at a later date. Leads can fracture or malfunction and impedance rise. If revision is required, then dissection of the lead off of the nerve can be done safely. In such cases, the implanted coils can be left in place if there is enough proximal nerve exposed to facilitate placement of a new lead.

When a pulse generator is replaced, the compatibility between dual or single pin models should be checked. The Model 105 and 106 generators are not compatible with the dual pin lead, and in those instances, the Model 102 R or 104 must be implanted. The 103 Demipulse® and 104 Demipulse® Duo are advantageous due to their much smaller size than the standard 102 and 102 R models. The model 106 AspireSR® is the newest model and is equipped with heart rate sensing capability that can provide stimulation in response to rapid elevations in heart rate that may precede a seizure.

25.4 Morbidity

Patients are at risk for airway compromise from a hematoma and for laryngeal nerve injury. The most frequently cited complications are wound infections, transient vocal cord paralysis causing hoarseness, and lead fracture. In rare instances, bradycardia has been reported. Meta-analysis of multiple clinical trials has shown a 3% infection rate with only 1% of cases requiring explantation. Deep infection rates forcing device removal have been reported in 4% of children. Vocal cord paralysis, if it occurs, is transient and has been reported in only 1% of cases of adults and children. Lead malfunction leading to high impedance values thus necessitating revision occurs in 2–7% of cases and can occur from weeks to years after surgery.

25.5 Conclusion

Vagus nerve stimulation can be an effective palliative option in patients with pharmacoresistant epilepsy in whom seizure foci are surgically unresectable.

Suggested Readings

[1] Zabara J. Inhibition of experimental seizures in canines by repetitive vagal stimulation. Epilepsia. 1992; 33(6):1005–1012

[2] Fisher RS, Handforth A. Reassessment: vagus nerve stimulation for epilepsy: a report of the Therapeutics and Technology Assessment Subcommittee of the American Academy of Neurology. Neurology. 1999; 53(4):666–669

[3] Tatum WO, Johnson KD, Goff S, Ferreira JA, Vale FL. Vagus nerve stimulation and drug reduction. Neurology. 2001; 56(4):561–563

[4] Handforth A, DeGiorgio CM, Schachter SC, et al. Vagus nerve stimulation therapy for partial-onset seizures: a randomized active-control trial. Neurology. 1998; 51(1):48–55

[5] The Vagus Nerve Stimulation Study Group. A randomized controlled trial of chronic vagus nerve stimulation for treatment of medically intractable seizures. Neurology. 1995; 45(2):224–230

[6] You SJ, Kang H-C, Ko T-S, et al. Comparison of corpus callosotomy and vagus nerve stimulation in children with Lennox-Gastaut syndrome. Brain Dev. 2008; 30(3):195–199

[7] Nei M, O'Connor M, Liporace J, Sperling MR. Refractory generalized seizures: response to corpus callosotomy and vagal nerve stimulation. Epilepsia. 2006; 47(1):115–122

[8] McGregor A, Wheless J, Baumgartner J, Bettis D. Right-sided vagus nerve stimulation as a treatment for refractory epilepsy in humans. Epilepsia. 2005; 46(1):91–96

[9] Espinosa J, Aiello MT, Naritoku DK. Revision and removal of stimulating electrodes following long-term therapy with the vagus nerve stimulator. Surg Neurol. 1999; 51(6):659–664

[10] Bruce D, Li M, Fraser R, Alksne J. The Neuro-Cybernetic prosthesis (NCP) system for the treatment of refractory partial seizures: surgical technique and outcomes. Epilepsia. 1998; 39 Suppl 6:92–93

[11] Smyth MD, Tubbs RS, Bebin EM, Grabb PA, Blount JP. Complications of chronic vagus nerve stimulation for epilepsy in children. J Neurosurg. 2003; 99(3):500–503

[12] Asconapé JJ, Moore DD, Zipes DP, Hartman LM, Duffell WH, Jr. Bradycardia and asystole with the use of vagus nerve stimulation for the treatment of epilepsy: a rare complication of intraoperative device testing. Epilepsia. 1999; 40(10):1452–1454

[13] Révész D, Rydenhag B, Ben-Menachem E. Complications and safety of vagus nerve stimulation: 25 years of experience at a single center. J Neurosurg Pediatr. 2016; 18(1):97–104

26 Neuroethics Essentials in Functional Neurosurgery for Neurobehavioral Disorders

Cynthia S. Kubu

Abstract

This chapter outlines the ethical considerations in clinical research, risk benefit analyses, inclusion/exclusion, autonomy, and patient perception of benefit in functional neurosurgery for patients with neurobehavioral disorders.

Keywords: ethics, neuroethics, neurobehavioral disorders, functional neurosurgery, psychosurgery

26.1 Introduction

The brain is the neuroanatomical substrate that determines our unique selves. Surgery on this remarkable structure always has the potential to alter neurobehavioral function. Functional neurosurgery most often involves the treatment of movement disorders or epilepsy. Such patients have a variety of neurobehavioral symptoms and/or potential side effects that must be considered in the ethical analyses of risks and benefits of proceeding with surgery. There are, for example, risks of dementia and/or altered memory function. Functional procedures that target neurobehavioral symptoms present additional ethical considerations. The goals of this chapter are to outline the relevant ethical issues in functional neurosurgery for the treatment of neurobehavioral disorders.

This chapter will especially address the ethical issues surrounding the treatment of neurobehavioral disorders. Such disorders include those that directly alter cognition, mood, personality, or engender repetitive complex behavioral symptoms such as self-injurious behavior. Ethical safeguards are particularly important in this population because of the nature and severity of symptoms that may confer additional vulnerabilities. And, of course, psychosurgery has a history of abuse in the past century.

> Neurobehavioral disorders include those entities that alter cognition mood or personality, or engender repetitive complex behavioral patterns.

26.2 Due Diligence with Respect to Science

Good ethics depend on good science. All neurosurgical interventions that treat neurobehavioral disorders must be based on robust science. Such prior investigation involves the development of animal models, use of functional neuroimaging studies, and human pilot study data with reliable and valid measures.[1] Despite the long history of prior neurosurgical interventions to treat severe neurobehavioral disorders,[2] there is a paucity of data from randomized, controlled clinical trials. Such data is needed.

Furthermore, it is morally imperative to incorporate good clinical research methodologies in future applications of novel or innovative neurosurgical interventions for the treatment of neurobehavioral disorders. At a minimum, the methodology should include the use of valid and accepted measures to assess changes over time, a clearly defined protocol, and specific safety measures.[1,3,4] All investigational trials for the neurosurgical treatment of neurobehavioral disorders require the involvement of an independent Ethics Committee and/or Institutional Review Board (IRB) to provide ethical and regulatory oversight to safeguard patients.[1] Current recommended guidelines also advocate for the adoption of independent, randomized and blinded controlled trials with minimized conflicts of interest or bias.[1,5] Results from these trials should be shared with the wider scientific community, preferably in a shared registry. Finally, if there is the intention to publish the outcomes of an innovative trial or even a single case study, this constitutes IRB defined research and appropriate research guidelines should be followed. Such processes maintain transparency and provide the best protection to patients, the neurosurgical team, science, the field, and the public.

> Good ethics requires good science.

26.3 Risk/Benefit Analyses

There are few guidelines to identify patients who will benefit from a surgery for a specific neurobehavioral disorder or to identify those who are at higher risk for injury. Given this uncertainty, neurosurgical teams must proceed cautiously and rely on their knowledge of the underlying functional neuroanatomy of the disorder and surgical target(s) to identify potential neurobehavioral outcomes (both positive and negative) including changes in mood, motivation, cognition, and behavior. Assessment of risk also includes those known surgical risks as bleeding, infection, or implanted equipment failure. Given the uncertainty associated with many neurosurgical procedures for severe neurobehavioral disorders, the level of patient suffering must be high to ethically justify the surgery.

> Given the uncertainty with the functional treatment of neurobehavioral disorders, patient suffering must be high to ethically justify any surgery.

26.4 Inclusion/Exclusion Analyses

Neurobehavioral disorders are among the leading causes of disability. They entail considerable suffering for the patients and their family members.[6] Despite well-established evidence based treatments, a significant number of patients continue to suffer and do not respond to these established therapies in a sustained manner or suffer unacceptable side effects. Neurosurgery for neurobehavioral disorders should be reserved for these patients.[1,7]

The current consensus is that neurosurgery to treat neurobehavioral disorders should be limited to the treatment of adults.[7] It is possible, however, to make an ethical argument to intervene in late adolescence for specific patients to maximize the opportunity for them to form appropriate peer relationships, complete their education, and be maximally successful in their transition to adulthood.

Neurobehavioral disorders are among the most complex disorders we treat and include mood, personality, motivational, cognitive, motor, sensory, and physiological symptoms.[8] Consequently, an interdisciplinary expert neurosurgical team is essential. Such a team includes trained functional neurosurgeons, psychiatrists, neurologists, and neuropsychologists with the relevant expertise in the target disorder/procedure. Partnership with a dedicated bioethicist and ties to other mental health and rehabilitation specialists is also advisable.[1,7] Best clinical practice dictates that surgical candidacy is determined by a consensus decision involving all relevant specialists.[2] This "consensus conference" provides a forum for varied perspectives to be incorporated into the decision to offer a patient surgery and to proactively identify concerns so as to maximize benefit and minimize harm.[9]

There are a limited number of centers with the requisite expertise in neurosurgical treatment of neurobehavioral disorders. Patients may need to travel long distances for surgery and follow-up visits. There has been some discussion in the deep brain stimulation (DBS) literature on the importance of family support when determining candidacy for surgery. There is a real need for support in post-operative care and transportation to follow-up appointments.[9,10] This practical consideration may lead to concerns about justice in patient selection. To exclude patients without social support or easy access to DBS centers would "create additional disparities in the level of care of these patients, further disadvantaging them."[10] It may be the case that ablative procedures might be associated with greater risk, but still provide substantial benefit. Ablation may then be ethically justifiable when it is too burdensome for the patient to return for regular programming sessions when neuromodulatory procedures are performed.[9]

> Surgical candidacy should be a consensus decision amongst all relevant specialists.

26.5 Autonomy

Autonomy is an integral consideration in the informed consent process and includes the assurance that the patient and family have a clear understanding of all aspects of the surgery and treatment. This includes the need for long-term follow-up for patients with implanted devices.[11] There are several potential challenges to autonomy associated with neurosurgical treatment of neurobehavioral disorders. First, cognitive impairments may limit the patients' ability to provide informed consent. Second, many patients view neurosurgery as a "last resort" which can lead to a sense of desperation and increased vulnerability.[10] Not all patients, however, indicate that desperation drives their desire to consider DBS for severe depression.[12] Other challenges to autonomy are associated with media depictions of DBS or other surgical procedures that imply a "miracle cure" and can lead to inappropriate expectations.[13]

Challenges to autonomy may ensue when patients and family members disagree about pursuing surgery. Family members may push a patient toward a surgery they do not want or, dissuade a patient from surgery out of a selfish desire to maintain their caregiver role.[9,10,11,14] No patient should undergo surgery against their will, but there is not any data regarding outcome in those cases in which the patient wants to proceed with surgery and the family is opposed to it. Assessment of the family's level of support for the patient's decision to have surgery provides an opportunity to identify interpersonal dynamics that might impact care and a need for further education on surgical risks and benefits.

Finally, there has been considerable interest in the bioethics literature on the concept of autonomy when the goal of surgery is to alter behavior that may be integral to a person's identity. Although these philosophical considerations are important, from a pragmatic clinical perspective concerns regarding autonomy arise primarily from isolated case reports documenting dramatic and undesirable changes in behavior after a functional neurosurgical procedure. For example, hypomania may develop as a consequence of sub-thalamic stimulation for the treatment of Parkinson's disease. Such a behavioral change should be weighed against the large pool of data that demonstrates few changes in personality after such surgery.[15,16,17] However, for many disorders, there is insufficient available data on behavioral changes. This thorny topic requires interdisciplinary research since the implications for legal responsibility are significant.

> The concept of autonomy is an important ethical consideration when the goal of surgery is to alter behavior that may be integral to a one's identity.

26.6 Patient's Quality of Life and Perception of Benefit

Functional neurosurgery is elective surgery with the goal of improving quality of life. Life quality is a concept that is inherently individualized and value-laden. There has been considerable discussion of a "satisfaction gap" in which the patient is unhappy with the surgical outcome, but the surgeon is pleased with it.[18] It is important to inquire systematically about the patient's goals for the procedure and to clarify how a reduction in specific symptoms will improve *their* quality of life.[19] For example, a patient with Parkinson's disease may say that their primary goal is to reduce their tremor, yet they may have an unexpressed, unrealistic, underlying goal to return to a surgical practice. A clear understanding of the patient's expectations for the outcome of surgery is an essential element of the informed consent process. It minimizes the possibility of such a "satisfaction gap."

> The goal of functional neurosurgery is to improve quality of life, but this is a value-laden concept that risks a gap between surgeon and patient expectations.

26.7 Conclusion

The relevant clinical ethical considerations for the neurosurgical treatment of neurobehavioral disorders are complex and require careful consideration and deliberation. Neurosurgical teams have the privileged opportunity to ease human suffering, but they also have the responsibility to proceed in an ethical and scientific manner that maximally benefits patients, their families, and the field of medicine as a whole.

References

[1] Nuttin B, Wu H, Mayberg H, et al. Consensus on guidelines for stereotactic neurosurgery for psychiatric disorders. J Neurol Neurosurg Psychiatry. 2014; 85(9):1003–1008

[2] Mashour GA, Walker EE, Martuza RL. Psychosurgery: past, present, and future. Brain Res Brain Res Rev. 2005; 48(3):409–419

[3] Kubu CS, Ford PJ. Beyond mere symptom relief in deep brain stimulation: An ethical obligation for multi-faceted assessment of outcome. AJOB Neurosci. 2012; 3(1):44–49

[4] Bell E, Leger P, Sankar T, Racine E. Deep brain stimulation as clinical innovation: An ethical and organizational framework to sustain deliberations about psychiatric deep brain stimulation. Neurosurgery. 2016; 79(1):3–10

[5] Fins JJ, Schlaepfer TE, Nuttin B, et al. Ethical guidance for the management of conflicts of interest for researchers, engineers and clinicians engaged in the development of therapeutic deep brain stimulation. J Neural Eng. 2011; 8(3): 033001

[6] NIMH. U.S. Leading categories of diseases/disorders. Retrieved June 4, 2017 from: https://www.nimh.nih.gov/health/statistics/disability/us-leading-categories-of-diseases-disorders.shtml

[7] Rabins P, Appleby BS, Brandt J, et al. Scientific and ethical issues related to deep brain stimulation for disorders of mood, behavior, and thought. Arch Gen Psychiatry. 2009; 66(9):931–937

[8] Heimer L, Van Hoesen GW. The limbic lobe and its output channels: implications for emotional functions and adaptive behavior. Neurosci Biobehav Rev. 2006; 30(2):126–147

[9] Kubu CS, Ford PJ. Clinical ethics in deep brain stimulation for movement disorders Submitted

[10] Bell E, Mathieu G, Racine E. Preparing the ethical future of deep brain stimulation. Surg Neurol. 2009; 72(6):577–586, discussion 586

[11] Clausen J. Ethical brain stimulation - neuroethics of deep brain stimulation in research and clinical practice. Eur J Neurosci. 2010; 32(7):1152–1162

[12] Christopher PP, Leykin Y, Appelbaum PS, Holtzheimer PE , III, Mayberg HS, Dunn LB. Enrolling in deep brain stimulation research for depression: influences on potential subjects' decision making. Depress Anxiety. 2012; 29(2): 139–146

[13] Racine E, Waldman S, Palmour N, Risse D, Illes J. "Currents of hope": neurostimulation techniques in U.S. and U.K. print media. Camb Q Healthc Ethics. 2007; 16(3):312–316

[14] Ford PJ, Henderson JM. Functional neurosurgical intervention: neuroethics in the operating room. In: Illes J, ed. Neuroethics: Defining the Issues in Theory, Practice, and Policy. Oxford: Oxford University Press; 2006:213–228

[15] Leentjens AF, Visser-Vandewalle V, Temel Y, Verhey FR. [Manipulation of mental competence: an ethical problem in case of electrical stimulation of the subthalamic nucleus for severe Parkinson's disease]. Ned Tijdschr Geneeskd. 2004; 148(28):1394–1398

[16] Mandat TS, Hurwitz T, Honey CR. Hypomania as an adverse effect of subthalamic nucleus stimulation: report of two cases. Acta Neurochir (Wien). 2006; 148(8):895–897, discussion 898

[17] Funkiewiez A, Ardouin C, Caputo E, et al. Long term effects of bilateral subthalamic nucleus stimulation on cognitive function, mood, and behaviour in Parkinson's disease. J Neurol Neurosurg Psychiatry. 2004; 75(6): 834–839

[18] Agid Y, Schüpbach M, Gargiulo M, et al. Neurosurgery in Parkinson's disease: the doctor is happy, the patient less so? J Neural Transm Suppl. 2006; 70(70): 409–414

[19] Kubu CS, Cooper SE, Machado A, Frazier T, Vitek J, Ford PJ. Insights gleaned by measuring patients' stated goals for DBS: More than tremor. Neurology. 2017; 88(2):124–130

27 Depression

Gaddum Duemani Reddy, Nir Lipsman and Clement Hamani

Abstract

Depression is a prevalent condition that may be very disabling. While medications and psychotherapy are often effective, approximately 30% of patients do not respond to conventional treatments. These patients may be managed with combinations of medications, augmentation regimens and sometimes electroconvulsive therapy. It is estimated that 10% of patients will not be responsive and comprise a population of treatment refractory depression. Ablative procedures and more recently vagus nerve stimulation, motor cortex stimulation and deep brain stimulation (DBS) have been proposed as therapies for this population. Several DBS targets have been investigated. Overall, results of initial open label reports have not been corroborated by blinded randomized clinical trials. In this chapter we discuss surgical therapies for treatment refractory depression.

Keywords: depression, deep brain stimulation, vagus nerve stimulation, cingulate gyrus, internal capsule

27.1 Introduction

Depression is a common condition with a one-year prevalence in the United State of 5-10%. A third of patients do not respond to combinations of medical and psychotherapy, and even electroconvulsive therapy is ineffective 30% of the time. Ablative neurosurgical procedures have been used for decades to treat depression. More recently, neuromodulatory therapies have been introduced. This chapter will discuss the most common neurosurgical procedures used to treat depression, their indications, outcome and morbidity.

27.2 Ablative Procedures

27.2.1 Anterior Cingulotomy

In anterior cingulotomy a lesion is made in a region corresponding to Brodmann Area 24 and a portion of the anterior cingulate gyrus. Anterior cingulotomy is useful both in obsessive-compulsive disorder and depression. Clinical outcomes may correlate more with anterior lesion position than with lesion volume and microelectrode recordings can be helpful to identify the dorsal and ventral regions of the gyrus. In a prospective review of thirty-three patients with refractory depression treated by cingulotomy, seventeen patients needed no further treatment. A third of these had at least a 50% reduction in the Beck Depression Inventory and another 42% had reductions of between 35% and 50%.

27.2.2 Subcaudate Tractotomy

In subcaudate tractotomy a lesion is made in the tracts below the caudate nucleus, in the region of the substania innominata. The operation was initially done by craniotomy but the procedure is now done stereotactically and the lesion made using thermocoagulation. In more than a thousand cases performed since 1961, the estimated overall undefined success rate was 40–60%. A 1995 prospective study of 23 patients with either major depression or bipolar affective disorder treated by tractotomy showed lowered Hamilton Rating Scale for Depression Scores (HAMD) at six months that correlated with improved global outcome as measured by multiple scales. Most reports describing this technique are over a decade old, but in a 2017 case report, gamma knife radiofrequency ablation reduced HAM-D scores from twenty-three to four, an improvement that was sustained for 2 years.

27.2.3 Limbic Leucotomy

The combination of anterior cingulotomy and subcaudate tractotomy is known as limbic leucotomy. In a 2002 study of twenty-one patients who had leucotomy for either obsessive-compulsive disorder or major depressive disorder, there was benefit in approximately half of all patients with a few adverse events observed over the two-year evaluation period. In a study of 16 patients who had undergone radiofrequency limbic leucotomy for major depressive disorder over 7 years, depression scores, as measured by the HAM-D or BDI, declined by about 50%.

27.2.4 Anterior Capsulotomy

In anterior capsulotomy, the anterior limb of the internal capsule is lesioned. While primarily described for the treatment of obsessive-compulsive disorder or anxiety disorders, there have been a few reports on the use of anterior capsulotomy for the treatment of depression. In a 2011 study, twenty patients treated with anterior capsulotomy were evaluated for a mean of seven years. Half of the patients had at least a 50% reduction in HAM-D scores.

27.3 Deep Brain Stimulation

27.3.1 Subcallosal Cingulate

The subcallosal cingulate (SCG) region was the first identified potential target for deep brain stimulation of medically refractory depression. Patients who responded to antidepressant medications also had increased anterior cingulate gyral glucose metabolism. Those who did not respond had an inverse metabolic pattern. PET studies identified the subcallosal cingulate region (including Broadmann 25) as hypermetabolic in normal subjects in a transient sad state as well as in treatment responsive depression patients. A similar decrease in metabolism within this region was found following electroconvulsive therapy. In depressed patients that benefitted from anterior cingulotomy, improvement in BDI correlated with pre-operative level of metabolism in this subcallosal cingulate region. Treatment with the selective serotonin reuptake inhibitor paroxetine was associated with a decrease in subcallosal hypermetabolism in treatment responsive depression patients, a finding that was not present in patients who were responsive to cognitive brain therapy.

Some of this work spurred the use of SCG as a DBS target. In 2005, six patients with treatment resistant depression underwent a six-month trial of chronic stimulation with electrodes implanted in the SCG. In these subjects, presurgical PET imaging revealed a pattern characterized by elevated blood flow in the subgenual region and reduced flow in the dorsolateral prefrontal cortex. Four of six (66%) patients responded to treatment (≥ 50% reduction in HAM-D scores compared to baseline). Postoperative PET imaging studies at 3 and 6 months in treatment responders also showed a reversal in the pattern of blood flow observed in the preoperative period.

Several ensuing case reports demonstrated benefit. A 2008 case report described a long-term benefit in a patient with medically refractory depression who had been previously treated with radiofrequency cingulotomy. A clinical benefit in a 2010 study following right-sided SCG DBS, prompted the study of asymmetrical effects of right versus left hemispheric stimulation. Lozano, Kennedy and colleagues published long-term follow up data on 20 patients implanted with SCG DBS electrodes. Improvement at 1–3 years ranged from 45–75%. Holtzheimer et al., reported their results on 7 patients with bipolar II disorder and 10 patients with major depressive disorder showing a trend towards an increase in stimulation efficacy over time, with 36% remission and 36% response rate at 1 year and up to a 58% remission rate and a 92% response rate after 2 years. Lozano et al., also published initial results of a three center prospective open-label trial, with a 57% response rate (> 50% decrease in HAM-D scores) at 1 month, a 48% at 6 months and a 29% at a year. When responders were defined as patients having > 40% reduction in HAM-D, response rate at one year increased to 62%.

With the success of these initial studies, a multicenter randomized control trial was initiated to study Broadman area DBS. It was discontinued after a futility analysis predicated the probability of success being no greater than 17.2%. Despite these findings, several groups have been conducting clinical trials to improve the therapy. Newly proposed strategies include characterizing predictors of response to SCG DBS, refining surgical targeting and clarification of surgical candidacy. Electrode locations in patients who did or did not respond to surgery are fairly similar. In a recent study, however, diffusion tensor imaging (DTI) and the volume of tissue activated by stimulation revealed that DBS responders shared bilateral pathways from their activation volumes to the medial frontal cortex, rostral and dorsal cingulate cortex via the cingulum bundle, and subcortical nuclei (▶ Fig. 27.1). In a 2015 trial, 8 patients were implanted with SCG electrodes. Five responders were randomized to undergo a double-blinded active vs. sham stimulation study. In these subjects, active stimulation was shown to be more efficacious than sham, suggesting that in candidates who respond to the therapy DBS may indeed be exerting a beneficial effect.

27.3.2 Ventral Capsule/Ventral Striatum

The ventral anterior limb of the internal capsule and the associated ventral striatum (VC/VS) was the first approved target of deep brain stimulation for a psychiatric illness—obsessive-compulsive disorder—by the U.S. Food and Drug administration. In studies that contained the cumulative experience of different centers, the average decrease in the Yale-Brown Obsessive Compulsive Scores at three years was approximately 40%. In some of the patients reported in the literature, DBS induced an associated decrease in the HAM-D Score of 43.2%, suggesting a

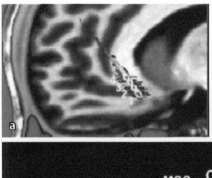
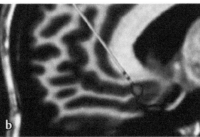
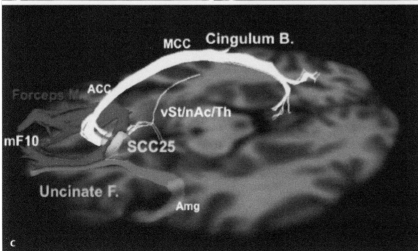

Fig. 27.1 Subgenual cingulum. **(a)** Postsurgical computed tomography image superimposed on the presurgical T1 image in a patient treated with SCG DBS. Contacts are numbered inferior to superior, 1 to 4. **(b)** Activation volume using contact 1 and typical parameters for a sample subject. **(C)** Optimal SCG DBS fiber bundle target template. Red: forceps minor. Blue: uncinate fasciculus. Yellow: cingulate bundle. ACC, anterior cingulate cortex; Amg, amygdala; Cingulum B., cingulum bundle; Forceps M., forceps minor; MCC, middle cingulate cortex; mF10, medial frontal (Brodmann area 10); nAc, nucleus accumbens; SCC25, subcallosal cingulate cortex (Brodmann area 25); Th, thalamus; Uncinate F., uncinate fasciculus; vSt, ventral striatum. *Adapted and reprinted from Riva-Posse et al. with permission from Elsevier.*

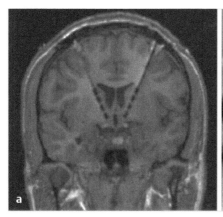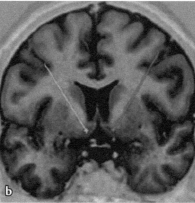

Fig. 27.2 Ventral capsule/ Ventral Striatum (VC/VS) and nucleus accumbens. **(a)** Magnetic resonance images from a representative patient showing postoperative deep brain stimulation (DBS) lead position. **(b)** Location of nucleus accumbens in a coronal plane with projections of the left and right electrode path in the surgical planning stage. *Reprinted from Malone et al with permission from Elsevier and Schlaepfer et al by permission from Macmillan Publishers.*

concomitant improvement in comorbid depression. This prompted an open label trial of VC/VS DBS in which fifteen patients with severe chronic medically refractory depression underwent bilateral chronic implantation (▶ Fig. 27.2). This trial showed an initial response rate of 40% at 6 months and 53.3% at the last follow up. The remission rate, characterized by a reduction in the HAM-D to below 10, was in the range of 20% at 6 months and 40% at the last follow up.

The success of these initial trials led to a randomized prospective multi-center sham-controlled study that was published in 2015. Thirty patients with treatment resistant depression underwent a 16-week blinded active versus sham stimulation course. For the stimulation group, optimal settings were determined prior to the stimulation phase. Results of this portion of the trial were negative, with 3 out of 15 patients (20%) in the stimulation group responding to treatment, versus 2 out of 14 (14.3%) in the control group. The study then preceded to an open label extension phase, during which response rates at 12, 18 and 24 months were found to be 20%, 26.7% and 23.3%, respectively.

In contrast, a recently published sham-controlled randomized control trial of 25 patients with medically resistant depression did show a benefit of active over sham stimulation. This study used a longer optimization phase of up to 52 weeks, after which 16 patients (9 responders and 7 non-responders) participated in a randomized crossover phase. Stimulation in this setting resulted in a significant difference in HAM-D scores between sham and stimulation arms in patients who responded to treatment.

27.3.3 Nucleus Accumbens

In 2008, Schlaepfer and colleagues published their initial results on three patients with medically resistant depression implanted with bilateral DBS electrodes in the nucleus accumbens. This target has overlap with the VC/VS, with dorsal electrodes located in the region of the ventral capsule (Fig. 27.2). One of the implanted sites is located within the ventral capsule. The nucleus accumbens has a role in reward processing and as a gateway between emotional and motor brain centers. The results of this initial study showed a drop in the average HAM-D score from 33.7 at baseline to 19.7 after 1 week of stimulation and a return to 29.3 after 1 week of discontinuation. PET

imaging showed increased activation in the ventral striatum, the dorsolateral and dorsomedial prefrontal cortex, the cingulate cortex and the bilateral amygdala. In a study published in 2010, ten patients were implanted of which half had a positive response at 12 months. Long-term studies showed a durable effect of DBS in these patients with no substantial relapses over four years.

27.3.4 Medial Forebrain Bundle

The medial forebrain bundle (MFB) is the connection pathway for several prominent structures in the "reward" pathway, including the nucleus accumbens, the ventral tegmental area of the midbrain, the ventromedial and lateral nuclei of the hypothalamus, and the amygdala. Schlaepfer et al., targeted the supero-lateral branch of the MFB in seven patients with refractory depression (▶ Fig. 27.3). Six of these individuals had prominent acute responses, characterized by a 50% reduction in Montgomery-Asberg Depression Rating Scale (MADRS) scores. In addition to short-term results, positive outcomes were registered at the last clinical follow up, up to four years after surgery.

In an interim analysis of an ongoing pilot study conducted by different investigators, the efficacy of MFB-DBS was assessed in four TRD patients over a 52-week period. Study design included a four-week single-blinded sham stimulation period prior to stimulation initiation. While there were no significant mean changes in mood during the sham stimulation phase, 75% of patients had > 50% decrease in MADRS scores at 7 days post-stimulation initiation relative to baseline. At 26 weeks, two patients had a > 80% decrease in MADRS scores, whereas one patient did not respond to DBS. In contrast to responders, this subject had reduced connectivity between the targeted region and the frontal cortex.

27.3.5 Inferior Thalamic Peduncle (ITP)

Velasco et al., initially suggested the ITP as a potential target for stimulation to treat depression in 2005. They successfully treated one patient with major depressive disorder using bilateral ITP DBS. In 2007, the same group published additional patients treated with DBS in this target.

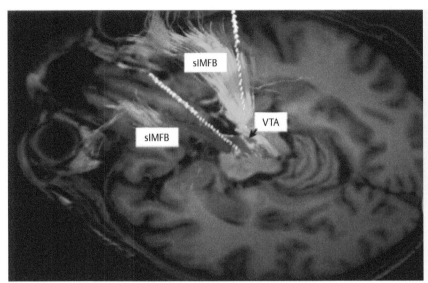

Fig. 27.3 Medial Forebrain Bundle. Diffusion tensor imaging–based patient individual planning of bilateral supero-lateral medial forebrain bundle (slMFB) deep brain stimulation. Three-dimensional rendering as seen from posterior and superior left includes final DBS electrode positions (white rods). VTA, ventral tegmental area. *Reprinted from Schlaepfer et al; with permission from Elsevier.*

27.3.6 Lateral Habenula

In 2010, Sartorius et al., described their experience with bilateral lateral habenula DBS in a 64 year old female suffering from treatment resistant depression. Though the patient had no immediate response, after approximately 4 weeks she experienced an improvement in depressive symptoms. Accidental discontinuation of stimulation resulted in a severe relapse, further suggesting a DBS effect.

27.3.7 Vagus Nerve Stimulation

Vagus nerve stimulation (VNS) for the treatment of depression has been proposed based on the observation that it alters norepinephrine and serotonin concentrations in cerebrospinal fluid and changes the functional connectivity of regions involved in the circuitry of mood disorders. In addition, patients with epilepsy treated with VNS sometimes have improvements in depressive symptoms.

In an initial open label study, 30 patients with TRD received VNS for 10 weeks with 40% of response. At one year, 28 of these patients were assessed and 46% were characterized as responders. In contrast to DBS, VNS is associated with a high incidence of stimulation-induced side effects at short-term, including voice changes (53%), cough (13%), dyspnea (17%) and neck pain (17%). These, however, tend to subside at one year (voice changes 21%, cough 0%, dyspnea 7%, and neck pain 7%).

In a second series of publications, out of sixty patients treated (including the original 30) 30.5% were responders at 10 weeks. At 1–2 years, this number increased to 42–44%. In these studies, patients who had fewer antidepressant treatment trials had a better response to VNS.

A multicenter, placebo controlled study performed a blinded assessments of patients receiving VNS or sham stimulation for 10 weeks. No significant differences were found between sham and treatment groups in most scores (including HAMD and MADRS). Overall, 15.2% of the patients in the experimental group and 10% of sham treated patients had a positive response. After the 10th week of stimulation, patients underwent an open label phase and received stimulation for 1 year. At that time point, 29.8% of patients were considered to be responders.

27.3.8 Epidural Cortical Stimulation

Nahas and colleagues in 2010 implanted bilateral epidural cortical stimulation paddle leads over the anterior frontal poles and midlateral prefrontal cortex in five patients. Under blinded conditions, acute post-surgical stimulation was associated with significant mood changes. Patients were then followed for 7 months, showing an average improvement in HAMD scores from pre implant baseline of 55%. These results were sustained at long-term with 41%, 54% and 45% improvements being recorded at 1, 2 and 5 years, respectively. In a different set of studies, Kopell et al. implanted twelve patients with epidural cortical electrodes over the left dorsolateral prefrontal cortex in a single blind, sham-controlled study. During a sham-controlled phase, no significant differences were noticed when patients receiving sham or active stimulation were compared. In a subsequent open label phase, a significant improvement was observed in HDRS and MADRS scores. Contacts leading to a greater degree of improvement were located in lateral and anterior regions of the dorso lateral pre-frontal cortex.

27.4 Conclusions

After a controversial history, surgery for psychiatric disorders has regained interest. Studies are now conducted in experienced health care centers under strict ethical control. Appropriate surgical management of these conditions, including depression, requires multidisciplinary patient evaluations and an adequate follow-up documenting response to surgical treatment.

After the success of initial open label studies and the failure of blinded trials, it is clear that more study is required to identify surgical approaches and targets, appropriate candidates and predictors of a good outcome.

Suggested Readings

[1] Mayberg HS, Lozano AM, Voon V, et al. Deep brain stimulation for treatment-resistant depression. Neuron. 2005; 45(5):651–660

[2] Holtzheimer PE, Kelley ME, Gross RE, et al. Subcallosal cingulate deep brain stimulation for treatment-resistant unipolar and bipolar depression. Arch Gen Psychiatry. 2012; 69(2):150–158

[3] Riva-Posse P, Choi KS, Holtzheimer PE, et al. Defining critical white matter pathways mediating successful subcallosal cingulate deep brain stimulation for treatment-resistant depression. Biol Psychiatry. 2014; 76(12):963–969

[4] Malone DA , Jr, Dougherty DD, Rezai AR, et al. Deep brain stimulation of the ventral capsule/ventral striatum for treatment-resistant depression. Biol Psychiatry. 2009; 65(4):267–275

[5] Dougherty DD, Rezai AR, Carpenter LL, et al. A Randomized Sham-Controlled Trial of Deep Brain Stimulation of the Ventral Capsule/Ventral Striatum for Chronic Treatment-Resistant Depression. Biol Psychiatry. 2015; 78(4):240–248

[6] Bergfeld IO, Mantione M, Hoogendoorn ML, et al. Deep Brain Stimulation of the Ventral Anterior Limb of the Internal Capsule for Treatment-Resistant Depression: A Randomized Clinical Trial. JAMA Psychiatry. 2016; 73(5):456–464

[7] Schlaepfer TE, Cohen MX, Frick C, et al. Deep brain stimulation to reward circuitry alleviates anhedonia in refractory major depression. Neuropsychopharmacology. 2008; 33(2):368–377

[8] Rush AJ, Marangell LB, Sackeim HA, et al. Vagus nerve stimulation for treatment-resistant depression: a randomized, controlled acute phase trial. Biol Psychiatry. 2005; 58(5):347–354

[9] Williams NR, Short EB, Hopkins T, et al. Five-Year Follow-Up of Bilateral Epidural Prefrontal Cortical Stimulation for Treatment-Resistant Depression. Brain Stimul. 2016; 9(6):897–904

[10] Schlaepfer TE, Bewernick BH, Kayser S, Mädler B, Coenen VA. Rapid effects of deep brain stimulation for treatment-resistant major depression. Biol Psychiatry. 2013; 73(12):1204–1212

28 Functional Neurosurgery for Obsessive-Compulsive Disorder

Nicole C.R. McLaughlin

Abstract

Obsessive-compulsive disorder (OCD) affects two to three percent of the population, and a third of OCD patients are poorly responsive to all conventional treatments. For a subgroup of such OCD patients, psychiatric neurosurgery- lesions or deep brain stimulation (DBS)- is an option. This chapter provides an overview of the most common neurosurgical techniques for OCD, with a focus on outcomes and safety. In addition, detailed information about the typical processes used to evaluate potential patients is included.

Keywords: obsessive-compulsive disorder, psychiatric neurosurgery, ablation, neuromodulation, anxiety

Obsessive-compulsive disorder (OCD) affects two percent of the population, and the World Health Organization ranks OCD as one of the 10 most disabling conditions.[1] OCD is characterized by *obsessions*, which are intrusive, persistent, repetitive thoughts that cause distress, as well as *compulsions*, which are physical or mental acts that are carried out in an aim to reduce the distress associated with the obsessions. A third of OCD patients are poorly responsive to all conventional treatments.[2] For a subgroup of such OCD patients, neurosurgery- lesioning or deep brain stimulation (DBS) are an option.

28.1 OCD Neurocircuitry and Relation to Neurosurgery

Abnormalities in the cortico-striato-thalamo-cortical circuitry are evident in multiple psychiatric disorders, including OCD.[3] These neuroanatomical models of OCD that have been developed from functional neuroimaging are consistent with the empirically-developed targets chosen for lesions or DBS. Decades of research have consistently demonstrated that lesions within CSTC circuitry reduce OCD symptoms. While studies have shown clinical improvement after these procedures, the mechanism for such improvement remains unknown.

28.2 Patient Selection

Standards for psychiatric neurosurgery have included strict criteria for patient selection. Approval is completed through a multi-disciplinary committee after an extensive psychiatric and medical evaluation, including review of all prior treatments. In some countries, governmental approval is required before surgery. Though exact guidelines may differ slightly across sites, approval for surgery is generally based upon: (1) Patients with severe, treatment-resistant OCD, of at least 5 years in duration, which has caused functional interference and poor quality of life. Severity is based on the YBOCS, with a score over 26 to 30; (2) Patients who have failed all conventional treatments, and prior treatment trials must be clearly documented and judged

as adequate, which often requires interviews with prior treating clinicians. Medication trials (duration of at least two months) include trials of a serotonin reuptake inhibitor (often high dose trials are needed in OCD), as well as a neuroleptic trial and trials of clomipramine and clonazepam. These should also include at least 20 sessions of exposure and response/ritual prevention (ERP) (3) Patients with current comorbid substance abuse or severe personality disorders may not be appropriate candidates. The ability to comply with follow-up treatments should also be judged, particularly with DBS, where the pulse generators require frequent charging and patients need to return for frequent post-surgical visits; (4) Significant neurological conditions (e.g. extensive white matter disease, stroke) may be a contraindication. Medical conditions that may increase surgical risks may also be a contraindication. Pre-operative work-up includes an MRI, neurological exam, and neuropsychological assessment; (5) With both ablative and neuromodulatory procedures, patients should continue to receive treatment with a psychiatrist and a therapist skilled in ERP. The majority of patients remain on psychiatric medications post-surgery, though there may be a decrease in the number of prescribed medications. In the case of DBS, access to specialized psychiatric neurosurgery teams is recommended for clinical monitoring and device adjustment. Patients will need continued pulse generator replacements, and future costs, particularly of DBS, should be considered. Long-term follow-up is essential to track clinical change and adverse effects; (6) Patients should always be able to provide appropriate consent for a neurosurgical procedure. Presently, these procedures are reserved for those 18 years of age or older; (7) Though not mandatory, family support is recommended and likely contributes to improved outcomes after surgery.

28.3 Ablative Procedures

Ablative procedures were largely developed empirically, with targets often derived from early work on animals. There are four most commonly used ablative procedures: subcaudate tractotomy (SCT), anterior cingulotomy (ACG), limbic leucotomy (LL), and anterior capsulotomy. All procedures use stereotactic methods, though with different techniques. Thermolesions involve craniotomy, insertion of an electrode, and radiofrequency heating of the tip to cause a lesion. Approximately two decades ago gamma knife radiosurgery was also introduced.

28.3.1 Subcaudate Tractotomy

In SCT, lesions are placed in the substantia inominata, ventral to the caudate, and is intended to interrupt tracts between the OFC and subcortical limbic structures. The procedure is not commonly used except as part of a LL (discussed below), and is usually done with thermocoagulation. Outcomes vary considerably, and success rates range from 33 to 67 percent.[4] Complications include transient disorientation, seizures, fatigue, and weight gain. There has been one reported death due to a neurosurgical complication.[4] Post-operative cognitive impairments have not been reported, but research is limited.[5]

28.3.2 Anterior Cingulotomy

ACG has been the most widely used neurosurgical method for the treatment of OCD in the US. Lesions are placed within the dorsal ACC impinging on the cingulum bundle, in an aim to modify cingulo-striatal projections, and disinhibit the pregenual ACC. Clinical improvement for ACG ranges from 25 to 57 percent.[4] Complications include medication-responsive seizures, hemiplegia, headache, transient dizziness, urinary retention, and subdural hematoma.[4] Cognitive assessments have shown no significant long-term decline, and occasional improvement in post-surgical functioning.[6]

28.3.3 Limbic Leucotomy

LL is the combination of a SCT and an ACG, expecting that this technique would produce better results than either lesion alone.[7] Success rates range from 36 to 69 percent improvement.[4,7,8,9] Given that there are dual lesions, adverse effects may be more prevalent than other procedures, but are transient and include short-term memory deficits, headache, confusion/delirium, lethargy, perseveration, urinary incontinence, seizure, and enduring lethargy. As with the other procedures detailed above, there are no reports of significant cognitive impairment after surgery, though there are some notes of disinhibition and apathy.[10,11,12]

28.3.4 Anterior Capsulotomy

Anterior capsulotomies are currently one of the most commonly used psychiatric neurosurgery procedures, and are traditionally performed using thermolesion by radiofrequency or gamma knife stereotactic radiosurgery. Portions of the anterior arm of the internal capsule are lesioned, and fibers connecting the dorsomedial thalamus to the prefrontal cortex and subgenual anterior cingulate are sectioned. Research has shown a 38 to 100 percent improvement rate.[4] The first controlled study of a lesion procedure in psychiatry was carried out through GK capsulotomy, and in the long-term, 7 out of 12 patients were considered responders. A recent comparison between capsulotomy by thermolesioning and GK noted no significant difference between procedures, and lasting improvement in 48 percent of patients.[13] Adverse effects included weight gain, transient headache, transient postoperative confusion, fatigue, incontinence, and convulsions.[4] GK capsulotomy may cause less discomfort and have more rapid recovery, as it is less invasive. However, potential side effects from radiation exposure include cerebral edema, small asymptomatic caudate infarctions, and cysts·.[14] As with other procedures, long-term cognitive decline is rare, though increased impulsivity/aggression has been reported, as well as decline in short-term memory/executive functioning after larger lesions.[13,15,16,17]

28.3.5 Deep Brain Stimulation

Current targets for OCD have included the ventral capsule/ventral striatum, subthalamic nucleus (STN), nucleus accumbens, and the inferior thalamic peduncle. Electrodes are inserted (usually bilaterally) and are connected to a pulse generator placed in the chest wall. Neurostimulation can be adjusted through several parameters, including the activation of different contacts on a lead, intensity, polarity, and frequency. DBS may be considered reversible and more optimizable than lesion generation; however, additional risks are incurred when compared to GK radiosurgery. Success rates have ranged from 35 to 70 percent.[18,19] Adverse effects include asymptomatic hemorrhage, seizure, superficial infection, and hypomanic/manic symptoms (which may be reversible). Battery depletion may lead to worsened depression and OCD.[19]

28.4 Discussion

Though neurosurgical treatments for psychiatric indications have been performed for centuries, the field has become more rigorous. In the past ten to twenty years there has been a resurgence of interest in the field. Though research has indicated that both DBS and ablative procedures lead to comparable clinical improvement, there are advantages and disadvantages for each option that should be thoroughly discussed with the surgical candidate. Close screening and follow-up is always essential. In addition, our understanding of the mechanism of action contributing to clinical improvement is incomplete, and this understanding may lead to more individualized treatments and improved outcome. Thus, although our first steps into the examination of this complex subject have provided some direction, we continue to require extensive, collaborative research in order to answer some of these remaining questions.

References

[1] Veale D, Roberts A. Obsessive-compulsive disorder. BMJ. 2014; 348(348): g2183

[2] Jenike MA, Rauch SL, Baer L, Rasmussen SA. Neurosurgical treatment of obsessive-compulsive disorder. In: Jenike MA, Baer L, Minichiello WE, eds. Obsessive-compulsive disorders: Practical Management. St. Louis, MO: Mosby; 1998

[3] Greenberg BD, Rauch SL, Haber SN. Invasive circuitry-based neurotherapeutics: stereotactic ablation and deep brain stimulation for OCD. Neuropsychopharmacology. 2010; 35(1):317–336

[4] Lopes AC, de Mathis ME, Canteras MM, Salvajoli JV, Del Porto JA, Miguel EC. [Update on neurosurgical treatment for obsessive compulsive disorder]. Br J Psychiatry. 2004; 26(1):62–66

[5] Broseta J, Barcia-Salorio JL, Roldan P, et al. Stereotactic subcaudate tractotomy: long term results and measuring the effects on psychiatric symptoms. In: Hitchcock ER, Meyerson BA, eds. Modern Concepts in Psychiatric Surgery. Amsterdam: Elsevier/North Holland Biomedical Press; 1979:241–252

[6] Jung HH, Kim CH, Chang JH, Park YG, Chung SS, Chang JW. Bilateral anterior cingulotomy for refractory obsessive-compulsive disorder: Long-term follow-up results. Stereotact Funct Neurosurg. 2006; 84(4):184–189

[7] Kelly D, Mitchell-Heggs N. Stereotactic limbic leucotomy–a follow-up study of thirty patients. Postgrad Med J. 1973; 49(578):865–882

[8] Hay P, Sachdev P, Cumming S, et al. Treatment of obsessive-compulsive disorder by psychosurgery. Acta Psychiatr Scand. 1993; 87(3):197–207

[9] Montoya A, Weiss AP, Price BH, et al. Magnetic resonance imaging-guided stereotactic limbic leukotomy for treatment of intractable psychiatric disease. Neurosurgery. 2002; 50(5):1043–1049, discussion 1049–1052

[10] Kelly D, Richardson A, Mitchell-Heggs N. Stereotactic limbic leucotomy: neurophysiological aspects and operative technique. Br J Psychiatry. 1973; 123 (573):133–140

[11] Mitchell-Heggs N, Kelly D, Richardson A. Further exploration of limbic leucotomy. In: Hitchcock ER, Ballantine HT, Myerson BA, ed. Modern Concepts in Psychiatric Surgery. Amsterdam Elsevier; 1979

[12] Smith JS, Kiloh LG, Cochrane N, Kljajic I. A prospective evaluation of open prefrontal leucotomy. Med J Aust. 1976; 1(20):731–733, 735

[13] Rück C, Karlsson A, Steele JD, et al. Capsulotomy for obsessive-compulsive disorder: long-term follow-up of 25 patients. Arch Gen Psychiatry. 2008; 65(8):914–921

[14] Nakajima H, Yamanaka K, Ishibashi K, Iwai Y. Delayed cyst formations and/or expanding hematomas developing after Gamma Knife surgery for cerebral arteriovenous malformations. J Clin Neurosci. 2016; 33:96–99

[15] Nyman H, Mindus P. Neuropsychological correlates of intractable anxiety disorder before and after capsulotomy. Acta Psychiatr Scand. 1995; 91 (1):23–31

[16] Oliver B, Gascón J, Aparicio A, et al. Bilateral anterior capsulotomy for refractory obsessive-compulsive disorders. Stereotact Funct Neurosurg. 2003; 81 (1–4):90–95

[17] Mindus P, Nyman H. Normalization of personality characteristics in patients with incapacitating anxiety disorders after capsulotomy. Acta Psychiatr Scand. 1991; 83(4):283–291

[18] Greenberg BD, Gabriels LA , D.A. M, et al. Deep Brain Stimulation of the Ventral Internal Capsule/Ventral Striatum for Obsessive-Compulsive Disorder: Worldwide Experience. Mol Psychiatry. 2008(May):20:; e-pub ahead of print

[19] Greenberg BD, Malone DA, Friehs GM, et al. Three-year outcomes in deep brain stimulation for highly resistant obsessive-compulsive disorder. Neuropsychopharmacology. 2006; 31(11):2384–2393

29 Neurosurgery Treatment for Anorexia Nervosa

Chen-Cheng Deng, Guo-Zhn Lin, Tao Wang, Dian-You Li, Shikun Zhan, Bo-Min Sun

Abstract

Anorexia nervosa (AN) is one of the most challenging of the psychiatric disorders to treat. However, the poor clinical outcome of medical therapy in severe cases warrants the consideration of novel treatment modalities. Magnetic resonance imaging-guided bilateral anterior capsulotomy has been a longstanding approach for patients with severe obsessive-compulsive disorder (OCD). Because of the homogeneity between OCD and AN, and their comorbidity, capsulotomy has been used for enduring cases of AN. Deep brain stimulation (DBS) of the nucleus accumbens/ventral capsule and subcingulate region has also been used in a few cases. DBS's implantable requirement, however, limits its use in patients with low bodyweight as is seen in AN. Capsulotomy can enable those patients in life threatening condition, with refractory AN, to normalize their weight. While it may be an acceptable life-saving treatment, it is indicated only when patients fulfill strict criteria, given the complications and irreversibility of surgery.

Keywords: psychosurgery, capsulotomy, deep brain stimulation, anorexia nervosa, neuromodulation

29.1 Patient Selection

1. Patients are diagnosed by independent psychiatrists, according to the DSM-IV criteria rather than DSM-5 criteria. The latter provides a broader definition of the disease entity.[1,2] If AN persists longer than seven years, it is likely that the disease has plateaued.[3] Thus, in the authors' series, disease duration prior to surgery was usually more than 3 years, though the degree of disability was also considered

2. Patients must be eighteen years or older.

3. Patients are resistant to standard medicine and to psychotherapy treatments. Adequacy is defined as having been treated with at least two selective serotonin re uptake inhibitors, with anti-psychotics as augmentation, for at least twelve weeks at maximum tolerable dosage, and evidence-based psychotherapy conducted by an experienced therapist for three months.[4]

4. Patients are in a life-threatening situation, defined as a physiological state with a BMI ≤ 13, or if they have attempted suicide.

5. Patients, together, with/without their legal representative, have the ability and willingness to provide informed consent.

6. Patients have normal fluid and electrolyte balance, and do not have a coagulopathy as measured by activated partial thromboplastin time and international normalized ratio.

Exclusion Criteria:
1. Medical contraindication to neurosurgery.
2. Inability to undergo MR imaging study.
3. Presence of a metabolic disease, such as diabetes, rather than an idiopathic psychiatric disorder alone.

29.2 Preoperative Preparation

Because of long-term malnutrition, general anesthesia or surgery may be contraindicated. Anorexia Nervosa (AN) patients are prone to electrolyte disturbances, cardiac failure, abnormal liver function, and coagulation abnormalities.[5,6] For such patients, extensive preoperative screening that should include electrocardiograms and coagulopathy testing is essential. Hypokalemia and hypoalbuminemia are the most common electrolyte disorders and these should be normalized. Most patients with AN have psychiatric comorbidities such as OCD, depression, anxiety, and even suicidal ideation. The mental status of AN patients is often unstable and patients frequently present with major depression. Thus, patients must be closely monitored throughout the entire procedure.

29.2.1 Intraoperative Management

Local anesthesia is recommended so as to avoid hypervolemia and excessive electrolytes dilution. For DBS, when general anesthesia is required, doses of anesthetic drugs should be adjusted for weight and, during the operation, electrocardiographic changes and potassium levels should be monitored carefully to minimize the risk of arrhythmias.

Because the skull of AN patients is usually thinned from bone rarefaction, burr holes can be dangerous and lead to epidural hematomas. To avoid excessive cerebrospinal fluid drainage, fibrin glue should be applied immediately after opening the dura. A warm air blower is helpful during surgery to maintain normal body temperature. Appropriate padding should be applied to all pressure points to avoid the higher risk of skin sores in these patients.

29.3 Operative Procedure

29.3.1 Capsulotomy

A stereotactic frame is mounted on the patient's head under local anesthesia or mild sedation. Following frame placement, a 1.5 Tesla MRI is obtained. The targeted internal capsule is identified on the stereotactic MRIs. Target coordinates are calculated and the trajectory angle measured. Bilateral burr holes are drilled anterior to the coronal suture based on the measured entrance trajectory. The anterior capsule target is located between the anterior and middle third of the anterior limb of the internal capsule, as defined in MR images at the approximate level of the foramen of Monro. After dural opening and cauterization of the pia-arachnoid, a 2-mm diameter radiofrequency electrode with a 2-mm uninsulated tip is used for impedance measurement, followed by a stimulation test and lesioning. The radiofrequency lesions are generated by ablation at 75 degrees centigrade for 60 seconds. During lesioning, neurological examination is repeated to ensure that there is no impairment of motor or sensory functions. After adequate

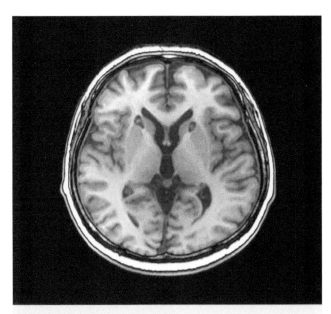

Fig. 29.1 6-month post capsulotomy.

cooling, the electrode is withdrawn by 2 mm and the ablation procedure is repeated 4–5 times to ensure complete ablation of the anterior limb of the internal capsule. A lesion 4–5 mm in diameter and 10–12 mm in length along the contoured target is thus produced (▶ Fig. 29.1). Post-operative MRIs are obtained one week after surgery to confirm the lesion sites.

29.3.2 Deep Brain Stimulation

Surgical Procedure

Electrodes are implanted bilaterally in the ventral striatum/ventral capsule (VC/VS) using a frame-based, magnetic resonance imaging-guided stereotactic technique. Targeting is based on prior experience with DBS for OCD.[7] Leads are implanted following the dorso-ventral trajectory of the anterior limb of the internal capsule (AIC), with an anterior angle of approximately 90° to the intercommissural line. The target for contact 0 is the VS below the level of the anterior commissure. The intention is to position contact 1 near the junction of the VS and VC, with contacts 2 and 3 located more dorsal within the AIC. Nominal target coordinates for the electrode tip are 6–7 mm lateral to midline (X), 1–2 mm anterior to the posterior border of the anterior commissure (Y), and 3– 4 mm inferior to the anterior commissure–posterior commissure line (Z). Microelectrode recordings are not used for identifying ultimate target location within VC/VS. Final targeting is based on individual anatomical landmarks and intra-operative responses to test stimulation. Intra-operative test stimulation is performed after lead implantation, with the patient awake and able to respond to questions. The goal of test stimulation is to identify contact locations that produce acute improvements in mood and anxiety, without significant adverse effects. Common observations during intra-operative stimulation include acute mood improvement, spontaneous smiling, reduced anxiety, and increased energy and awareness. Adverse effects include tachycardia, increased anxiety, a sense of warmth/sweating, speech perseveration, and facial motor effects. Qualitative symptom improvement and/or lack of adverse effects to stimulation of at least one contact are indicative of proper targeting. Nevertheless, the response rate and pattern is not well established. Postoperative imaging is done to verify lead placement. Leads are later connected by subcutaneous extensions to implantable neurostimulators placed bilaterally in an infraclavicular location under general anesthesia.

Stimulation Procedures

After a postoperative recovery phase of two to four weeks, patients undergo several hours of outpatient stimulation parameter titration and these sessions continue for many months, as described for OCD and major depression,[7,8] All electrodes are tested first in a monopolar configuration to determine the effects elicited at each contact. Next, bipolar contact pairs are selected while the patients are blinded to the stimulation settings. This requires two to four hours for each survey session. Chronic stimulation parameters are selected because of improved mood in the absence of adverse effects. Other effects that help determine the optimal parameters include increased eye contact, facial expressiveness, and interpersonal spontaneity. These are similar to those that are used during intra-operative testing. Once the appropriate settings are identified, the patients enter a chronic stimulation phase in which they return at least monthly for device interrogation. During this phase modifications to the stimulation settings, usually to the amplitude or pulse width, can be made to mitigate adverse effects and to optimize efficacy.

29.4 Postoperative Management (Including Complications)

29.4.1 Postoperative Management

As patients with AN have very low body weight, careful control of rehydration fluids is important. Mannitol should not be infused given the high risk of intracranial hemorrhage. Electrolytes need to be closely monitored. Pharmacological therapy for the disorder can restart on the second day after surgery, but the dosage should now be adjusted to the patients' symptoms. Psychiatric intervention can be re started two weeks after surgery.

29.4.2 Adverse Events Associated with Surgery for Anorexia Nervosa

Operative Complications

Intracranial hematomas represent the most severe complications of this surgery. In 216 cases of stereotactic surgery at this institution, epidural hematomas occurred in four patients. One patient died as a result of disseminated intravascular coagulation. Hematomas occur more frequently in AN patients than in other disorders treated with stereotactic surgery, Wound infections are more common after DBS treatment than in lesioning procedures as a result of subcutaneous fluid collections and hematomas. In this center, the wound infections incidence is 2%, which is similar to other medical centers.

Neuropsychological Complications

Short-term neuropsychological side effects include incontinence, disorientation, sleep disturbance, and headache. These usually resolve within two months of the operation. A number of patients experience long-term side effects that include memory loss, fatigue, excessive weight gain, and personality changes.

DBS System-associated Complications

DBS hardware complications include wire or lead fracture or migration, hardware rejection and malfunction of the pulse-generator. Bhatia et al., had a 4% incidence of hardware-associated morbidity after treating 191 patients who underwent 330 procedures.[9] The mean duration between implantation and onset was two years.[10]

Alterations in weight were observed in some patients who underwent sub-thalamic DBS for movement disorders. The cause was thought not to be simply the elimination of involuntary movement. In a three-year longitudinal study published in 2012, Sun et al., found that patients with AN benefited from chronic DBS stimulation of the nucleus accumbens.[5] In 2013, Lozano also reported that continuous DBS stimulation of the subcallosal cingulate gurus improves the BMI and other psychiatric symptoms of patients with AN.[6]

DBS has some disadvantages in the treatment of AN when compared to capsulotomy. Patients with AN usually are in poor physical condition and muscle atrophy may be a contraindication to pulse-generator placement. Young women with AN may reject DBS treatment because of the prominence of the implantable pulse generator (IPG) in the chest wall, altering their body appearance. Other patients do not wish to commit to a life of device programming and maintenance. Finally, DBS is expensive, more expensive than capsulotomy. This high cost might be the chief obstacle to DBS implantation in China and in developing countries, though smaller and less expensive IPGs may make DBS a more accessible option in the future.[11]

29.5 Conclusions

Capsulotomy is an invasive and irreversible operation. Bilateral capsulotomy can cause short-term side effects such as incontinence, disorientation, sleep disorders, and refeeding syndrome. These symptoms usually disappear within one month. However, it's safety and efficacy based on longitudinal data must continue to be explored. Considering the adverse effects and complications that can occur, strict inclusion criteria and treatment guidelines must be used before proceeding with such surgery.[12,13]

References

[1] Association AP, Association AP. Diagnostic and Statistical Manual-Text Revision (DSM-IV-TRim, 2000). American Psychiatric Association; 2000

[2] American Psychiatric Association. Association D-5 AP. Diagnostic and Statistical Manual of Mental Disorders; 2013. doi:10.1176/appi.books.9780890425596.744053

[3] Touyz S, Hay P. Severe and enduring anorexia nervosa (SE-AN): in search of a new paradigm. J Eat Disord. 2015; 3:26

[4] Zipfel S, Giel KE, Bulik CM, Hay P, Schmidt U. Anorexia nervosa: aetiology, assessment, and treatment. Lancet Psychiatry. 2015; 2(12):1099–1111

[5] Wu H, Van Dyck-Lippens PJ, Santegoeds R, et al. Deep-brain stimulation for anorexia nervosa. World Neurosurg. 2013; 80(3–4):29.e1–29.e10

[6] Lipsman N, Woodside DB, Giacobbe P, et al. Subcallosal cingulate deep brain stimulation for treatment-refractory anorexia nervosa: a phase 1 pilot trial. Lancet. 2013; 381(9875):1361–1370

[7] Denys D, Mantione M, Figee M, et al. Deep Brain Stimulation of the Nucleus Accumbens for Treatment-Refractory Obsessive-Compulsive Disorder. Arch Gen Psychiatry. 2010; 67(10):1061–1068

[8] Bergfeld IO, Mantione M, Hoogendoorn MLC, et al. Deep brain stimulation of the ventral anterior limb of the internal capsule for treatment-resistant depression: A randomized clinical trial. JAMA Psychiatry. 2016; 73(5):456–464

[9] Bhatia S, Zhang K, Oh M, Angle C, Whiting D. Infections and hardware salvage after deep brain stimulation surgery: a single-center study and review of the literature. Stereotact Funct Neurosurg. 2010; 88(3):147–155

[10] Zhang J, Wang T, Zhang CC-CCCC, et al. The safety issues and hardware-related complications of deep brain stimulation therapy: a single-center retrospective analysis of 478 patients with Parkinson's disease. Clin Interv Aging. 2017; 12:923–928

[11] Zhang C, Li D, Zeljic K, Tan H, Ning Y, Sun B. A Remote and Wireless Deep Brain Stimulation Programming System. Neuromodulation. 2016; 19(4):437–439

[12] Nuttin B, Wu H, Mayberg H, et al. Consensus on guidelines for stereotactic neurosurgery for psychiatric disorders. J Neurol Neurosurg Psychiatry. 2014; 85(9):1003–1008

[13] Oudijn MS, Storosum JG, Nelis E, Denys D. Is deep brain stimulation a treatment option for anorexia nervosa? BMC Psychiatry. 2013; 13(1):277

30 Anterior Capsulotomy for Treatment of Refractory Schizophrenia

Chen-Cheng Deng, Guo-Zhn Lin, Tao Wang, Dian-You Li, Shikun Zhan, Bo-Min Sun

Abstract

Schizophrenia is a psychiatric disorder that may be associated with functional and structural impairments in the cortico-striato-thalamic circuitry.[1] It is a debilitating, disabling, and heterogeneous disorder that affects 1% of the population and is characterized by three symptomatic domains: There are positive symptoms such as hallucinations and delusions; negative symptoms include depression and apathy, and there are cognitive deficits. Conventional approaches to treatment have not yet been fully successful because of its symptom diversity and unclear etiology. First and second generation antipsychotics have been helpful for mild to moderate schizophrenia, but drug resistance, extrapyramidal side effects, and tardive dystonia complicate their use. Twenty to thirty percent of patients suffer a relapse during maintenance treatment.[2,3] Electroconvulsive therapy is the most rapidly effective treatment of refractory schizophrenia, but the cognitive deficits and memory impairments from it are still a major concern.[4] Repetitive transcranial magnetic stimulation is a promising therapy for the negative symptoms of schizophrenia and for auditory hallucinations.[5] It has not solved the issue of the heterogeneity of schizophrenic symptoms, and controlled trials will be required to validate its safety and effectiveness. Cognitive behavior therapy has moderate benefit, but it is time consuming.[6,7] Given the absence of an obvious answer for patients who are refractory to known treatment options, stereotactic surgery could be considered as an alternative treatment.

Keywords: schizophrenia, psychiatric neurosurgery, stereotactic operation, capsulotomy, deep brain stimulation

30.1 Patient Selection

An Ethics Committee should oversee all candidates for surgery. Informed consent must be obtained. In our practice immediate relatives can give consent for patients incapable of doing so.

This is an obvious ethically sensitive field. All candidates for neurosurgical treatment of schizophrenia must meet strict, accepted clinical criteria for severity, chronicity, disability, and treatment refractoriness. The risk of suicide should be considered when evaluating all of these individuals.[8]

30.2 Inclusion Criteria

Candidates must be 18–60 years old, examined by two separate psychiatrists, and diagnosed as schizophrenic according to the DSM-IV.[9]

Their Brief Psychiatric Rating Scale (BPRS) score must be ≥ 35 and the Clinical Global Impression (CGI) score must be > 4.[9] As such, their condition must impact their quality of life and prevent participation in normal activities, as clarified by a score of less than 60 on the Social and Occupational Functioning Scale.

Candidates must have failed at least two adequate treatment trials with different antipsychotic drugs.[10] Each drug must be tried for at least six weeks, and the dosage must have been equivalent to 600 mg or more of chlorpromazine daily.

Finally, patients must be intolerant to further nonsurgical approaches, and patients or their representatives must have the ability and willingness to give informed consent.

30.3 Exclusion Criteria

Candidates are excluded if there are cerebral anatomic abnormalities or impairments seen on 1.5 T MRI that would impact the risks of surgery or cannot undergo an MRI. They are excluded if they have other organic problems that prevent them from undergoing surgery, are pregnant, or have severe suicidal ideations. For those patients who hallucinate, or have aggressive behavior and refuse an MRI scan, neuroleptics such as haloperidol or chlorpromazine can be used to assist them in completing the MRI.

30.4 Surgery

Surgical approaches for schizophrenia include anterior capsulotomy, cingulotomy, and amygdalectomy.[9,10,11,12,13] Bilateral anterior capsulotomy is the most common treatment, and DBS is rarely done.(▶ Fig. 30.1)

RF lesions are made at 75 °C for 60 sec, after which the depth electrode is withdrawn 2 mm to allow for cooling. Another

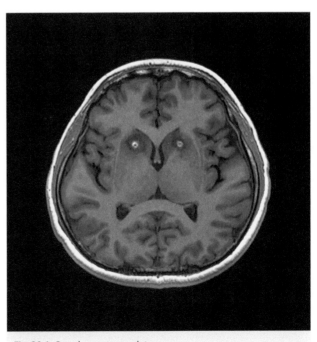

Fig. 30.1 One day post capsulotomy.

lesion is generated, the needle withdrawn again, and the process is repeated 4–5 times. The final lesion is 4–5 mm wide and 10–12 mm long.

30.5 Results

Patients are encouraged to participate in social activities as soon as feasible. In one study in which 100 patients who underwent bilateral anterior capsulotomy were followed with the social disability screening schedule, positive and negative symptom, brief psychiatric rating, activities of daily living, and global assessment scales, aggressive behavior, hallucinations, and delusions responded best as measured two-years after surgery.[9]

Aggressive behavior, hallucinations, and delusions responded best as measured two-years after bilateral anterior capsulotomy.

30.6 Acute Complications

The most severe complication is a 1% incidence of intracranial hemorrhage. Postoperative epilepsy also occurs with a 1% incidence. Depakote 500 mg for 1–3 months is recommended prophylactically. Urinary incontinence, disorientation, fatigue, and sleep disorders have been observed and last up to three months.

30.7 Long-term Side Effects

Memory loss, personality changes, lazy behavior, and hypererotism are observed. Hypererotism can be treated with estradiol valerate, however, other complications usually persist for up to two years.

30.8 Antipsychotics Adjustment

All patients should continue to take their antipsychotics for at least 2 years. Usually a 30%–50% reduction of preoperative dosage is recommended. Postoperative patients should be strictly followed. The suggestions for adjustment should be made after a comprehensive evaluation for psychiatric status postoperatively. Antipsychotic medication may be discontinued if psychiatric symptoms are absent after two years of follow-up.

30.9 Alternative Surgery

DBS is a well-accepted method for Parkinson's disease and dystonia treatment, however, there have been no rigorous clinical trials showing its safety and effectiveness in the treatment of schizophrenia.[14]

30.10 Conclusions

Schizophrenia is a heterogeneous disorder with varying expression of cognitive impairment as well as positive and negative symptoms that poses a therapeutic conundrum for physicians and their patients. Many of them are refractory to standard antipsychotic therapy, leaving functional treatment as an option. Stereotactic bilateral anterior capsulotomy is effective for treatment-refractory schizophrenia, but because the lesions generated are irreversible, major ethical concerns remain.[9] DBS for schizophrenia is an option for refractory schizophrenia. More clinical trials are warranted, however, and more effective therapeutic targets should be sought.

References

[1] Sui J, Pearlson GD, Du Y, et al. In search of multimodal neuroimaging biomarkers of cognitive deficits in schizophrenia. Biol Psychiatry. 2015; 78(11):794–804
[2] Lieberman J, Jody D, Geisler S, et al. Time course and biologic correlates of treatment response in first-episode schizophrenia. Arch Gen Psychiatry. 1993; 50(5):369–376
[3] Conley RR, Buchanan RW. Evaluation of treatment-resistant schizophrenia. Schizophr Bull. 1997; 23(4):663–674
[4] Andrade C, Arumugham SS, Thirthalli J. Adverse Effects of Electroconvulsive Therapy. Psychiatr Clin North Am. 2016; 39(3):513–530
[5] He H, Lu J, Yang L, et al. Repetitive transcranial magnetic stimulation for treating the symptoms of schizophrenia: A PRISMA compliant meta-analysis. Clin Neurophysiol. 2017; 128(5):716–724
[6] Gould RA, Mueser KT, Bolton E, Mays V, Goff D. Cognitive therapy for psychosis in schizophrenia: an effect size analysis. Schizophr Res. 2001; 48(2–3):335–342
[7] Sarin F, Wallin L, Widerlöv B. Cognitive behavior therapy for schizophrenia: a meta-analytical review of randomized controlled trials. Nord J Psychiatry. 2011; 65(3):162–174
[8] Nuttin B, Wu H, Mayberg H, et al. Consensus on guidelines for stereotactic neurosurgery for psychiatric disorders. J Neurol Neurosurg Psychiatry. 2014; 85(9):1003–1008
[9] Liu W, Hao Q, Zhan S, et al. Long-term follow-up of mri-guided bilateral anterior capsulotomy in patients with refractory schizophrenia. Stereotact Funct Neurosurg. 2014; 92(3):145–152
[10] Howes OD, McCutcheon R, Agid O, et al. Treatment-Resistant Schizophrenia: Treatment Response and Resistance in Psychosis (TRRIP) Working Group Consensus Guidelines on Diagnosis and Terminology. Am J Psychiatry. 2017; 174(3):216–229
[11] Tow PM, Armstrong RW, Oxon MA. Anterior cingulectomy in schizophrenia and other psychotic disorders; clinical results. J Ment Sci. 1954; 100(418):46–61
[12] Escobar JI, Chandel V. Nuclear symptoms of schizophrenia after cingulotomy: a case report. Am J Psychiatry. 1977; 134(11):1304–1306
[13] Chitanondh H. Stereotaxic amygdalotomy in the treatment of olfactory seizures and psychiatric disorders with olfactory hallucination. Confin Neurol. 1966; 27(1):181–196
[14] Corripio I, Sarró S, McKenna PJ, et al. Clinical Improvement in a Treatment-Resistant Patient With Schizophrenia Treated With Deep Brain Stimulation. Biol Psychiatry. 2016; 80(8):e69–e70

31 Alzheimer's Disease: Epidemiology, Pathophysiology and Surgery

Andres Lozano, Davis Xu

Abstract

Deep brain stimulation of the fornices is a promising surgical therapy for the treatment of Alzheimer's disease that aims to modulate dysfunctional neural networks and delay disease progression. Data from a recent Phase II clinical trial found fornix DBS to be safe and associated with better cognitive outcomes in patients older than 65 years. Further studies need to be conducted to assess the significance of clinical response and optimal patient population for treatment.

Keywords: Alzheimer's disease, deep brain stimulation, neuromodulation, dementia

31.1 Epidemiology

Alzheimer's disease is the most common age-related neurodegenerative disease, accounting for over 80% of the global incidence of dementia.[1] Currently, within the United States the Alzheimer's disease patient population includes approximately 200,000 individuals younger than 65 years and more than 5 million people 65 years-of-age or older.[2] Age is the predominant risk factor for Alzheimer's disease, with a doubling of disease incidence seen every 5-years after age 65. The resulting risk of diagnosis exceeds 1 in 3 for those older than 85 years. Based on current population demographics, the World Health Organization estimates that the global prevalence of disease will more than triple by 2050, surpassing 115 million cases.[1]

31.2 Pathophysiology

Since 1907, when Alois Alzheimer first described amyloid plaques and neurofibrillary tangles as the neuropathological hallmarks of his eponymous disease, these pathological hallmarks have come to highlight the central theme in Alzheimer's disease pathophysiology – an abnormal accumulation of misfolded proteins that leads to cellular dysfunction, synaptic loss, and neural network failure. Currently, a unifying model of Alzheimer's disease pathogenesis remains elusive, but within the past two decades, multiple lines of investigation implicate amyloid-β and tau, the components of amyloid plaques and neurofibrillary tangles respectively, as the seminal agents of disease pathogenesis and cellular injury.[3] On a macroscopic level, disease progression occurs as a consequence of progressive synaptic dysfunction that increasingly disrupts the activity of neural networks involved with memory, executive function, and language. Evidence of these disturbances is reflected by the incremental decline of regional glucose metabolism as well as structural and functional degradation of neural connectivity visualized through positron emission tomography (PET) and investigative magnetic resonance imaging (MRI) sequences.[4,5]

31.3 Treatments

31.3.1 Deep Brain Stimulation (DBS)

DBS has emerged as a promising surgical therapy for Alzheimer's disease, aiming to modulate the activity of dysfunctional neural networks by directly driving electrical activity and increasing neural circuit viability through trophic effects associated with stimulation.[6] Two DBS targets have been described for Alzheimer's disease. One of these, the nucleus basalis of Meynert (nBM), we will discuss only briefly due to limited literature data. The nBM is the primary relay of cholinergic projections to the neocortex and medial temporal lobes. DBS of the nBM for Alzheimer's disease has been described in 7 patients across 2 studies, and has been shown to increase subsequent global cerebral glucose metabolism in 4 patients at follow-up under 12 months.[7,8]

The other DBS target is the fornix, the principle output tract of the hippocampus and projection path within the circuit of Papez. Early studies with fornix DBS in rodents and epilepsy patients demonstrated improved memory of test subjects.[6,9] In patients with mild Alzheimer's disease, fornix DBS was recently evaluated by the ADvance trial, a phase II clinical study that yielded mixed results.[10] In ADvance, 42 patients underwent bilateral fornix DBS in a double-blinded fashion. Global cerebral glucose metabolism was statistically greater in patients receiving stimulation versus the sham group at 6-months, but did not remain statistically significant at 12 months.[10] On *post-hoc* analysis, age was found to be a significant discriminate of response with patients older than 65-years having improved clinical and metabolic outcomes in contrast to patients younger than 65 years who tended to have worse results with stimulation.[10] This age discrepancy has been found across other Alzheimer's disease studies, including multiple drug trials, suggesting that younger patients may represent a different disease phenotype.[11]

31.3.2 Patient Selection

The patients with AD that are most likely to respond are still undetermined. Preliminary evidence suggests that patients with early stages of disease in accordance with guidelines from the National Institute of Aging and Alzheimer Association may be the most appropriate candidates (▸ Table 31.1). Such early stage patients should demonstrate only mild dementia based on a score of 0.5 or 1 on the global Clinical Dementia Rating Sum of Boxes (CDR-SB) and a score of 12–24 on the Alzheimer's Disease Assessment Scale-13 (ADAS-Cog 13). Patients should be evaluated for neuropsychiatric symptoms through the Neuropsychiatric Inventory and excluded if their total score is ≥ 10 or any sub-domain score, except apathy, is ≥ 4. All patients should already be optimized on pharmacologic therapy before surgery and be free of medical contraindications for surgery or MR imaging. They should have a Modified Hachinski ischemia rating less than 4 to exclude those with possible co-existant vascular dementia. Age of eligibility remains a controversial topic with some suggestion that early onset patients (less than 65 years old) may be less likely to benefit with DBS.

31.4 Preoperative Preparation

All patients should undergo baseline neurocognitive testing and high resolution MR-imaging of the brain. An evaluation of cerebral glucose metabolism through PET is useful to evaluate the cerebral metabolic disturbance.

31.5 Operative Procedure

Placement of the electrodes can be done while the patient is awake or asleep, similar to the technique used for DBS in Parkinson's disease. Awake patients have a stereotactic frame placed under local anesthesia and then undergo high-resolution MR-imaging. Asleep patients are put under general anesthesia

Table 31.1 Clinical eligibility criteria for fornix DBS in the phase II clinical trial

Age	65-years or older
Global Clinical Dementia Rating Sum of Boxes (CDR-SB)	0.5–1
Alzheimer's Disease Assessment Scale-13 (ADAS-Cog 13)	12–24
Neuropsychiatric Inventory	Total ≤ 10, any subdomain ≤ 4 except apathy
Modified Hachinski ischemia rating scale	< 4
Adjuvant therapies	Must be on anticholinergic medication for at least 2 months before surgery

and then the stereotactic frame is co-registered to a pre-operative planning MRI through an intraoperative CT-scan (▶ Fig. 31.1).

Stereotactic targeting of the fornix proceeds with a skull entry generally 2 cm lateral to midline at the coronal suture, with aiming of the electrodes 2 mm anterior and tangential to the columns of the fornix and having the distal contacts just proximal to the mammillary bodies. Verification of lead placement can be performed through an intraoperative CT-scan that is then co-registered and blended with the planning MRI to allow projection of the actual lead position over their planned location. Patients who undergo surgery awake can have test stimulation of the deepest lead contacts that should elicit autonomic signs such as alterations in blood pressure, pulse, and diaphoresis. Approximately a third of patient may also experience autobiographical memories when the most superficial lead is stimulated, usually above 7V. After placement of the electrodes, a dual channel pulse generator is then implanted subcutaneously below the clavicle and connected by an extension channel.

31.6 Postoperative Management (Including Complications)

31.6.1 Complications

Post-operatively, all patients should undergo a follow-up CT or MRI scan to verify electrode placement as well as screen for intracranial complications. Data from large patient series reveal that the rate of adverse events associated with DBS surgery is low. The most dangerous complication is intraparenchymal hemorrhage, which occurs approximately 2% of the time, but is generally asymptomatic and rarely requires additional surgical management.[12] Long-term adverse events are more common and include wound infection (1.7–5.6% risk) and failure or malfunction of the hardware (< 5% risk).[12,13] Behavioral or

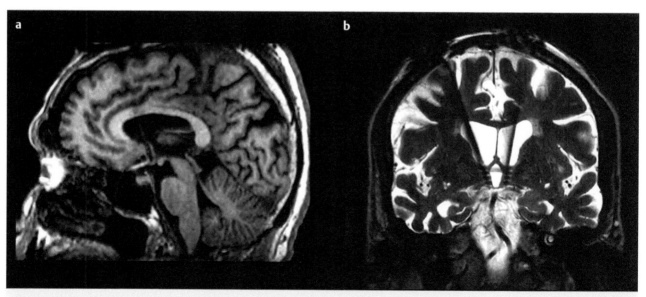

Fig. 31.1 Placement of fornix electrodes. **(a)** Sagittal T1-weighted and **(b)** coronal T2-weighted magnetic resonance imaging demonstrates placement of the electrodes ~2 mm anterior to the fornix with the distal contact just proximal to mammillary bodies.

psychiatric disturbances have not been shown to be elicited by stimulation.

31.6.2 Stimulation Programming

The identification of the optimal stimulation parameters is an area of ongoing investigation. Patients usually begin undergoing electrode activation and programming 2 weeks after surgery. The default stimulation is run at either the top or second from the top electrode contact and is delivered at an amplitude of 3.0–3.5 V, a frequency of 130 Hz, and a pulse width of 90 μsec.[10]

31.7 Conclusion

Alzheimer's disease remains a complex neurocognitive disorder with unclear underpinnings. Fornix DBS has been shown to be safe and offers some potential benefit in delaying the clinical progression of disease. Further analysis of larger patient cohorts is needed to define the significance of clinical response as well as identify the optimal patient population and most appropriate stimulation parameters.

References

[1] Alzheimer's Association. Alzheimers Dement. 2014; 10(2):47–92

[2] Querfurth HW, LaFerla FM. Alzheimer's disease. N Engl J Med. 2010; 362(4): 329–344

[3] Bloom GS. Amyloid-β and tau: the trigger and bullet in Alzheimer disease pathogenesis. JAMA Neurol. 2014; 71(4):505–508

[4] Jacobs HI, Radua J, Lückmann HC, Sack AT. Meta-analysis of functional network alterations in Alzheimer's disease: toward a network biomarker. Neurosci Biobehav Rev. 2013; 37(5):753–765

[5] Smith GS, de Leon MJ, George AE, et al. Topography of cross-sectional and longitudinal glucose metabolic deficits in Alzheimer's disease. Pathophysiologic implications. Arch Neurol. 1992; 49(11):1142–1150

[6] Hao S, Tang B, Wu Z, et al. Forniceal deep brain stimulation rescues hippocampal memory in Rett syndrome mice. Nature. 2015; 526(7573):430–434

[7] Kuhn J, Hardenacke K, Lenartz D, et al. Deep brain stimulation of the nucleus basalis of Meynert in Alzheimer's dementia. Mol Psychiatry. 2015; 20(3):353–360

[8] Turnbull IM, McGeer PL, Beattie L, Calne D, Pate B. Stimulation of the basal nucleus of Meynert in senile dementia of Alzheimer's type. A preliminary report. Appl Neurophysiol. 1985; 48(1–6):216–221

[9] Suthana N, Haneef Z, Stern J, et al. Memory enhancement and deep-brain stimulation of the entorhinal area. N Engl J Med. 2012; 366(6):502–510

[10] Lozano AM, Fosdick L, Chakravarty MM, et al. A Phase II Study of Fornix Deep Brain Stimulation in Mild Alzheimer's Disease. J Alzheimers Dis. 2016; 54(2): 777–787

[11] Schneider LS, Kennedy RE, Wang G, Cutter GR. Differences in Alzheimer disease clinical trial outcomes based on age of the participants. Neurology. 2015; 84(11):1121–1127

[12] Fenoy AJ, Simpson RK , Jr. Risks of common complications in deep brain stimulation surgery: management and avoidance. J Neurosurg. 2014; 120(1):132–139

[13] Bjerknes S, Skogseid IM, Sæhle T, Dietrichs E, Toft M. Surgical site infections after deep brain stimulation surgery: frequency, characteristics and management in a 10-year period. PLoS One. 2014; 9(8):e105288

32 Normal Pressure Hydrocephalus

Jonathan Melius and Tyler J. Kenning

Abstract

Normal pressure hydrocephalus (NPH) is a progressive, chronic disorder that can often be treated with a ventriculoperitoneal shunt. NPH most commonly presents with a "magnetic gait" in the setting of ventricular enlargement. The classic NPH triad, which also includes cognitive impairment and urinary incontinence, is only seen in 60% of cases. Ventricular enlargement is thought to result from decreased cerebrospinal fluid (CSF) absorption and must be documented radiographically. Temporary CSF removal, often referred to as a tap test, helps to determine appropriate surgical candidacy for ventriculoperitoneal shunting.

Keywords: Ventriculomegaly, Normal pressure hydrocephalus, Magnetic gait, Cognitive impairment, Urinary incontinence, Cerebrospinal fluid tap test, Ventriculoperitoneal shunt

Normal pressure hydrocephalus (NPH) is an insidiously progressive, chronic disorder that lacks an identifiable antecedent cause. Normal cerebrospinal fluid (CSF) pressures accompany the radiographic finding of ventricular enlargement on cranial imaging. The clinical presentation includes gait and balance impairments and may involve disturbances in cognition and control of urination. The classic triad of symptoms is seen in only 60% of cases.

NPH is a disease of older adults, most commonly afflicting those over 60 years of age. There is an estimated 0.2% prevalence of probable NPH in adults age 70–79 and 6% in those over 80 years old. Asymptomatic ventriculomegaly, however, is estimated to occur in 1% of the elderly. It is unclear if this entity represents an NPH precursor or represents a normal anatomical variant.[1]

32.1 Clinical Presentation

The most common symptom of NPH is that of gait disturbance and is described as "a magnetic" gait as patients take slow, short, shuffling steps with outward rotated feet, a wide base, and diminished step height. Patients have difficulty with tandem gait, display en-bloc turning (requiring 3 or more steps to turn 180 degrees) and often have impaired balance. There is often a history of repeated falls. This is the most likely symptom to improve with treatment.

The cognitive impairment of NPH is likely a result of subcortical/frontal dysfunction. It manifests as psychomotor slowing, daytime sleepiness, inattention, decreased concentration and apathy. While executive functions are impaired, there is an absence of aphasia, agnosia and apraxia. Additionally, in the early stages of the disease process, patients may experience urinary urgency and frequency without incontinence. Later on, however, bladder and even bowel incontinence can occur.

32.2 Pathophysiology

The pathophysiology of normal pressure hydrocephalus remains somewhat unclear, but there is believed to be decreased CSF absorption at the arachnoid villi that transiently result in increased CSF pressures and pulsatility. As greater force is applied to the brain in normal-sized ventricles, ventricular enlargement results and CSF pressures return to normal. With dilatation of the ventricles, periventricular axons and subependymal vessels are stretched causing microvascular ischemia and white matter damage.

32.3 Diagnosis

The diagnostic sensitivity of NPH is reduced by the variability that exists in its clinical presentation and course. It requires convergent date from the clinical history, physical examination and cranial imaging. Clinical symptomatology must include gait/balance disturbance and some degree of impairment in either cognition or urinary continence, or both. The onset of symptoms should be insidious in onset with an origin after age 40 and a minimal duration of at least 3–6 months. Symptoms should progress over time and there should be no antecedent event or other neurological or medical conditions as potential causes of the presenting symptoms.

In addition to the clinical symptoms, an NPH diagnosis requires the documentation of ventricular enlargement on either CT or MRI that is not entirely attributable to cerebral atrophy or a result of CSF obstruction. A commonly used radiographic marker is the Evans' index, which is the ratio of the maximal width of the frontal horns of the lateral ventricles to the maximal inner diameter of the skull at the same level (▶ Fig. 32.1). Although with the Evan's index, the ratio can vary

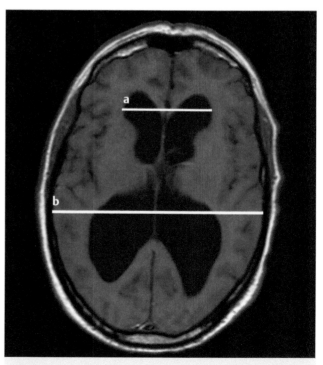

Fig. 32.1 Evans ratio: ratio of the maximum width of the frontal horns of the lateral ventricles (**a**) and maximal internal diameter of the skull at the same level (**b**). Ventriculomegaly defined as > 0.3.

with age and gender and is dependent on the location and angle of the CT image. A value greater than 0.3 is considered abnormal.

Potentially incapacitating symptoms of NPH can be improved or even reversed by permanent cerebrospinal fluid diversion with a ventriculoperitoneal shunt (VPS). Ataxia, dementia and incontinence associated with more advanced stages of NPH tend to be less responsive than symptoms of less than two years duration, emphasizing the utility of early diagnosis. Overall up to two-thirds of patients suspected of having NPH based on clinical symptoms and imaging alone will have a favorable response to shunting. Those patients with the complete symptom triad likely will demonstrate the greatest improvement. As the complication rate with shunting of NPH patients has been reported to be as high as 35% in some series, adjunctive testing should be performed to improve the diagnostic accuracy.

With supplemental testing, the ability to predict a positive response to VPS for NPH can potentially be increased to greater than 80%. This testing usually replicates the removal of CSF in some form. The performance of a high volume (35–50 ml) lumbar puncture (i.e., cerebrospinal fluid tap test) and the subsequent assessment of symptomatic improvement can improve the sensitivity of the testing to almost 80%. A "pre-tap" and "post-tap" objective assessment of cognitive and gait function yields a better determination of surgical candidacy than relying on subjective improvement alone.

Placement of a lumbar drain and an inpatient trial of continual CSF removal over a period of up to three days may increase the sensitivity closer to 90%.[2] This technique, however, is associated with a much higher cost associated with an inpatient hospital stay and complication rate (e.g., infection, extraaxial hematoma formation, drain disconnection) in this elderly population and may not be worth the additional risk. For more difficult cases, CSF outflow resistance can be assessed through infusion studies, but these can often be difficult to interpret and may be of questionable clinical utility.[3]

We advocate for a more structured outpatient assessment in which an initial consultation is performed with a comprehensive history, physical exam, and review of all available cranial imaging. The examination focuses on cognitive function and ambulation, as it is difficult to reliably assess urinary incontinence in the outpatient neurosurgical office. Our cognitive evaluation consists of rapid and delayed memory testing, the

Folstein mini-mental status exam (FMMSE), and timed cognitive testing. Ambulation status is assessed with a modified Timed Up and Go (TUG) test and a 25-foot walk. The patient then has a high volume (ideally 40 ml CSF removal) lumbar puncture with a follow-up appointment approximately 24 hours for repeat testing. Pre- and post-LP scores are compared and VPS is recommended if there is 1) a > 20% overall improvement, 2) a > 25% improvement in any two single parameters (excluding FMMSE), and 3) a > 50% improvement in a single parameter (excluding FMMSE), or 4) the FMMSE score improves by ≥ 8 points.

32.4 Treatment

The treatment of NPH is permanent CSF diversion with a ventriculoperitoneal shunt (VPS) and a programmable valve. Favorable prognostic factors for VPS placement include symptoms for less than six months and, perhaps more significantly, gait disturbance as the earliest and dominant symptoms. Poor prognostic factors include more prolonged symptoms (> 2 years) and dementia preceding or being present without accompanying gait disturbance. Gait abnormalities are the most likely to respond to shunting, followed by cognitive function and urinary incontinence.

Although shunting can completely alleviate symptoms in some patients, more often these are only partially improved. Patients often experience a dramatic improvement immediately postoperatively, but then tend to deteriorate over time. This raises the question as to whether the correct diagnosis was made or is this regression simply a part of the natural aging process. One study found 75% of shunted NPH patients to have definite documented gait improvement after 3–6 months, but this number dropped to 50% at 1 year and to 33% at 3 years postoperatively.[4]

The risks of shunting include an approximately 3% rate of intracerebral hematoma formation, 2–17% rate of subdural hematomas, 3–6% risk of infection, 3–11% incidence of resultant seizures, and a 20% shunt revision rate over 5 years (▶ Fig. 32.2).[5] Therefore, the risk-to-benefit ratio must be individualized for each patient. The suspicion of shunt-responsive NPH must exist with reasonable certainty based on preoperative testing. There must be a low surgical risk rate related to a

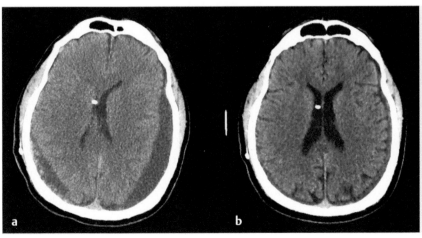

Fig. 32.2 Axial CT images after VPS placement with a programmable valve for NPH. **(a)** 1 month postoperatively showing over drainage and the formation of bilateral subdural hematomas. **(b)** 3 months postoperatively with adjustment in programmable valve showing improvement in extraaxial collections.

patient's comorbidities. Finally, the degree of NPH-related morbidity must warrant the shunt-related risks.

Although any neurosurgical intervention, including ventriculoperitoneal shunting, is associated with the potential for significant morbidity, some have cited the exorbitant estimated lifetime costs of custodial care, which have been estimated to be \$110,000–125,000, as enough reason to offer VPS to anyone suspected of having NPH.[6] Forgoing ancillary testing and proceeding to shunt insertion based on history, examination and imaging alone has been advocated. The reasons cited for such practice are that no screening test by itself is sufficiently specific and sensitive, testing is expensive, progressive dementia is devastating to patients and their caregivers, the cost of long-term institutional care is high, and the risk-benefit atio of modern shunt insertion is acceptably low.[7]

32.5 Conclusion

Suspicion for the presence of normal pressure hydrocephalus requires the identification of the classic triad of symptoms (gait disturbances, urinary incontinence, and dementia) but the realization that they are often not all present. The diagnosis must be confirmed through clinical exam and radiologic findings. Finally, surgical candidacy should be evaluated with a CSF withdrawal trial and some form of objective testing before and after the procedure. If treatment is deemed appropriate, ventriculoperitoneal shunting with a programmable valve is the intervention of choice.

References

[1] Iseki C, Kawanami T, Nagasawa H, et al. Asymptomatic ventriculomegaly with features of idiopathic normal pressure hydrocephalus on MRI (AVIM) in the elderly: a prospective study in a Japanese population. J Neurol Sci. 2009; 277 (1–2):54–57

[2] Chotai S, Medel R, Herial NA, Medhkour A. External lumbar drain: A pragmatic test for prediction of shunt outcomes in idiopathic normal pressure hydrocephalus. Surg Neurol Int. 2014; 5:12

[3] Eklund A, Smielewski P, Chambers I, et al. Assessment of cerebrospinal fluid outflow resistance. Med Biol Eng Comput. 2007; 45(8):719–735

[4] Klassen BT, Ahlskog JE. Normal pressure hydrocephalus: how often does the diagnosis hold water? Neurology. 2011; 77(12):1119–1125

[5] Toma AK, Papadopoulos MC, Stapleton S, Kitchen ND, Watkins LD. Systematic review of the outcome of shunt surgery in idiopathic normal-pressure hydrocephalus. Acta Neurochir (Wien). 2013; 155(10):1977–1980

[6] Stein SC, Burnett MG, Sonnad SS. Shunts in normal-pressure hydrocephalus: do we place too many or too few? J Neurosurg. 2006; 105(6):815–822

[7] Kameda M, Yamada S, Atsuchi M, et al. SINPHONI and SINPHONI-2 Investigators. Cost-effectiveness analysis of shunt surgery for idiopathic normal pressure hydrocephalus based on the SINPHONI and SINPHONI-2 trials. Acta Neurochir (Wien). 2017; 159(6):995–1003

33 Principles of Chronic Nociceptive and Neuropathic Pain

Michael D. Staudt and Jennifer A. Sweet

Abstract

In this chapter, we will briefly review the relevant anatomy of pain signal processing, as well as the gate control theory of pain. We will also discuss the transition from acute to chronic pain, the difference between nociceptive and neuropathic pain, and the principles of peripheral and central sensitization.

Keywords: acute pain, chronic pain, gate control theory, nociceptive pain, neuropathic pain, peripheral and central sensitization, pain transmission

33.1 Introduction

The pathophysiology of pain transmission and processing is complex and involves numerous peripheral and central components. Of course the physiological sensation of acute pain is an important protective response. Chronic pain no longer serves this physiological function. It is the result of plastic changes in the peripheral and central nervous system. As such, chronic pain can be considered a pathological disease state and not a symptom. In this chapter, we will briefly review the relevant anatomy of pain processing and the gate control theory, as well as discuss the differences between acute and chronic pain, nociceptive and neuropathic pain, and peripheral and central sensitization.

33.2 Pain Anatomy & The Gate Control Theory

Pain signals arise from free nerve endings and thermal receptors of the peripheral nervous system. It is transmitted by Aδ and C fibers, to the dorsal root ganglia, where the information is first processed. From the dorsal root ganglia, signals pass to the dorsolateral tract of Lissauer to synapse in the substantia gelatinosa of dorsal horn. Pain signals ultimately reach the brain through ascending pathways, most notably the anterior and lateral spinothalamic tracts, for cortical processing. Through different feedback mechanisms descending modulatory systems may alter these signals.

Acute pain protects the body from damaging stimuli. Chronic pain does not serve the same purpose. Can we understand how it comes about? Can we stop it from developing?

Much of our modern understanding of pain originates from the gate control theory of pain. The theory posits that interneurons within the substantia gelatinosa of the dorsal horns modulate pain signals before they are transmitted to the brain.[1] This revolutionary idea powered the development of neuromodulation for chronic pain. Spinal cord stimulation works, yet, the concept behind it does not adequately explain why or how chronic pain develops.[2]

33.3 Nociceptive and Neuropathic Pain

Nociceptive pain, or the detection of and response to noxious stimuli, refers to the peripheral pathway in which signals conveying non-neuronal tissue damage are transmitted to the central nervous system.[3] Primary afferent receptors, or nociceptors, are classified as somatic or visceral. Somatic nociceptors are located in cutaneous tissue, bone, joints and muscles, whereas visceral nociceptors are located in visceral structures and surrounding hollow organs. These primary afferents transmit signals to the dorsal horn of the spinal cord by two fiber types: Myelinated Aδ fibers conduct signals quickly and are responsible for pinprick sensation. Unmyelinated C fibers conduct signals slower. They signal burning, dull or itching pain.[4] Nociceptive information is then conducted to the brain via lateral and medial ascending pathways to reach the thalamus. The lateral thalamic relay projects to the somatosensory cortex and is involved in the sensory-discriminative component of pain, whereas the medial thalamic relay projects to the insula and cingulate cortex and is involved in the affective component of pain.[5]

Neuropathic pain derives from damage to nervous system structures or the nerves themselves. As such, pathological processes such as vascular and autoimmune diseases, malignancies and infections can lead to the onset of neuropathic pain.[6] Lesions that produce neuropathic pain invariably involve nociceptive pathways, resulting in aberrant pain signaling to various pain centers in the absence of ongoing noxious stimuli. In response to nervous system injury, microglia become activated and release various pro-inflammatory cytokines that alter normal synaptic function, causing disorganized connectivity and the ectopic generation of action potentials.[7]

33.4 The Transition from Acute to Chronic Pain

The transition from acute to chronic pain can be clinically defined as the ongoing presence of pain despite resolution of the initial tissue injury.[8] Traditionally, acute and chronic pain conditions were distinguished by fixed durations of time. These varied by practitioner definition and disease pathologies.[8] Such an approach is insufficient. It does not consider potential triggering mechanistic or cognitive factors, or the patient experience. Depressed mood, exposure to previous trauma, and negative pain beliefs all contribute to the development of chronic pain and disability.[9] Although targeting the cognitive factors of pain perception remain an essential component of multi-modal pain management, our understanding of the cellular and molecular mechanisms underlying chronic pain states is essential in the development of new therapeutic agents.

33.5 Peripheral and Central Sensitization

Pain signaling may become pathological as a result of continued stimulation and inflammation, leading to the development of allodynia (pain response secondary to a normally innocuous stimulus) or hyperalgesia (exaggerated pain response to stimulation).[10] The development of pathological pain and chronic pain states is dependent on plasticity at both the peripheral and central level, referred to as sensitization.

Peripheral sensitization is the result of tissue injury or inflammation, and refers to the decreased threshold for nociceptor activation and subsequent increased responsiveness to stimuli. Tissue injury results in the alteration of the local chemical environment of peripheral nociceptors, with an upregulation of inflammatory mediators including bradykinin, prostaglandins, and substance P. These mediators can directly sensitize nociceptors or induce downstream changes that potentiate receptor signaling and prolong nociceptor firing.[11] As the pain elicited by peripheral sensitization represents nociceptor activation, its effects are restricted to the site of injury.[11] It also has a primary role in thermal, but not mechanical sensitivity.[12]

Central sensitization refers to the increased excitability of central pain transmission pathways, most commonly involving the dorsal horn of the spinal cord. Glutamate, an excitatory neurotransmitter, is strongly expressed following injury and has an important role in pain signaling and the development of central sensitization.[4] Glutamate, in addition to co-regulatory neuropeptides and growth factors, is released from the presynaptic terminals (in this case primary afferent nociceptors) and binds to both ionotropic and metabotropic postsynaptic receptors, which depolarizes secondary afferents and causes a massive influx of intracellular calcium.[4,13] Calcium is a second messenger that contributes to the activation of downstream signaling; along with other transcriptional factors and protein kinase activation, their action subsequently alters gene expression and forms the molecular basis underlying central sensitization.[14] Both short and long-term sensitization mechanisms are responsible for inducing plasticity and the rearrangement of the spinal cord connections which relay pain signals.[4,6]

33.6 Conclusion

The processes described above are the beginnings of an explanation for the development of chronic pain conditions, both nociceptive and neuropathic in etiology. Understanding these mechanisms will be critical for discovering medical and surgical solutions. While the gate control theory was in many ways a launch pad for the field of neuromodulation, more descriptive theories of pain transmission must pave the way for future successes in the treatment of chronic pain.

References

[1] Melzack R, Wall PD. Pain mechanisms: a new theory. Science. 1965; 150 (3699):971–979

[2] Melzack R. Pain: past, present and future. Can J Exp Psychol. 1993; 47(4): 615–629

[3] Sherrington CS. The integrative action of the nervous system. New York: C. Scribner's Sons; 1906

[4] Woolf CJ, American College of Physicians, American Physiological Society. Pain: moving from symptom control toward mechanism-specific pharmacologic management. Ann Intern Med. 2004; 140(6):441–451

[5] Treede RD, Kenshalo DR, Gracely RH, Jones AK. The cortical representation of pain. Pain. 1999; 79(2–3):105–111

[6] Campbell JN, Meyer RA. Mechanisms of neuropathic pain. Neuron. 2006; 52 (1):77–92

[7] Costigan M, Scholz J, Woolf CJ. Neuropathic pain: a maladaptive response of the nervous system to damage. Annu Rev Neurosci. 2009; 32:1–32

[8] Reichling DB, Levine JD. Critical role of nociceptor plasticity in chronic pain. Trends Neurosci. 2009; 32(12):611–618

[9] Young Casey C, Greenberg MA, Nicassio PM, Harpin RE, Hubbard D. Transition from acute to chronic pain and disability: a model including cognitive, affective, and trauma factors. Pain. 2008; 134(1–2):69–79

[10] Treede RD, Meyer RA, Raja SN, Campbell JN. Peripheral and central mechanisms of cutaneous hyperalgesia. Prog Neurobiol. 1992; 38(4):397–421

[11] Hucho T, Levine JD. Signaling pathways in sensitization: toward a nociceptor cell biology. Neuron. 2007; 55(3):365–376

[12] Latremoliere A, Woolf CJ. Central sensitization: a generator of pain hypersensitivity by central neural plasticity. J Pain. 2009; 10(9):895–926

[13] Dougherty PM, Palecek J, Zorn S, Willis WD. Combined application of excitatory amino acids and substance P produces long-lasting changes in responses of primate spinothalamic tract neurons. Brain Res Brain Res Rev. 1993; 18(2): 227–246

[14] Kawasaki Y, Kohno T, Zhuang ZY, et al. Ionotropic and metabotropic receptors, protein kinase A, protein kinase C, and Src contribute to C-fiber-induced ERK activation and cAMP response element-binding protein phosphorylation in dorsal horn neurons, leading to central sensitization. J Neurosci. 2004; 24(38):8310–8321

34 Neuromodulation for Neuropathic Pain

Michael D. Staudt and Jonathan P. Miller

Abstract

Neuromodulation refers to the modification of normal nervous system activity by electrical stimulation or delivery of a pharmacological agent to the brain, spinal cord or peripheral nerves. It is the management of neuropathic pain that has benefited most from this innovation and spinal cord stimulation (SCS) is the most commonly used neuromodulation modality. Additional modes include intrathecal drug infusion, peripheral nerve, deep brain and motor cortex stimulation. This chapter provides a brief overview of neuromodulation in the treatment of chronic neuropathic pain, with a focus on the clinical indications and relevant evidence to support its use.

Keywords: neuromodulation, spinal cord stimulation, peripheral nerve stimulation, deep brain stimulation, motor cortex stimulation, intrathecal drug delivery, neuropathic pain

34.1 Introduction

The mechanistic basis of neuromodulation derives from the gate control pain theory, by which a non-noxious stimulus suppresses pain signaling.[1] The understanding that pain pathways can be modified in this manner has altered the focus of chronic pain treatment. The publication of two seminal studies has led to reversible neuromodulation replacing ablation as a standard of care. Shealy et al., published their work on dorsal column or spinal cord stimulation in 1967.[2] That same year Wall and Sweet introduced the concept of peripheral nerve stimulation (PNS).[3] Additional therapeutic modes that have since been studied are: deep brain stimulation (DBS), motor cortex stimulation (MCS), and intrathecal (IT) drug delivery. The technology behind neuromodulation continues to improve and the indications for its use have expanded and diversified.

34.2 Spinal Cord Stimulation

SCS is most effective in the treatment of neuropathic extremity pain. It is generally ineffective for nociceptive pain, except for ischemic injury pain. The benefit in ischemic pain may be from improved blood flow and not altered pain pathways.[4] SCS improves quality-of-life and pain levels in patients with failed back surgery syndrome, or complex regional pain syndrome.[5,6] Most studies of SCS are retrospective and show time related diminishing effectiveness.[7] Yet, at least 50% of patients remain satisfied with the quality of their pain relief.[8]

SCS use in the treatment of chronic pain is FDA-approved in the United States. The stimulus source is either a percutaneously placed epidural lead or surgically-placed paddle (▶ Fig. 34.1). Standard stimulation is at a tonic frequency of 40–80 Hz. Paresthesia-free stimulation is a recently introduced concept in the field. It has the potential to improve the treatment of axial neuropathic pain and salvage patients who do not respond to conventional SCS.[9,10] Dorsal root ganglion stimulation also has the potential to provide targeted modulation in the treatment of focal neuropathic or nociceptive pain.[11]

34.3 Peripheral Nerve Stimulation

The most common PNS modality is percutaneous occipital nerve stimulation (ONS) for occipital neuralgia.[12] Although most studies contain small patient populations without a control or comparison group, significant and sustained pain alleviation is consistently described.[13] Additional indications for the use of PNS include ONS for chronic migraine, sphenopalatine ganglion stimulation for cluster headaches, trigeminal neuralgia, post-stroke central pain and post-herpetic neuralgia.[14,15,16] Peripheral nerve field stimulation, or the targeting of a non-dermatomal areas of pain with a subcutaneously inserted electrode has been described in the treatment of low back, chest and abdominal wall and joint pain.[16]

PNS implantation is done by percutaneous insertion techniques that are relatively simple procedures with a low risk of injuring neurovascular structures and few absolute contraindications. There is great interest in the development of new such stimulation devices and to define appropriate and broad clinical indications. However, most PNS devices are not FDA-approved and are used off-label.

34.4 Deep Brain Stimulation

The most common targets for intracranial stimulation with DBS are the sensory thalamus and periventricular-periaqueductal gray (PVG-PAG), which are targeted for the treatment of neuropathic and nociceptive pain respectively.[17,18] Patients may have electrodes directed to both targets concurrently. Sensory thalamus stimulation has been used for facial anesthesia dolorosa, post-stroke central pain and phantom limb pain.[17,19] However, the early effects of stimulation eventually wane, suggesting that the initial therapeutic effect may be related to electrode insertion.[20] The therapeutic effects of PVG-PAG stimulation on antinociception has been hypothesized to be mediated by endorphin release, but likely encompass both opioid and non-opioid mechanisms.[18]

The clinical efficacy of DBS as a pain treatment modality has been debated, although results may be dependent on clinical indication and appropriate patient selection.[21,22] PVG-PAG stimulation is susceptible to the phenomenon of tolerance, and higher stimulation parameters are necessary over time to achieve the same therapeutic effect.[23] Also, nociceptive pain responds better than deafferentation or neuropathic pain.[22] Currently, the use of DBS in the treatment of pain is not FDA-approved and is considered off-label.

34.5 Motor Cortex Stimulation

MCS was developed in response to the inadequacy of DBS in treating central deafferentation pain syndromes, including

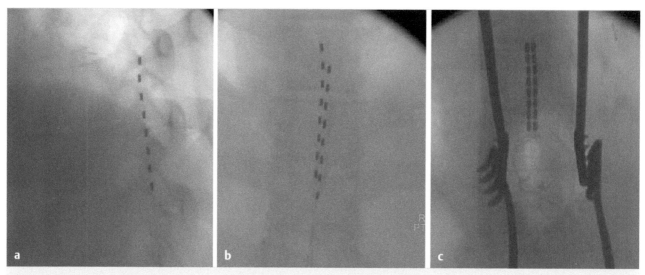

Fig. 34.1 Intraoperative fluoroscopy demonstrating placement of thoracic epidural spinal cord stimulator electrodes for the treatment of post-laminectomy syndrome. Lateral (**a**) and anteroposterior (**b**) radiographs demonstrate percutaneouselectrode placement at the top of the T8 vertebral body during a trial (**a**; single electrode confirmed in a dorsal position) and for permanent implantation (**b**; two electrodes). Anteroposterior radiograph demonstrating placement of 2 × 8 epidural paddle lead overlying the T7–8 vertebra via thoracic laminotomy (**c**).

post-stroke central pain and trigeminal neuropathic pain.[24,25] These are refractory to most conservative and interventional management paradigms. Additional indications include phantom limb pain, and pain related to peripheral nerve injury or spinal cord injury.[26]

MCS is one of the few effective treatment paradigms for central deafferentation pain. 50% to 75% of patients achieve significant pain relief.[27] However, the benefit is often lost over time, and restoration of adequate stimulation parameters requires reprogramming.[28] Accordingly, the maintenance of long-term pain relief is inconsistent.[29] Stimulus amplitude and frequency, pulse width adjustment should be adjusted with care, since seizures may be induced when energy input is increased during programming.[28] Similar to DBS for pain, the use of MCS for pain relief is an off-label application of a device otherwise approved for human implantation, and not FDA-approved.

34.6 Intrathecal Drug Delivery

IT drug therapy is widely used for the treatment of chronic refractory neuropathic or nociceptive pain. The FDA has approved two IT agents for pain treatment. These are: the opioid, morphine, and a non-opioid calcium channel antagonist, ziconotide. Baclofen (a $GABA_B$ receptor agonist) is FDA-approved for the treatment of spasticity, but is used off-label by some practitioners in a multi-modal pain treatment strategy. Numerous other IT drug therapies such as local anesthetics, other opioids and adrenergic agonists are used off-label as monotherapies or in combination therapy to synergistically target differing pain receptors.[30]

IT morphine has fewer and less serious side effects than systemic opioids.[30] Normally, IT morphine infusion is first tried alone. Other agents are added in steps if the initial pain control is inadequate. Ziconotide may be used as a first line drug or as an adjunct. It is often useful in patients with neuropathic pain

that is refractory to opioid therapy.[31] Its use in combination with IT morphine to treat cancer and non-cancer related pain is safe and efficacious.[32] When using multiple agents, it is important to carefully consider the dosing of each individual drug due to their unique therapeutic window and complication profile.

34.7 Conclusion

Indications for neuromodulation have expanded to encompass a variety of neuropathic pain syndromes. Implantable technology has become more sophisticated. Smaller and easier to use devices now exist and this has led to further clinical interest and wider use by a variety of practitioners. However, the field requires more well designed, prospective studies to best define the clinical indications and patient populations to achieve the greatest benefit from this innovative technology

References

[1] Melzack R, Wall PD. Pain mechanisms: a new theory. Science. 1965; 150 (3699):971–979

[2] Shealy CN, Mortimer JT, Reswick JB. Electrical inhibition of pain by stimulation of the dorsal columns: preliminary clinical report. Anesth Analg. 1967; 46(4):489–491

[3] Wall PD, Sweet WH. Temporary abolition of pain in man. Science. 1967; 155 (3758):108–109

[4] Cook AW, Oygar A, Baggenstos P, Pacheco S, Kleriga E. Vascular disease of extremities. Electric stimulation of spinal cord and posterior roots. N Y State J Med. 1976; 76(3):366–368

[5] Kumar K, Taylor RS, Jacques L, et al. Spinal cord stimulation versus conventional medical management for neuropathic pain: a multicentre randomised controlled trial in patients with failed back surgery syndrome. Pain. 2007; 132(1–2):179–188

[6] Kemler MA, Barendse GA, van Kleef M, et al. Spinal cord stimulation in patients with chronic reflex sympathetic dystrophy. N Engl J Med. 2000; 343 (9):618–624

[7] Kemler MA, de Vet HC, Barendse GA, van den Wildenberg FA, van Kleef M. Effect of spinal cord stimulation for chronic complex regional pain syndrome

Type I: five-year final follow-up of patients in a randomized controlled trial. J Neurosurg. 2008; 108(2):292–298

[8] Kumar K, Hunter G, Demeria D. Spinal cord stimulation in treatment of chronic benign pain: challenges in treatment planning and present status, a 22-year experience. Neurosurgery. 2006; 58(3):481–496, discussion 481–496

[9] Van Buyten JP, Al-Kaisy A, Smet I, Palmisani S, Smith T. High-frequency spinal cord stimulation for the treatment of chronic back pain patients: results of a prospective multicenter European clinical study. Neuromodulation. 2013; 16 (1):59–65, discussion 65–66

[10] de Vos CC, Bom MJ, Vanneste S, Lenders MW, de Ridder D. Burst spinal cord stimulation evaluated in patients with failed back surgery syndrome and painful diabetic neuropathy. Neuromodulation. 2014; 17(2):152–159

[11] Liem L, Russo M, Huygen FJ, et al. One-year outcomes of spinal cord stimulation of the dorsal root ganglion in the treatment of chronic neuropathic pain. Neuromodulation. 2015; 18(1):41–48, discussion 48–49

[12] Weiner RL, Reed KL. Peripheral neurostimulation for control of intractable occipital neuralgia. Neuromodulation. 1999; 2(3):217–221

[13] Sweet JA, Mitchell LS, Narouze S, et al. Occipital Nerve Stimulation for the Treatment of Patients With Medically Refractory Occipital Neuralgia: Congress of Neurological Surgeons Systematic Review and Evidence-Based Guideline. Neurosurgery. 2015; 77(3):332–341

[14] Saper JR, Dodick DW, Silberstein SD, McCarville S, Sun M, Goadsby PJ, ONSTIM Investigators. Occipital nerve stimulation for the treatment of intractable chronic migraine headache: ONSTIM feasibility study. Cephalalgia. 2011; 31(3):271–285

[15] Schoenen J, Jensen RH, Lantéri-Minet M, et al. Stimulation of the sphenopalatine ganglion (SPG) for cluster headache treatment. Pathway CH-1: a randomized, sham-controlled study. Cephalalgia. 2013; 33(10):816–830

[16] Deer TR, Krames E, Mekhail N, et al. Neuromodulation Appropriateness Consensus Committee. The appropriate use of neurostimulation: new and evolving neurostimulation therapies and applicable treatment for chronic pain and selected disease states. Neuromodulation. 2014; 17(6):599–615, discussion 615

[17] Hosobuchi Y, Adams JE, Rutkin B. Chronic thalamic stimulation for the control of facial anesthesia dolorosa. Arch Neurol. 1973; 29(3):158–161

[18] Richardson DE, Akil H. Long term results of periventricular gray self-stimulation. Neurosurgery. 1977; 1(2):199–202

[19] Mazars G, Merienne L, Cioloca C. [Treatment of certain types of pain with implantable thalamic stimulators]. Neurochirurgie. 1974; 20(2):117–124

[20] Hamani C, Schwalb JM, Rezai AR, Dostrovsky JO, Davis KD, Lozano AM. Deep brain stimulation for chronic neuropathic pain: long-term outcome and the incidence of insertional effect. Pain. 2006; 125(1–2):188–196

[21] Coffey RJ. Deep brain stimulation for chronic pain: results of two multicenter trials and a structured review. Pain Med. 2001; 2(3):183–192

[22] Bittar RG, Kar-Purkayastha I, Owen SL, et al. Deep brain stimulation for pain relief: a meta-analysis. J Clin Neurosci. 2005; 12(5):515–519

[23] Kumar K, Toth C, Nath RK. Deep brain stimulation for intractable pain: a 15-year experience. Neurosurgery. 1997; 40(4):736–746, discussion 746–747

[24] Tsubokawa T, Katayama Y, Yamamoto T, Hirayama T, Koyama S. Chronic motor cortex stimulation for the treatment of central pain. Acta Neurochir Suppl (Wien). 1991; 52:137–139

[25] Meyerson BA, Lindblom U, Linderoth B, Lind G, Herregodts P. Motor cortex stimulation as treatment of trigeminal neuropathic pain. Acta Neurochir Suppl (Wien). 1993; 58:150–153

[26] Brown JA, Barbaro NM. Motor cortex stimulation for central and neuropathic pain: current status. Pain. 2003; 104(3):431–435

[27] Monsalve GA. Motor cortex stimulation for facial chronic neuropathic pain: A review of the literature. Surg Neurol Int. 2012; 3 Suppl 4:S290–S311

[28] Henderson JM, Boongird A, Rosenow JM, LaPresto E, Rezai AR. Recovery of pain control by intensive reprogramming after loss of benefit from motor cortex stimulation for neuropathic pain. Stereotact Funct Neurosurg. 2004; 82 (5–6):207–213

[29] Sachs AJ, Babu H, Su YF, Miller KJ, Henderson JM. Lack of efficacy of motor cortex stimulation for the treatment of neuropathic pain in 14 patients. Neuromodulation. 2014; 17(4):303–310, discussion 310–311

[30] Deer TR, Pope JE, Hayek SM, et al. The Polyanalgesic Consensus Conference (PACC): Recommendations on Intrathecal Drug Infusion Systems Best Practices and Guidelines. Neuromodulation. 2017; 20(2):96–132

[31] Staats PS, Yearwood T, Charapata SG, et al. Intrathecal ziconotide in the treatment of refractory pain in patients with cancer or AIDS: a randomized controlled trial. JAMA. 2004; 291(1):63–70

[32] Alicino I, Giglio M, Manca F, Bruno F, Puntillo F. Intrathecal combination of ziconotide and morphine for refractory cancer pain: a rapidly acting and effective choice. Pain. 2012; 153(1):245–249

35 Spinal Cord Stimulation Using High Frequency and Burst Waveform Variation

Jeffrey E. Arle

Abstract

This chapter will review the burst and high frequency waveform patterns that may be used during spinal stimulation for pain, their mechanisms of action and clinical basis for use. Also to be reviewed will be closed loop systems that are based on evoked compound action potentials.

Keywords: waveform, burst, high frequency, ecaps, spinal cord stimulation

35.1 Introduction

Spinal cord stimulation (SCS) is widely used to treat chronic neuropathic pain disorders and to a lesser extent heart failure, cardiac arrhythmia, paraplegia, and peripheral vasculopathy. In 1967 C. Norman Shealy, MD published a preliminary study on the treatment of pain by dorsal column stimulation. He described stimulation frequencies of 10–50 Hz, a pulse width of 400 µs and an amplitude of 1V. Waveforms have varied little in the half century since that initial paper and consist of charge-balanced biphasic square-waves at frequencies of 40–200 Hz. Pulse-widths have ranged between 50 and 300 µs. Class I studies have confirmed that such waveforms are effective for the treatment of what has been labeled as failed back surgery syndrome (FBSS) and complex regional pain syndrome (CRPS). However, additional work performed in the past decade has shown that other patterns may be more efficacious and engage other features of the underlying neural circuitry.

First- why does SCS treat neuropathic and not nociceptive pain?

SCS is thought to activate larger axons (> 10µm) located in the periphery of the dorsal columns. The retrograde action potentials generated by stimuli in these larger fibers then reverberate into the dorsal horn circuitry. They activate dorsal horn inter-neuronal pools that inhibit the wide dynamic range neurons carrying pain signals. When nociceptive fibers are activated in the periphery, the circuitry activated by SCS is inhibited, allowing the nociceptive pain signals to continue cephalad.

When larger axons are activated by SCS waveforms, anterograde action potentials are generated. These fibers are responsible for vibration sensation and activation of them is the basis for the perception of paresthesias. While this general mechanistic theory explains the majority of the findings in SCS, it does not explain why SCS may fail to relieve pain. Large fibers represent only one percent of the dorsal column fiber population. Capturing enough of them in the target dermatomes may not be possible with typical programming paradigms if, for example, localized scar tissue is extensive or the cerebrospinal fluid space is wider. Adjacent, untargeted areas may be also be stimulated causing unintended sensations.

35.1.1 Burst Stimulation

Before 2007, Dirk De Ridder, MD in Antwerp, Belgium had only used burst stimulation directed towards the auditory cortex for the treatment of intractable tinnitus. Tonotopic lemniscal auditory pathways fire with tonic signaling. The physiologic response to tonic signalling is slow and possibly graded. Action potentials may be produced throughout the period of stimulation. Extra-lemniscal auditory pathways use signaling bursts. Burst firing is a more powerful activation of the cerebral cortex than tonic firing. Bursting techniques are now being adapted to SCS based on how medial and lateral pain pathways use tonic and burst signaling at the thalamic level. The burst SCS signal (Burst-DR™ St. Jude Medical, Inc., St. Paul, MN) consists of five rectangular pulses at 500 Hz with a PW of one msec and bursting every 25 msec, (40 Hz). The bursts have a shaped envelope and charge balanced portion (▶ Fig. 35.1). The 1 msec pulse-width is much longer more than typical neuromodulation signals. It has been clinically compared to tonic 500 Hz signals. However, if the tonic signal has a < 500µsec pulse-width and subthreshold stimulation is used, it is thought to be comparable to 10,000 Hz high frequency stimulation. Such stimulation appears to be at least equal to traditional SCS parameters and can recover benefit in patients who have failed traditional SCS. Burst stimulation with epidural SCS, does not cause vibratory paresthesias at therapeutic amplitude levels. Paresthesia-free stimuli seem to be better tolerated and the mechanism for its effectiveness and how that mechanism could be optimized is yet to be known.

35.1.2 High Frequency Stimulation

High frequency stimulation, using 10 kHz (HF10, Senza system; Nevro Corp., Redwood City, CA) has been shown to give equal or superior results for pain relief when compared to traditional, lower frequency stimulation. In the large randomized controlled trial (SENZA-RCT) twice as many patients responded to HF-10 than to traditional SCS for back and leg pain. Patients also do not feel paresthesias with high frequency stimulation.

Is the reason for the absence of paresthesias the same with Burst and HF-10?

Are the mechanisms of pain relief the same between Burst and HF-10?

These are fundamental and unanswered questions for which answers need be sought in order to optimize their use and to develop new opportunities for the use of these waveforms in SCS treatment.

35.2 Burst and Burst-DR

▶ Fig. 35.1 shows the waveform for Burst-DR™. There are several unique features to it. The biphasic square wave is charge balanced between bursts and not during the burst. This allows

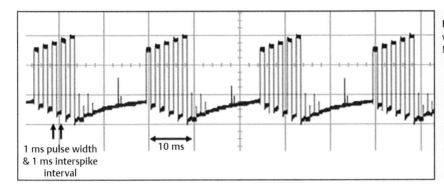

Fig. 35.1 Waveform for burst-DRTM. Reproduced with permission from De Ridder et al, 2010, Neurosurgery; and 2013, World Neurosurgery.

1 ms pulse width & 1 ms interspike interval

10 ms

for a cathodic offset during the burst. This may be important because of the lengthy, one msec, pulse width present. Traditional SCS pulse width ranges from 100–300µs. The anodic and cathodic amplitudes of the pulses progressively increase within each burst. It is not known how much such elements affect pain relief. In one study Nathan Crosby, PhD, at The University of Pennsylvania, analyzed recordings from high-threshold and wide dynamic range neurons (WDR) in the rat dorsal horn. WDR neurons can undergo "wind up" a phenomenon that allows response intensity to increase with increasing stimulus frequency. Crosby varied burst stimuli parameters such as the number of burst pulses, pulse frequency, pulse-width, burst frequency, and amplitude. As pulse-width increased from 250µs to 1000µs greater reduction of WDR firing occurred. When the number of pulses per burst increased by up to seven pulses/burst, the firing rate of WDR neurons was further reduced. If pulse frequency was increased up to 500 Hz and amplitude increased up to 90% of threshold, WDR firing rate was progressively reduced. One can conclude that the pulse-width is a significant factor. However, Schu et al.. used a tonic stimulus of 500 Hz and varied the pulse-width based on what pulse-width was needed to maintain stimulation below threshold. This is important because it may be that the delayed charge-balancing of the burst and the longer pulse-width creates an effect on axons within the dorsal column that does not occur with tonic stimulation. Moreover, when patients were treated with tonic 500 Hz stimulation, the stimulation was also below threshold. This implies that activation of larger diameter fibers in the dorsal columns was inadequate, and they were unlikely to obtain adequate pain benefit. Those patients in the tonic group had less pain relief than the lower frequency tonic patients and almost equivalent relief to those in the placebo group. In further support of this analysis, a recent study by Kriek et al., compared 40 Hz, 500 Hz, 1200 Hz and Burst-DR paradigms to treat CRPS. Here, tonic stimuli were programmed to generate paresthesias in the painful areas when they activated larger axons. The study showed no difference between any of the groups in the ability to lessen pain, and there was no preference for the non-paresthesia, burst stimuli. Finally, another study in rats by Crosby et al,. suggested that there was a difference between tonic and burst stimulation using GABA circuitry to obtain pain reduction. GABA antagonists in tonic mode blocked the effects but not in burst conditions.

Clinical findings using the standard Burst-DR waveform have been more promising. Two-year evaluation period data are not available from the Sunburst study but earlier data presented at the 2016 North American Neuromodulation Society meeting, by Dr. Timothy Deer, indicated significant reductions in VAS pain scores over traditional SCS. The magnitude of that difference, though statistically significant, was only 5 mm on a 100 mm scale (43.5 vs 48.7). This is not appreciable to the average patient. Studies have shown that a pain reduction by13 points or less on the scale is not clinically discernible. The original premise of DeRidder that the medial pain pathways, synapsing more predominantly in the anterior insula, might respond better to bursts of action potentials rather than more regular patterns, is to some degree borne out by standardized low resolution brain electromagnetic tomography analysis (sLORETA) study data. sLORETA is an accurate brain localization tool. These data show that patients treated with these waveforms seem to activate centers in the brain within those pathways, but those centers are not activated using non-burst patterns of stimuli. These findings are thought to support the idea that the subjective aspects of pain may be modulated more by burst stimuli. There were only five patients and none of the patients achieved the minimum of 50% pain reduction with either tonic or burst paradigms. Moreover, although each paradigm produced pain improvement, burst had a greater effect. It could be that the sLORETA changes occurred because of the amount of pain benefit and were not related to the pathways activated by the stimuli.

There remain unanswered questions regarding the underlying mechanisms of action for Burst-DR, and while some subjective aspects of pain processing may account for effects of burst, it is likely there are influences from activation of the dorsal column axons and their effect on the dorsal horn circuitry, just as with traditional SCS. These potential effects need to be further elucidated.

35.2.1 High Frequency Stimulation

High frequency refers to SCS at frequencies above 2–3 kHz. Traditional, tonic stimulation has been used at frequencies below 1 kHz. For purposes of this discussion, even frequencies up to the limits of many implanted pulse generators (1200 Hz) will not be considered to be high frequencies. The rationale for this distinction is that there are likely fundamental differences in what occurs at the axonal membrane in dorsal column fibers at these multi-kilohertz oscillations since such rapid alterations of the field encroach on the time constants of the ionic channels themselves. Currently, the only system available for this form of stimulation is the HF-10 system from Nevro, Inc. It uses a charge-balanced 10 kHz waveform. The waveform itself is not a

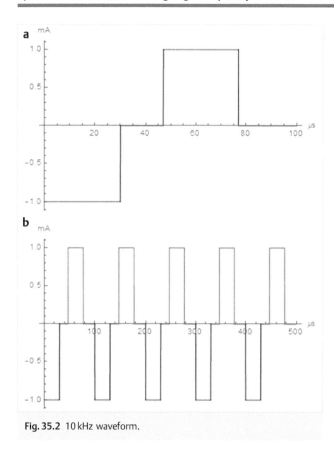

Fig. 35.2 10 kHz waveform.

simple, iterative charge-balanced square-wave, however, but instead has two flat pauses, differing in the amount of time and also separating cathode and anode phases (▶ Fig. 35.2).

The HF-10 therapy yields a paresthesia-free stimulus like Burst-DR, but has several other properties. Unlike tonic stimulation paradigms, HF-10 doesn't lead to pain relief until about 24–72 hours after the onset of stimulation. Amplitudes are in the 0.5–2mA range (most other SCS paradigms utilize between 2 and 5mA), and there is little correlation between where the electrode is located in the medial to lateral plane and how much benefit the patient obtains. Moreover, the best results seem to come from using a longitudinal bipole electrode configuration straddling the T9–10 disk space, regardless of whether the patient has mostly back pain or leg pain or where their spinal cord ends (e.g. within T12-L2). None of these characteristics are either observed or required of the other stimulus types (i.e. traditional tonic or Burst-DR).

The Senza-RCT study consisted of a prospective, randomized review of results with a two-year evaluation period in which 77% of patients had 70% relief in back pain and 73% had 65% relief of leg pain. Despite expert programming of the traditional stimulation patients, the responders with traditional stimulation achieved only 49% relief for back or leg coverage. In responders using traditional stimulation, the benefit only reached 41% and 46% pain reduction for back and leg, respectively. This suggests that traditional stimulation is less than 50% successful, yet the criteria for even placing the permanent system following a trial of stimulation is at least 50% pain relief. Thus, either the patient selection criteria were particularly stringent in this study or patients were not selected well at all. This would

undermine either the credibility of the results, or the programming of the patients. Neither of these conclusions seems likely. These results were after two-years of treatment, so one might expect that some benefit from traditional SCS may have been lost. However, analyzing the first year follow-up results shows this was not the case. Results at one year were virtually identical with traditional stimulation, yielding less than 50% benefit; for back or leg, 44% and 49%, respectively. In general, pain relief decreases between 60 and 85% are to be expected with stimulation for back and leg pain,

These concerns notwithstanding, HF-10 does seem to be comparable to traditional stimulation and should be considered as a reasonable alternative or first-line offering. Many patients would prefer not to feel paresthesias. Moreover, it may turn out that some patients respond to one type of therapy, and not as well or at all to others. Even in the same patient, over time, one therapy type may work for a while and then be supplanted by a different one, possibly even avoiding the significant potential of 'tolerance' to therapy by cycling through the different waveforms more rapidly, by the minute, hour, day, or longer cycle timeframes.

The mechanism by which HF-10 therapy does yield pain relief, like Burst-DR, is not well understood. The stimulation has either a direct or indirect effect on neurons within the dorsal horn, somehow then affecting the WDR neurons or other dorsal horn processing of pain. The indirect hypothesis suggests that, like traditional SCS mechanisms, there is a modification of dorsal column axons, both suppression and excitation, which leads to eventual 'indirect' inhibition of WDR neurons. There may be a combination of these mechanisms at work as well. Several questions need to be addressed by each hypothesis for further progress to be made. These are:

For the 'direct' hypothesis:

1. If electrodes are used only at the T9–10 disk interspace, given the weak field generated by HF-10, how can the dorsal horn neurons affected by the stimulation account for pain relief in other regions not involving neurons at the T9–10 dorsal horn (e.g. foot or lower leg, whose cells are generally located at segments below the T9–10 area and in the conus medullaris)?

2. For the same reason, how would an electrode over the right T9–10 dorsal horn have much affect at all on the *left* dorsal horn neurons? Current findings with HF-10, clinically, suggest that using paresthesia mapping of the electrode shows it can be predominantly on one side of the spinal cord and yet yield bilateral pain relief.

3. How is activity in the dorsal horn using HF-10 known to be 'direct' and not related to indirect effects of dorsal column axons, for example, modulating the dorsal horn neurons? Studies suggesting effects on dorsal horn neurons have not isolated them from the rest of the circuitry or eliminated the potential input from dorsal column axons, as occurs in the indirect theory. In fact, the activity of any dorsal horn neurons with HF-10 without such isolation would support either hypothesis.

4. What basis is there for such miniscule fields that HF-10 creates in the dorsal horn having any effect on neuronal cell bodies, ion channels, synapses or axons?

5. What basis would there be with a 'direct' effect to explain the delays seen in yielding pain benefit of typically over 24–48 hours?

For the 'indirect' hypothesis:

1. The effects of HF-10 on dorsal column axons suggest suppression of large diameter axons and excitation of medium and smaller axons, but only if there is a relatively monophasic field reaching the dorsal column. What is the basis for such a transformation given that the HF-10 waveform is essentially charge balanced?
2. If large fibers are used in traditional SCS to inhibit WDR neurons, what is the basis of medium and smaller fibers having the same final common pathway?
3. How can the lack of recordings in the nucleus gracilis during HF-10 stimulation be explained if some axons are thought to be firing action potentials?
4. How can the delay in therapeutic benefit with the 'indirect' hypothesis be explained?
5. How can broad dermatomal pain benefit be explained using an 'indirect' mechanism?
6. How can the low amplitudes used in HF-10 yield the activity in the dorsal column axons required for the 'indirect' hypothesis?

35.3 State of the Art and the Future of Waveform Development

While we are seeing some advantages of newer waveforms (Burst-DR and HF-10) it seems likely that those will be refined further and other paradigms will emerge in the marketplace. Closed loop systems, for example, where real-time variation in the delivered stimulus can be achieved with enhanced feedback from the activation of actual targeted axons in the dorsal column, could give even more robust and reliable therapeutic benefit. Such a system is already in development. The Evoke™ SCS system(Saluda Medical, Artarmon, Australia) uses evoked compound action potentials (ECAPs) recorded at the superior end of the epidural electrode for feedback (▶ Fig. 35.3).

Early results suggest that pain relief may extend into the 90% or greater range. Nonetheless by understanding the mechanisms by which these waveforms function we will continue to enhance the care of patients in chronic pain.

Suggested Readings

[1] Eldridge P, Simpson BA, Gilbart J. The Role of Rechargeable Systems in Neuromodulation. Eur Neurol Rev. 2011; 6(3):187–192

[2] Shils JL, Arle JE. Intraoperative neurophysiologic methods for spinal cord stimulator placement under general anesthesia. Neuromodulation. 2012; 15 (6):560–571, discussion 571–572

[3] Shealy CN, Mortimer JT, Reswick JB. Electrical inhibition of pain by stimulation of the dorsal columns: preliminary clinical report. Anesth Analg. 1967; 46(4):489–491

[4] Kumar K, Taylor RS, Jacques L, et al. Spinal cord stimulation versus conventional medical management for neuropathic pain: a multicentre randomised controlled trial in patients with failed back surgery syndrome. Pain. 2007; 132(1–2):179–188

[5] North RB, Kidd D, Shipley J, Taylor RS. Spinal cord stimulation versus reoperation for failed back surgery syndrome: a cost effectiveness and cost utility analysis based on a randomized, controlled trial. Neurosurgery. 2007; 61(2): 361–368, discussion 368–369

[6] Kemler MA, Raphael JH, Bentley A, Taylor RS. The cost-effectiveness of spinal cord stimulation for complex regional pain syndrome. Value Health. 2010; 13 (6):735–742

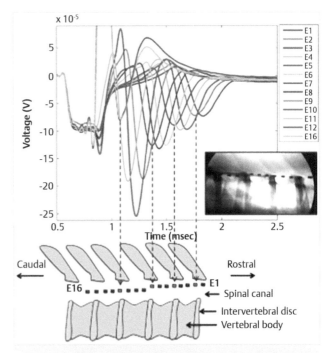

Fig. 35.3 The Evoke SCS systeme uses (ECAPs) recorded at the superior end of the epidural electrode for feedback.

[7] Arle JE, Carlson KW, Mei L, Iftimia N, Shils JL. Mechanism of dorsal column stimulation to treat neuropathic but not nociceptive pain: analysis with a computational model. Neuromodulation. 2014; 17(7):642–655, discussion 655

[8] Krauthamer V. Modulation of conduction at points of axonal bifurcation by applied electric fields. IEEE Trans Biomed Eng. 1990; 37(5):515–519

[9] Struijk JJ, Holsheimer J, van der Heide GG, Boom HBK. Recruitment of dorsal column fibers in spinal cord stimulation: influence of collateral branching. IEEE Trans Biomed Eng. 1992; 39(9):903–912

[10] Grill WM, Cantrell MB, Robertson MS. Antidromic propagation of action potentials in branched axons: implications for the mechanisms of action of deep brain stimulation. J Comput Neurosci. 2008; 24(1):81–93

[11] Arle JE, Mei L, Carlson KW, Shils JL. High-Frequency Stimulation of Dorsal Column Axons: Potential Underlying Mechanism of Paresthesia-Free Neuropathic Pain Relief. Neuromodulation. 2016; 19(4):385–397

[12] Arle JE, Carlson KW, Mei L, Shils JL. Modeling effects of scar on patterns of dorsal column stimulation. Neuromodulation. 2014; 17(4):320–333, discussion 333

[13] De Ridder D, van der Loo E, Van der Kelen K, Menovsky T, van de Heyning P, Moller A. Do tonic and burst TMS modulate the lemniscal and extralemniscal system differently? Int J Med Sci. 2007; 4(5):242–246

[14] Schu S, Slotty PJ, Bara G, von Knop M, Edgar D, Vesper J. A prospective, randomised, double-blind, placebo-controlled study to examine the effectiveness of burst spinal cord stimulation patterns for the treatment of failed back surgery syndrome. Neuromodulation. 2014; 17(5):443–450

[15] De Ridder D, Vanneste S, Plazier M, van der Loo E, Menovsky T. Burst spinal cord stimulation: toward paresthesia-free pain suppression. Neurosurgery. 2010; 66(5):986–990

[16] De Ridder D, Plazier M, Kamerling N, Menovsky T, Vanneste S. Burst spinal cord stimulation for limb and back pain. World Neurosurg. 2013; 80(5):642–649.e1

[17] de Vos CC, Bom MJ, Vanneste S, Lenders MW, de Ridder D. Burst spinal cord stimulation evaluated in patients with failed back surgery syndrome and painful diabetic neuropathy. Neuromodulation. 2014; 17(2):152–159

[18] Tiede J, Brown L, Gekht G, Vallejo R, Yearwood T, Morgan D. Novel spinal cord stimulation parameters in patients with predominant back pain. Neuromodulation. 2013; 16(4):370–375

[19] Van Buyten JP, Al-Kaisy A, Smet I, Palmisani S, Smith T. High-frequency spinal cord stimulation for the treatment of chronic back pain patients: results of a

prospective multicenter European clinical study. Neuromodulation. 2013; 16 (1):59–65, discussion 65–66

[20] Al-Kaisy A, Van Buyten JP, Smet I, Palmisani S, Pang D, Smith T. Sustained effectiveness of 10 kHz high-frequency spinal cord stimulation for patients with chronic, low back pain: 24-month results of a prospective multicenter study. Pain Med. 2014; 15(3):347–354

[21] Kapural L, Yu C, Doust MW, et al. Novel 10-kHz High-frequency Therapy (HF10 Therapy) Is Superior to Traditional Low-frequency Spinal Cord Stimulation for the Treatment of Chronic Back and Leg Pain: The SENZA-RCT Randomized Controlled Trial. Anesthesiology. 2015; 123(4):851–860

[22] Kapural L, Yu C, Doust MW, et al. Comparison of 10-kHz High-Frequency and Traditional Low-Frequency Spinal Cord Stimulation for the Treatment of Chronic Back and Leg Pain: 24-Month Results From a Multicenter, Randomized, Controlled Pivotal Trial. Neurosurgery. 2016; 79(5):667–677

[23] Crosby ND, Goodman Keiser MD, Smith JR, Zeeman ME, Winkelstein BA. Stimulation parameters define the effectiveness of burst spinal cord stimulation in a rat model of neuropathic pain. Neuromodulation. 2015; 18(1):1–8,–discussion 8

[24] Kriek N, Groeneweg JG, Stronks DL, de Ridder D, Huygen FJ. Preferred frequencies and waveforms for spinal cord stimulation in patients with complex regional pain syndrome: A multicentre, double-blind, randomized and placebo-controlled crossover trial. Eur J Pain. 2017; 21(3):507–519

[25] Crosby ND, Weisshaar CL, Smith JR, Zeeman ME, Goodman-Keiser MD, Winkelstein BA. Burst and Tonic Spinal Cord Stimulation Differentially Activate GABAergic Mechanisms to Attenuate Pain in a Rat Model of Cervical Radiculopathy. IEEE Trans Biomed Eng. 2015; 62(6):1604–1613

[26] Deer SUNBURST NANS. 2016 – results at https://clinicaltrials.gov/ct2/show/results/NCT02011893?sect=X01256#all

[27] Tashjian RZ, Deloach J, Porucznik CA, Powell AP. Minimal clinically important differences (MCID) and patient acceptable symptomatic state (PASS) for visual analog scales (VAS) measuring pain in patients treated for rotator cuff disease. J Shoulder Elbow Surg. 2009; 18(6):927–932

[28] Wolfe F, Michaud K. Assessment of pain in rheumatoid arthritis: minimal clinically significant difference, predictors, and the effect of anti-tumor necrosis factor therapy. J Rheumatol. 2007; 34(8):1674–1683

[29] De Ridder D, Vanneste S. Burst and Tonic Spinal Cord Stimulation: Different and Common Brain Mechanisms. Neuromodulation. 2016; 19(1):47–59

[30] Taylor RS, Desai MJ, Rigoard P, Taylor RJ. Predictors of pain relief following spinal cord stimulation in chronic back and leg pain and failed back surgery syndrome: a systematic review and meta-regression analysis. Pain Pract. 2014; 14(6):489–505

[31] Parker JL, Karantonis DM, Single PS, et al. Electrically evoked compound action potentials recorded from the sheep spinal cord. Neuromodulation. 2013; 16(4):295–303, discussion 303

36 Ablative Procedures for Trigeminal Neuralgia

Alp Ozpinar, Ronak H. Jani and Raymond F. Sekula, Jr

Abstract

Ablative procedures are important tools for the clinician involved in the care of the patient with facial pain to understand. For example, in patients with classical trigeminal neuralgia, ablative procedures should be reserved for those patients unsuited (i.e., without MRI-evidence of vascular compression of the trigeminal nerve), unfit (i.e., with comorbidities which preclude a general anesthetic), unable to realize the expected increased durability of microvascular decompression (i.e., with an expected short life-span typically less than five years), or in those patients who have failed microvascular decompression. With other types of facial pain (e.g., as a result of multiple sclerosis lesion/s), ablative treatments directed at the trigeminal ganglion or cisternal portion of the trigeminal nerve are the treatment of choice. In this chapter, the authors review the technical aspects as well as the intended benefits and expected risks of the various ablative procedures.

Keywords: ablation, glycerol rhizolysis, radiofrequency rhizolysis, balloon compression, radiosurgery, partial sensory rhizotomy, internal neurolysis

36.1 Patient Selection

Facial pain is a common and nonspecific symptom that is associated with known and unknown causes. Clinicians often use the term "trigeminal neuralgia" differently. In its most literal connotation, trigeminal neuralgia denotes pain emanating from within the three dermatomes of the trigeminal nerve. Many clinicians, however, reserve the term, trigeminal neuralgia (TN) to signify a more specific disorder, which primarily manifests as attacks of sudden, unilateral, and lancinating facial pain with characteristic triggers (e.g. light touch, cold air). These attacks often result from vascular compression of the intracisternal portion of the trigeminal nerve near its entry into the brainstem.[1,2,3] In recent years, vascular compression of the trigeminal nerve has been accepted as the most common cause of classical trigeminal neuralgia by the International Headache Society, the International Association for the Study of Pain, and the European Academy of Neurology.[4,5] Despite this long overdue acknowledgement, vascular compression of the trigeminal nerve is not involved in every case of classical TN, and incidental vascular compression of the trigeminal nerve can be found in patients without classical TN.[6] How does the clinician make sense of these seeming contradictions in an effort to properly select patients with classical TN for operative management?

Because patients with classical TN who are responding to carbamazepine or oxcarbazepine at the time of surgery, or responded to them in the past, have better outcomes with microvascular decompression (MVD) or any of the ablative procedures, patients should be asked about their past or current antiseizure responsiveness.[7] If they are responding, or have responded, this suggests that they will respond favorably to any of the available operations for classical TN. It is important to note that data regarding the use of ablation, when the diagnosis is not classical TN, is scarce, and that which does exist reveals poor short and long-term results.

36.1.1 Preoperative Evaluation

A patient who is medically fit to undergo MVD should undergo a gadolinium-enhanced MRI with thin-section multiplanar SSFP sequences that are heavily T2-weighted to determine if there is vascular compression, particularly severe compression or distortion along the centrally-myelinated portion of the trigeminal nerve.[8,9,10] If vascular compression exists, MVD should be considered for those patients presumed to have more than 5–10 years of life remaining.[8,11] An ablative procedure is a better option in patients with classical TN without MRI evidence of vascular compression. The early idea that, "There must be a vessel (intraoperatively), and it is my job to find it," no longer holds in an era of more detailed imaging.[12] Finally, an ablative procedure is likely a better option for those patients with failed or recurrent classical TN following a well-performed initial MVD when repeat MRI fails to identify missed or recurrent vascular compression

Although consensus guidelines for the surgical management of trigeminal neuralgia do not exist, ablative procedures are well indicated in: (a) patients with classical TN medically unfit for the anesthetic and operative rigors of MVD, (b) patients with classical TN without vascular compression, (c) patients with classical TN who have failed prior MVD, and (d) patients with classical TN who have a short life expectancy.

Percutaneous ablative procedures include glycerol rhizolysis of the trigeminal nerve and Gasserian ganglion (GR), radiofrequency rhizolysis of the trigeminal nerve and/or Gasserian ganglion (RF), balloon compression of the trigeminal nerve (BC), and radiosurgical (i.e., using the Leksell Gamma Knife® or Cyber Knife®) rhizolysis of the intracisternal portion of the trigeminal nerve. Open ablative procedures include partial sensory rhizotomy (PSR) (i.e., Dandy's procedure) and "internal neurolysis" (IN) of the intracisternal portion of the trigeminal nerve.

36.2 Operative Procedure

36.2.1 Percutaneous Ablative Procedures

Glycerol Rhizolysis of the Trigeminal Ganglion

In patients with cTN, recurrent cTN following a well-performed MVD, or in those medically unfit to undergo a posterior fossa exploration, GR is the most cost-effective treatment option.[13] When pain control occurs, it is usually within 24 hours from time of operation. Despite being the most cost-effective ablative treatment per quality-adjusted life year for TN, GR is the least-used treatment modality. GR is associated with a lower rate of dysesthesias as compared to other percutaneous procedures. It involves percutaneous penetration of the foramen ovale with a thin spinal needle using fluoroscopic guidance, and bathing of the trigeminal ganglion and nerve with injected sterile anhydrous glycerol. This procedure is often done under conscious sedation and can be repeated. In a study of 3370 patients undergoing GR, pain relief at 6 months and 3 years ranged from 78% to 88% and 53% to 54%, respectively.[14] Complications from GR include dysesthesias (23%) of which 19% were mild and 3% were moderate, herpes eruption (3%), bacterial meningitis (1%), chemical meningitis (3%), and mild hearing loss (2%).[15]

Radiofrequency Rhizolysis of the Trigeminal Ganglion

Sweet and Wepsic promoted the use of percutaneous radiotherapy rhizotomy based on their laboratory evidence that gradually increasing thermal injury of the trigeminal ganglion first injures unmyelinated pain fibers.[16] It has the advantage of leading to immediate pain relief, occurring in approximately 98% of cases. In one study, by Tang et al., that included 304 elderly patients (70 years or older) complete pain relief was observed in 100% patients at discharge, but the rate of pain relief dropped to 85%, 75%, and 49% at 1 year, 3 years, and 10 years, respectively.[17] The incidence of painful dysesthesias was greater when the thermal injury was made with temperatures higher than 79 °C. Although it is the most durable ablative procedure, this result is nearly always associated with sensory loss.[16]

Balloon Compression

Like glycerol rhizolysis and radiofrequency rhizotomy, BC involves a fluoroscopically guided percutaneous approach through the foramen ovale, and subsequent injury to the myelin of the trigeminal nerve, in this case by mechanical compression. Based on animal studies, this procedure has the advantage of selectively avoiding injury to small and unmyelinated fibers, sparing the fibers that mediate the corneal reflex. BC does not require patient interaction and is done under general anesthesia. Atropine or external pacemaker must be available during surgery to counteract the expected trigeminal depressor response.

Brown and Pilitsis demonstrated initial pain relief in 92% of 56 patients.[18] Actuarial rates of complete pain relief were 91% and 69% at 6 months and 3 years, respectively, and others have reported similar rates of pain relief. Complications from BC include dysesthesia (4%), herpes eruption (4%), masseter weakness (1%), and diplopia (3%).[15] Rates of masseter weakness, dysesthesia, and severe numbness can be reduced by balloon compression pressure monitoring and by limiting the duration of compression.[18]

36.2.2 Open Ablative Treatment Options

Internal Neurolysis

Internal neurolysis involves "brushing or combing" of the intracisternal segment (i.e., between the porus trigeminus and the root entry point of the trigeminal nerve into the pons) of the sensory bundle (i.e., Portio major) of the of the trigeminal nerve.[19,20] Recently, Ko et al. performed this procedure on 27

patients resulting in immediate relief of pain in 85% of patients.[20] Seventy-two percent of patients maintained significant pain relief without medications for 5 years. Ninety-six percent of the patients experienced numbness and one patient had anesthesia dolorosa (4%). The rate of dysesthesias or deafferentation pain was 16%.

Partial Sensory Rhizotomy

In 1929, Dandy reported his results of an open partial or complete sensory rhizotomy of the sensory bundle of the intracisternal segment of the trigeminal nerve at the pons.[21] In a comparative analysis, 4% of MVD and 20% of PSR patients were unsatisfied with the outcome of the respective procedure, whereas the final outcome was thought to be better than expected in 80% of MVD and 54% of PSR patients. Importantly, 22% of patients undergoing PSR felt that they were worse off.[22]

36.3 Conclusion

TN remains a challenging disorder to manage, but as our understanding of its pathogenesis improves, treatment options will also improve. For now, the clinician should carefully weigh the aforementioned factors for each patient, particularly considering a patient's life expectancy.

References

[1] Dandy WE. Concerning the cause of trigeminal neuralgia. Am J Surg. 1934; 24 (2):447–455

[2] Gardner WJ, Miklos MV. Response of trigeminal neuralgia to decompression of sensory root; discussion of cause of trigeminal neuralgia. J Am Med Assoc. 1959; 170(15):1773–1776

[3] Jannetta PJ. Arterial Compression of the Trigeminal Nerve at the Pons in Patients with Trigeminal Neuralgia. J Neurosurg. 1967; 26 1:159–162

[4] Cruccu G, Finnerup NB, Jensen TS, et al. Trigeminal neuralgia: New classification and diagnostic grading for practice and research. Neurology. 2016; 87 (2):220–228

[5] Headache Classification Committee of the International Headache Society (IHS). The International Classification of Headache Disorders, 3rd edition (beta version). Cephalalgia. 2013; 33(9):629–808

[6] Sekula RF, Hughes M, Mousavi H. 190 A Comparative Analysis of Operative and Radiographic Findings of Neurovascular Compression of the Trigeminal Nerve in Patients Without Trigeminal Neuralgia. Neurosurgery 2016;63 (Suppl 1):175

[7] Barker FG , II, Jannetta PJ, Bissonette DJ, Larkins MV, Jho HD. The long-term outcome of microvascular decompression for trigeminal neuralgia. N Engl J Med. 1996; 334(17):1077–1083

[8] Sekula RF , Jr, Frederickson AM, Jannetta PJ, Quigley MR, Aziz KM, Arnone GD. Microvascular decompression for elderly patients with trigeminal neuralgia: a prospective study and systematic review with meta-analysis. J Neurosurg. 2011; 114(1):172–179

[9] Maarbjerg S, Wolfram F, Gozalov A, Olesen J, Bendtsen L. Significance of neurovascular contact in classical trigeminal neuralgia. Brain. 2015; 138(Pt 2): 311–319

[10] Hughes MA, Frederickson AM, Branstetter BF, Zhu X, Sekula RF , Jr. MRI of the Trigeminal Nerve in Patients With Trigeminal Neuralgia Secondary to Vascular Compression. AJR Am J Roentgenol. 2016; 206(3):595–600

[11] Sekula RF, Marchan EM, Fletcher LH, Casey KF, Jannetta PJ. Microvascular decompression for trigeminal neuralgia in elderly patients. J Neurosurg. 2008; 108(4):689–691

[12] McLaughlin MR, Jannetta PJ, Clyde BL, Subach BR, Comey CH, Resnick DK. Microvascular decompression of cranial nerves: lessons learned after 4400 operations. J Neurosurg. 1999; 90(1):1–8

[13] Sivakanthan S, Van Gompel JJ, Alikhani P, van Loveren H, Chen R, Agazzi S. Surgical management of trigeminal neuralgia: use and cost-effectiveness from an analysis of the Medicare Claims Database. Neurosurgery. 2014; 75 (3):220–226, discussion 225–226

[14] Xu-Hui W, Chun Z, Guang-Jian S, et al. Long-term outcomes of percutaneous retrogasserian glycerol rhizotomy in 3370 patients with trigeminal neuralgia. Turk Neurosurg. 2011; 21(1):48–52

[15] Asplund P, Blomstedt P, Bergenheim AT. Percutaneous Balloon Compression vs Percutaneous Retrogasserian Glycerol Rhizotomy for the Primary Treatment of Trigeminal Neuralgia. Neurosurgery. 2016; 78(3):421–428, discussion 428

[16] Sweet WH, Wepsic JG. Controlled thermocoagulation of trigeminal ganglion and rootlets for differential destruction of pain fibers. 1. Trigeminal neuralgia. J Neurosurg. 1974; 40(2):143–156

[17] Tang YZ, Jin D, Bian JJ, Li XY, Lai GH, Ni JX. Long-term outcome of computed tomography-guided percutaneous radiofrequency thermocoagulation for classic trigeminal neuralgia patients older than 70 years. J Craniofac Surg. 2014; 25(4):1292–1295

[18] Brown JA, Pilitsis JG. Percutaneous balloon compression for the treatment of trigeminal neuralgia: results in 56 patients based on balloon compression pressure monitoring. Neurosurg Focus. 2005; 18(5):E10

[19] Ma Z, Li M. "Nerve combing" for trigeminal neuralgia without vascular compression: report of 10 cases. Clin J Pain. 2009; 25(1):44–47

[20] Ko AL, Ozpinar A, Lee A, Raslan AM, McCartney S, Burchiel KJ. Long-term efficacy and safety of internal neurolysis for trigeminal neuralgia without neurovascular compression. J Neurosurg. 2015; 122(5):1048–1057

[21] Dandy WE. An operation for the cure of tic douloureux: Partial section of the sensory root at the pons. AMA Arch Surg. 1929; 18(2):687–734

[22] Zakrzewska JM, Lopez BC, Kim SE, Coakham HB. Patient reports of satisfaction after microvascular decompression and partial sensory rhizotomy for trigeminal neuralgia. Neurosurgery. 2005; 56(6):1304–1311, discussion 1311–1312

37 Principles of Trigeminal Neuralgia

Jeffrey A. Brown

Abstract

Trigeminal neuropathic pain (TNP) is an umbrella term that encompasses pain syndromes that consist primarily of paresthesias (shooting pains), dysesthesias (constant burning pain) or a mixture of them. Surgical treatment is either by ablation or decompression. Ablative options are reserved for those patients with a predominance of paresthesias. Microvascular decompression is an option when there is an MRI demonstrated vascular association. Initial clinical benefit is comparable in appropriately selected patients with ablation and decompression. Benefit is less when decompression is done in patients with a predominance of dysesthesias. Neurosurgeons who treated TNP should be able to offer multiple options for treatment based on presentation, health and age.

Keywords: trigeminal neuropathic pain, trigeminal neuralgia, microvascular decompression, trigeminal rhizotomy, radiosurgery

Generations of physicians have described the stabbing, electric shock pains of trigeminal neuralgia but were frustrated by their inability to treat them. In fact, such shocks are the earliest signs and most treatable symptoms of a progressive neuropathic pain syndrome. Its later, more difficult to treat, manifestations consist of constant, burning, tingling pain that may also be associated with sensory loss.

Recent descriptions of neuropathic facial pain subdivide it into multiple entities. TN1 describes the "classic" elements of intermittent stabbing facial pain triggered by anything that elicits facial sensory input- talking, chewing, or touching one's face on the side of the pain. TN2 describes the entity in which there is a component of constant pain, best described as burning, tingling, or prickling. Other categories are used for pain that is a result of surgical injury, or the effect of a sclerotic plaque in the trigeminal pathway seen in multiple sclerosis.

A more basic understanding of trigeminal neuropathic pain is to describe it as dominated by paresthesias, by dysesthesias or by a mixture of the two.

Neuropathic pain describes that pain seen in the absence of detectable or ongoing tissue damage and is often located where there is a sensory deficit. Paresthesias are the paroxysmal, shooting, stabbing components to neuropathic pain. Dysesthesias are unfamiliar, unpleasant burning, often constant elements to the pain. An extensive descriptive vocabulary emerges from having patients complete a McGill pain questionnaire. It is validated for trigeminal neuralgia, multimodality, quantifiable and consists of twenty subcategories of terms that indicate progressively more severe discomfort. It can differentiate intertwined nociceptive from neuropathic pain elements.

Peter Jannetta's discovery, published first in 1967 as a case report, that trigeminal neuralgia is caused by a compressive vascular association of the trigeminal nerve with a loop of the superior cerebellar artery has defined the modern surgical treatment of trigeminal neuropathic pain.

Magnetic resonance imaging of the trigeminal nerve using thin cut FIESTA or CISS techniques should be done when considering the diagnosis, if possible, and allows accurate visualization of venous or arterial vascular association. This should eliminate any need for surgical exploration of the nerve. The only surgical exceptions are re- operations for recurrent pain in which imaging of the nerve is difficult.

Once the diagnosis is made, the first line of treatment consists of an adequate trial of anticonvulsants. Anticonvulsants work by slowing electrical conduction to the site of the "short circuit" in the nerve. Pathologic analysis of micro biopsies taken beneath the site of vascular compression definitively have shown dysmyelinization consistent with repeated injury to large myelinated fibers with failed efforts at healing leading to approximation of "naked" axons. Anticonvulsant drugs must be titrated slowly upwards, stopping when pain is adequately controlled or when symptoms of excessive dose are evident. Such symptoms included lethargy, difficulty with balance or other cognitive issues. Medical treatment has failed if these symptoms become dominant or if pain persists in the face of such symptoms becoming bothersome. Carbamazepine (Tegretol) is approved for the treatment of neuropathic pain. Other anticonvulsants used include gabapentin, oxcarbaxepine, Dilantin and extended release versions of these drugs.

The principles of neuropathic facial pain surgical treatment are:

1. Pain consisting primarily of paresthesias can be treated by microvascular decompression or a proven ablative technique.
2. Pain that consists primarily of constant dysesthesias should not be treated by an ablative technique.
3. Pain associated with multiple sclerosis should be treated by an ablative technique if there is a sclerotic plaque within the trigeminal pathway, but may be unrelated to multiple sclerosis if the disease is not active and there is a visible vascular compression.
4. Accepted, often used and well-documented ablative surgical treatments include: radiofrequency thermal rhizotomy, glycerol rhizotomy, gamma knife radiosurgery, LINAC or cyberknife radiosurgery and balloon compression rhizotomy. Peripheral neurectomies of the supraorbital or infraorbital branches of the trigeminal nerve are occasionally performed as secondary efforts.
5. Temporizing percutaneous efforts with Botox, nerve blocks and acupuncture are unproven.

Studies indicate that the best quality of life occurs after successful microvascular decompression and next, after balloon compression. Microvascular decompression is indicated if MR imaging shows a vascular association and the patient is a surgical candidate. When MR imaging cannot be done, a CT cisternogram can provide adequate imaging of the nerve. There is no age limit to the surgery, however anticoagulant drugs must be discontinuable for a variable period of time in the pre and perioperative period. MVD in older patients is technically easier than in younger patients, because of the larger size of the cerebellar cisterns, though the risk of stroke is higher.

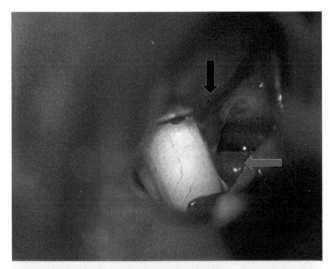

Fig. 37.1 Intraoperative image of the trigeminal nerve affected in a "sandwich" by a loop of the superior cerebellar artery (vertical arrow) compressing a distal vein close to Meckel's cave (horizontal arrow) and against the nerve. Neuropathic facial pain may derive from compression of the trigeminal nerve throughout its cisternal path, not only at the root entry zone

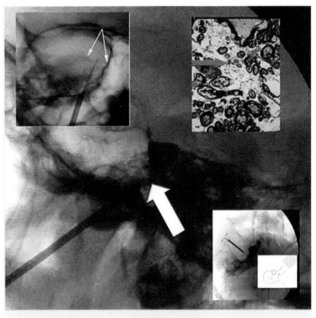

Fig. 37.2 Montage of fluoroscopic images that shows the proper placement of the balloon during balloon compression trigeminal rhizotomy. A modified submental view visualizes the foramen ovale medial to the mandible and lateral to the maxillary sinus (lower right frame). The balloon tip is then advanced to the midpoint in the dip in the petrous bone representing the point of passage of the trigeminal nerve from the posterior to anterior fossa where there is also a split in the tentorium (thin arrows). This can be identified when the petrous bone is positioned in the midpoint of the ipsilateral orbit radiographically. The inflated balloon lies on the petrous bone posterior to the clival line and has the appearance of a "pear shape." (large arrow) The balloon tip is then contained by the split in the tentorium that allows passage of the trigeminal nerve from the posterior fossa. Balloon compression selectively injures myelinated fibers and preserves unmyelinated pain fibers (upper right ultrastructual cross section image of a rabbit trigeminal nerve after balloon compression; upper arrow points to an uninjured unmyelinated fiber and lower arrowhead points to an injured myelinated fiber).

Principles of MVD surgery are:

1. Proper positioning is achieved either in a straight lateral position or supine with head rotation in younger more supple patients.
2. Cranial exposure should be to the margins of the juncture of the lateral and sigmoid sinuses. This can be done by use of a neuronavigation system.
3. Intra operative monitoring of auditory brainstem evoked potentials should be used in order to limit risk of hearing loss or injury to the facial nerve.
4. Opening of the arachnoid overlying the trigeminal nerve in order to achieve visualization of the full cisternal portion of the trigeminal nerve since compression may be at any point within the cistern. This may require coagulation and sectioning of the superior petrosal venous complex.
5. Decompression of compressive veins is preferable to coagulation and sectioning because there is risk of cerebellar swelling with sectioning of larger veins and injury to the trigeminal nerve during coagulation (▶ Fig. 37.1).
6. Reoperation should only be undertaken by neurosurgeons experienced in the procedure and, it should be expected that (a) the cerebellar hemisphere will be adherent to the suture line of the previous closure and (b) the Teflon fibers previously inserted will be adherent to the trigeminal nerve leading to a higher risk of nerve injury from the exposure.
7. Younger patients have a higher incidence of constant neuropathic pain, bilateral pain and a venous source of compression.

Pain relief after MVD for patients with predominant paresthesias is about 90%; with predominance of constant, burning dysesthesias, the success drops by 15%. Once successful the incidence of recurrent pain is 15% at 15 years as demonstrated by a Kaplan-Meyer survival curve for pain free days, or about 1%/year to that point.

The incidence of stroke, hearing loss, facial weakness or other cranial nerve injury is in the range of 1–3% in large published series.

The principles of ablative treatment are:

1. The goal of treatment is hypesthesia in the region of pain, not anesthesia.
2. Thermal and glycerol rhizotomy and gamma knife radiosurgery (when placing the frame) are performed under brief intravenous sedation. Cyberknife radiosurgery does not require sedation at any point. Balloon compression requires general anesthesia.
3. Ablative treatments target the retrogasserian portion of the trigeminal nerve.
4. Ablative treatments cause partial demyelination of the nerve proximal to the site of "short circuit" except in cases of multiple sclerosis.
5. Balloon compression is the only truly selective cause of injury and is specific for large myelinated fibers that mediate light touch. It preserves small and unmyelinated fibers that mediate pain. It is successful because it reduces the electrical input to the site of short circuit, not because it "stops" pain transmission (▶ Fig. 37.2).

6. Recurrence rates after ablative treatment are in the range of 30% within 3–5 years. This is because the goal of treatment is hypesthesia and this allows re-myelinization to occur with resultant possible pain recurrence.

If the predominant neuropathic pain is constant and MVD and medication have not been successful in alleviating the pain, then several forms of neuromodulation have been used. These are currently off label applications of devices approved for use in humans for other pain syndromes. Options include motor cortex stimulation and, more recently, peripheral branch trigeminal stimulation. Motor cortex stimulation has been repeatedly shown to provide 50–75% likelihood of reducing pain by 50–75%. More recent laboratory studies in rodents have confirmed the hypothesis that motor cortex stimulation works by inhibiting thalamic hyperactivity caused by the trigeminal nerve injury and secondary loss of sensory nerve input. The mechanism for peripheral stimulation effectiveness, its duration and likelihood of benefit has not been adequately studied. With motor cortex stimulation there are a number of long-term studies showing ongoing benefit.

Glossopharyngeal neuralgia may be caused by vascular compression of the IXth and upper Xth nerve fibers by a loop of the posterior inferior cerebellar artery. MVD of these fibers should be considered if there is MRI visualization of a compressive loop. Sectioning of the GPN can cause bothersome dysesthesias and should not be considered an early option. Specialized intraoperative monitoring of vagal motor function is required when operating on the GPN.

In summary, the surgical treatment of neuropathic facial pain requires that the neurosurgeon be able to perform multiple surgical options, as there is no single surgery appropriate to all patients. A clear understanding of the nature of the pain to be treated is essential in the surgical decision making process.[1,2,3,4,5,6,7,8,9,10,11]

References

[1] Jannetta PJ. Arterial compression of the trigeminal nerve at the pons in patients with trigeminal neuralgia. J Neurosurg. 1967; 26 1:159–162

[2] Barker FG , II, Jannetta PJ, Bissonette DJ, Jho HD. Trigeminal numbness and tic relief after microvascular decompression for typical trigeminal neuralgia. Neurosurgery. 1997; 40(1):39–45

[3] Taha JM, Tew JM , Jr, Buncher CR. A prospective 15-year follow up of 154 consecutive patients with trigeminal neuralgia treated by percutaneous stereotactic radiofrequency thermal rhizotomy. J Neurosurg. 1995; 83(6):989–993

[4] Zakrzewska JM, Thomas DG. Patient's assessment of outcome after three surgical procedures for the management of trigeminal neuralgia. Acta Neurochir (Wien). 1993; 122(3–4):225–230

[5] Brown JA, Pilitsis JG. Percutaneous balloon compression for the treatment of trigeminal neuralgia: results in 56 patients based on balloon compression pressure monitoring. Neurosurg Focus. 2005; 18(5):E10

[6] Brown JA, Pilitsis JG. Motor cortex stimulation for central and neuropathic facial pain: a prospective study of 10 patients and observations of enhanced sensory and motor function during stimulation. Neurosurgery. 2005; 56(2): 290–297, discussion 290–297

[7] Brown JA, Hoeflinger B, Long PB, et al. Axon and ganglion cell injury in rabbits after percutaneous trigeminal balloon compression. Neurosurgery. 1996; 38 (5):993–1003, discussion 1003–1004

[8] Hilton DA, Love S, Gradidge T, Coakham HB. Pathological findings associated with trigeminal neuralgia caused by vascular compression. Neurosurgery. 1994; 35(2):299–303, discussion 303

[9] Kondziolka D, Zorro O, Lobato-Polo J, et al. Gamma Knife stereotactic radiosurgery for idiopathic trigeminal neuralgia. J Neurosurg. 2010; 112(4):758–765

[10] Adler JR , Jr, Bower R, Gupta G, et al. Nonisocentric radiosurgical rhizotomy for trigeminal neuralgia. Neurosurgery. 2009; 64(2) Suppl:A84–A90

[11] Miller JP, Acar F, Burchiel KJ. Classification of trigeminal neuralgia: clinical, therapeutic, and prognostic implications in a series of 144 patients undergoing microvascular decompression. J Neurosurg. 2009; 111(6):1231–1234

38 Intraoperative Neurophysiologic Monitoring during Microvascular Decompression for Trigeminal Neuralgia

Denmark Mugutso, Charles Warnecke, and Marat Avshalumov

Abstract

Intraoperative neurophysiologic monitoring (INM) has become an integral part of microvascular decompression (MVD) surgery for trigeminal neuralgia (TN). Multimodality INM, emphasizing cranial nerve (CN) monitoring and often including somatosensory evoked potentials (SSEPs) to monitor patient positioning reduces the risk of permanent postoperative neurological deficits. CN V, VII and VIII are most frequently monitored during MVD procedures for TN. This chapter reviews basic INM techniques currently in widespread use during MVD procedures for TN.

Keywords: brainstem auditory evoked responses, microvascular decompression, cranial nerves

38.1 Somatosensory Evoked Potentials and Electromyography

The major risks of MVD are neurological injury to CN V, VII and, especially, VIII. An added concern is nerve injury from the lateral decubitus patient positioning most often used for the surgery. Such positioning allows for easier access to the retromastoid area. The cerebellum becomes displaced downward under gravity, requiring reduced retraction. However, this position may result in the compression of the contralateral arm, axilla and brachial plexus.[1] SSEP monitoring is widely used for detection of potential iatrogenic injury to neuronal structures. We monitor SSEPs before and after patient positioning to assess any potential changes to baseline waveforms and inform the surgeon of any necessary adjustments in positioning. SSEPs also detect global systemic changes such as body temperature, anesthetic equilibrium, and blood flow to the extremities and to vital neural structures (▶ Fig. 38.1).

During the procedure, retraction around the nerves, ischemia, and heat from electrocautery puts CN V and VII at risk of injury. Functional integrity of the motor portions of these CNs is evaluated by free-running electromyography (EMG) that detects real-time nerve activity from surgical manipulation. Triggered EMG with a hand-held probe also provides additional nerve health information to the surgeon.

To monitor free running EMG, two subdermal needle electrodes are placed in each muscle innervated by the respective CNs: the masseter/temporalis for the TN and the following muscles for the facial nerve: frontalis, orbicularis oculi, orbicularis oris, and mentalis (▶ Fig. 38.2a). Iatrogenic EMG activity can be classified, based on the response amplitude and duration, as spikes, bursts, and trains. Three types of trains, in decreasing severity, have been identified: A-trains are the most clinically significant and are usually associated with post-operative facial paresis.[2] They have a distinct sinusoidal waveform of high frequency sound, short or long duration, and amplitudes ranging from 100–200 µV (▶ Fig. 38.2c).

38.2 Brainstem Auditory Evoked Responses

Recordings of brainstem auditory evoked responses (BAER) measure the functional integrity of CN VIII. BAERs are obtained from broadband sound clicks delivered to the ear canal through ear inserts and plastic tubing (▶ Fig. 38.2b). Subdermal electrodes placed on the scalp, ear, and upper dorsal neck record the elicited waves, which are labeled in Roman numerals as waves I, II, III, IV, and V. These waves have different origin and generators along the auditory pathway (▶ Fig. 38.3a).[3] Although BAERs are acquired continuously during the procedure, the pre-incision baseline, baseline after dural opening, during arachnoid dissection and exposure of the nerves and vessels, during retraction of cerebellum, during manipulation of the offending vessel, and Teflon placement (▶ Fig. 38.3b).

The analysis of BAERs focuses mainly on waves I, III and V, with wave V being the most robust of all BAERs. In fact, wave V

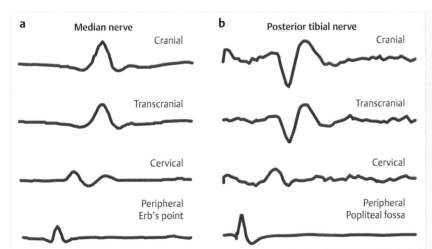

a Median nerve
Cranial
Transcranial
Cervical
Peripheral Erb's point

b Posterior tibial nerve
Cranial
Transcranial
Cervical
Peripheral Popliteal fossa

Fig. 38.1 Somatosensory Evoked Potentials. Typical SSEPs traces recorded along the medial-lemniscal pathway from cortical, transcortical, cervical, and peripheral locations (Erb`s point for the upper extremity and popliteal fossa for the lower: **(a)** upper extremity SSEPS elicited by stimulation of median nerve; **(b)** lower extremity SSEPs elicited by stimulation of posterior tibial nerve. Stimulation parameters: duration 200–500 µs, intensity 30–50mA, system bandpass 30 Hz-1 kHz, rate 2.71–3.41/s, repetitions per average 200–300.

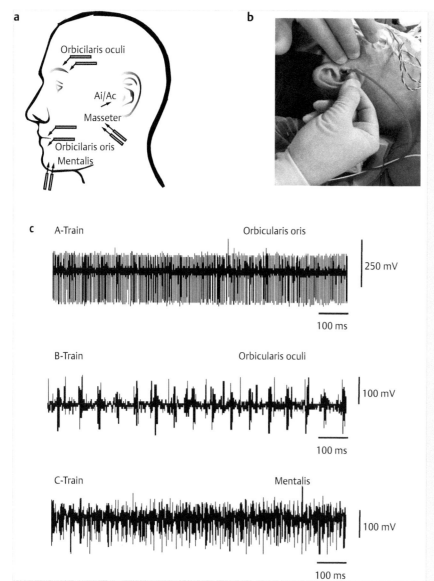

Fig. 38.2 EMG and BAERs electrode arrangements. (a) Schematic electrode placement for monitoring EMG responses from CN V, VII and auditory response from CNVIII (Ai/Ac); (b) practical placement of the stimulating ear insert for BAERs stimulation; c) different types of pathological train EMG activity recorded from CN VII as a result of surgical manipulation during MVD.

may be the only component recorded in patients with significant pre-operative conduction and sensorineural hearing loss.[4] Iatrogenic injury to CN VIII causes latency delay and an amplitude drop of Wave V. Changes in both the latency and amplitude of wave V and the rates of changes reliably predict postoperative hearing loss.[5] The commonly accepted alert criteria are 50% amplitude reduction and 0.5 msec increase in latency of wave V. Once alerted by the neurophysiologist, the surgeon should identify the cause and takes corrective action (▶ Fig. 38.3c). Persistence of the wave V amplitude regardless of latency delays correlates with hearing preservation after surgery.[6] More recent data suggests that loss of amplitude is a more reliable predictive factor than an increase in latency.[5,6]

A complementary alert criterion evaluates interpeak latencies (IPLs).[7] IPL increases for Waves I–V reflect slowing in total central auditory conduction from the distal part of CN VIII to the inferior colliculus. Changes in wave I-III IPLs might indicate impedance of peripheral conduction, whereas changes in

latencies between waves III-V strongly suggest a conduction compromise from cochlear nucleus to the inferior colliculus.

Changes in BAERs can be technical, physiological or from surgical manipulation.[3,4,5] BAER signals may deteriorate because of operator errors, dislodged electrodes, broken wires, or inadequate stimulation. Electrical artifacts and sound interference from electrocautery use or from drilling can also contribute to deterioration or loss of BAERs.

Physiological factors include the anesthetic regimen, ambient temperature changes, and ambient noise related to bone drilling. Anesthetic agents produce only minimal effect on BAERs, yet both interpeak latencies and latency of the wave I are progressively increased as the temperature cools. As a result, cold irrigation is undesirable during microvascular decompression while monitoring BAERs.[3,4]

Changes caused by surgical manipulation can be thermal, mechanical, or ischemic. Thermal injury comes from cauterization. Mechanical changes are attributed to moderate cerebellar

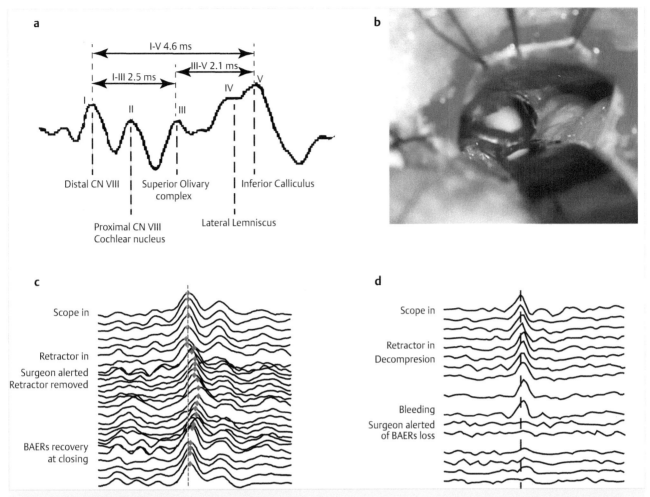

Fig. 38.3 Typical intraoperatrive BAERs. (a) BAERs traces showing auditory pathway generators for each Wave. The arrows indicate interpeak latencies. Absolute latencies for Wave I is 1.6–1.8 msec and 5.7–6 msec for Wave V. Stimulation parameters: stimulus rate 17.1 Hz, sound intensity 105 dB SpE, and filtering 30 Hz-3 kHz, repetitions per average 1200–1500; **(b)** Retractor placement; **(c)** BAERs traces showing latency delay of Wave V longer than 0.5 msec (red boxes) which improved to less than 0.5 msec from baseline latency (the grey dashed line); **(d)** BAERs traces showing a significant loss of Wave V responses without recovery by the end of the procedure.

retraction, usually gradual, prompting the neurophysiologist to alert the surgeon at 0.5 ms wave V latency delay. Aggressive retraction will show an immediate change. The surgeon should respond by adjusting, relaxing, or removing the retractor. Damage to the internal auditory artery causes cochlear ischemia and sudden loss of all BAERs (▶ Fig. 38.3d).[3,4,5]

Our experience has shown INM is of great value during MVD for TN in reducing the operative complications of hearing loss and facial weakness.

References

[1] Winfree CJ, Kline DG. Intraoperative positioning nerve injuries. Surg Neurol. 2005; 63(1):5–18, discussion 18

[2] Romstöck J, Strauss C, Fahlbusch R. Continuous electromyography monitoring of motor cranial nerves during cerebellopontine angle surgery. J Neurosurg. 2000; 93(4):586–593

[3] Legatt AD. BAEPs in surgery. In: Nuwer MR, Daube JR, Mauguirre F, eds. Intraoperative Monitoring of Neural Function Handbook of Clinical Neurophysiology. Vol. 8. Amsterdam, The Netherlands: Elsevier B.V.; 2008:334–349

[4] Moeller AR. Intraoperative Neurophysiologic Monitoring techniques for microvascular decompression procedures. In: Loftus CM, Biller J, Baron EM, eds. Intraoperative Neuromonitoring. McGraw Hill Education; 2014:273–284

[5] Simon MV. Neurophysiologic intraoperative monitoring of the vestibulocochlear nerve. J Clin Neurophysiol. 2011; 28(6):566–581

[6] Nadol JB, Jr, Chiong CM, Ojemann RG, et al. Preservation of hearing and facial nerve function in resection of acoustic neuroma. Laryngoscope. 1992; 102 (10):1153–1158

[7] Thirumala PD, Ilangovan P, Habeych M, Crammond DJ, Balzer J. Analysis of interpeak latencies of brainstem auditory evoked potential waveforms during microvascular decompression of cranial nerve VII for hemifacial spasm. Neurosurg Focus. 2013; 34(3):E6

39 Neuroprosthetics

Eric C Leuthardt, Wilson Z. Ray, Jarod L Roland

Abstract

Can a computer infer human intention or perception? It is now possible that it can.

Devices that convert brain signals, reflect its intentions, and then control an external device are known as neuroprosthetics. Their future development will have significant implications for the neurologically disabled. The greater our understanding of the cortical physiology underlying human intentions, the closer we will get to understanding the complexity of brain-derived control. This chapter summarizes the current status of the field of brain computer interface (BCI) and trends that may improve future clinical applications.

Keywords: electrodes, interface, EEG, ECoG, neuroprosthetics

39.1 Introduction

The expanding field of neuroprosthetics will substantially impact the future practice of neurosurgery. A neuroprosthetic device supplants or supplements the input and/or output of the nervous system. Neuroprosthetics can now bypass a deficit caused by disease or augment function to improve performance. Understand that there is varied terminology used to describe the development of this technology. Terms in use include brain computer interface (BCI), brain machine interface (BMI), neural interface system (NIS), direct neural interface (DNI), and mind-machine interface (MMI). These terms and others all describe the interface of the nervous system and external devices.

The field of neuroprosthetics integrates numerous disciplines. These include neuroscience, computer science, and engineering. Brain-machine interfacing research was actually conceived long before the advent of it as an organized academic field of study. Early questions were raised by Vidal, who in 1973 asked when studying electroencephalograms, "Can these observable electrical brain signals be put to work as carriers of information in man-computer communication or for the purpose of controlling such external apparatus as prosthetic devices or spaceships?" While his grander visions have not come to fruition, brain-driven operation of a prosthetic device is becoming commonplace in research labs across the world.

The field was stymied by the slow computation speeds of existing computers and software systems. Advances in microprocessor design/speeds and digital signal analysis enable computers to go far beyond current neuroprosthetic requirements. Computational speed is no longer a limiting factor. Technological advances in other relevant fields such as virtual reality, robotics, haptics, advanced imaging, and biomaterials also have provided the necessary tools for device development. This allows innovative introduction of motor, sensory, visual, auditory, speech, and other applications to the field. In this chapter we will review these applications and emphasize the role of neurosurgeons in its translation from fundamental research to clinical application.

39.2 Interface Modalities

The goal of a neuroprosthetic device is to replace or augment an individual's function by interfacing an external device with the nervous system. In the early phase of this field this was understood to be a device that detects brain signals to infer intentions, and then transforms those intentions to an external effector. Since the field's inception there have been many different types of signal inputs that have been used to achieve this goal. Each of these has distinct clinical considerations. The sources of signal input range from individual neuronal spiking, to field potential from cortical ensembles, or action potentials conducted by peripheral nerves. Output effectors are also wide-ranging. Classic and current examples include computer cursor control, robotic arm movement, and re-animation of paretic limbs. Neuroprosthetics are not unidirectional output devices. By reversing the direction of information transfer, an input device can provide simulated perceptions. Here the device records signals from the external environment and converts those signals into an appropriate stimulus delivered to the nervous system. These devices may thus use sensory input to provide tactile or proprioceptive feedback to assist with the control of robotic arm movements. It may also be an independent application. Cochlear implants record sounds and translate them into electrical stimuli. These are then delivered to the acoustic nerve and provide auditory perception to an otherwise deaf patient. In the broadest sense, neuroprosthetics can be categorized as "output neural interfaces" that convert the brain's intentions to external actions, or as "input neural interfaces" which take information from the environment and convert them into the brain's perceptions.

Neuroprosthetics may also be characterized by their mode of operation be it motor, somatosensory, speech, auditory and the source of neural interface (single unit neuron, cortical local field potential, peripheral nerve). The most successful neuroprosthesis to date is the cochlear implant. For neurosurgery the neuroprosthetics that are poised to impact the field are those that provide motor output. The goal of a motor output prosthesis is to be a device capable of interpreting an individual's movement intentions in real-time and direct the output to an effector such as a robotic limb. With these examples in mind, the various means of interfacing with the nervous system and their clinical implications will be explored.

39.3 Electroencephalography

Because it is non-invasive, electroencephalography (EEG) is still the most common means of studying cerebral electrophysiology. Electrodes are placed on a subject's scalp and electrical potentials from large cortical populations are recorded. Changes in neural rhythms are measured to evaluate various types of cognitive processes. The EEG, represents the summated electrical potentials from the electrochemical interaction of a vast number of cells, both neuronal and glial in origin. This

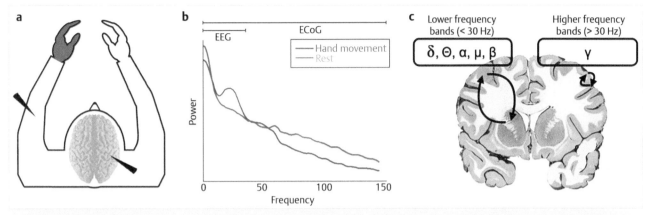

Fig. 39.1 Brain Signals. Brain Signals: **(a)** Volitional movement of right hand while electrode recording from contralateral cortex (EEG, ECoG, or intraparenchymal) or ipsilateral peripheral nerve. **(b)** Cortical field potentials with characteristic power decreases in low frequencies (Mu rhythm) and power increases in high Gamma range. **(c)** Thalamocortical and cortico-cortical rhythms. (Adapted from Leuthardt 2006 and Leuthardt 2009)

necessarily limits the complexity and precision of the information it provides.

Amplifiers and converters digitize the electrical signals that have been derived from the EEG. By sampling a continuous signal in brief, regular intervals, discrete values are obtained and stored in series, thereby converting the signal from an analog to a digital domain. The time-varying signal is then analyzed as the sum of multiple sinusoidal signals of varying frequency and amplitude. This process, using the Fourier transform, converts signals from a time domain to a frequency domain. In the frequency domain one can observe the change in power at a given frequency over time. This is known as time-frequency analysis. The distribution of signal power across a range of frequencies is the signal spectrum and its plot over time is the spectrogram. By time-locking the sampled signal to measured subject data, correlations are made between cortical activity and task performance. One such observation in signals measured over the motor homunculus is the reliably reproducible decrease in spectral power in the 8 to 13 Hz range. This occurs with overt or imagined movement of the hand contralateral to the side of the cortical recording.

Relevant physiologic signals in the EEG in humans is segmented into distinct components in the frequency domain and named by Greek alphabet characters. These are classically defined as the delta band below 4 Hz, theta band from 4 to 8 Hz, mu band from 8 to 13 Hz (also known as alpha), beta band from 13 to 30 Hz, and gamma band beyond 30 Hz. The mu rhythm is associated with motor electrophysiology and the Rolandic cortex (▶ Fig. 39.1a). Decreases in mu band spectral power with activity (▶ Fig. 39.1b) are thought to represent event related desynchronization. This release of synchronized cortical rhythms is thought to involve thalamocortical circuits modulating motor cortical systems (▶ Fig. 39.1c). Real-time measurements of power fluctuations in this frequency range provide a signal that represents motor movement intentions. Wolpaw and colleagues showed that these mu motor signals could be used to control a virtual cursor displayed on a computer screen using either real or imagined motor movements. In effect, the velocity of cursor movement was derived in real-time from changes in the mu spectral power volitionally modulated by the user. Similar modulations of EEG are observed in imagined

motor actions. This allows control without any peripheral activation of motor units.

EEG correlates of imagined motor movements are critical to the clinical application of BCIs in motor impaired patients. Real-world translation is impractical if overt motor function is required for the production of an adequate source control signal. Simply said, those who would need brain controlled prosthesis should not be required to move a limb to generate a control signal. It is thus essential that individuals affected by neurologic disorders such as amyotrophic lateral sclerosis (ALS), locked-in syndrome, or spinal cord injury (SCI) be capable of modulating cortical rhythms in the absence of end organ effect. Fortunately, preservation of this capability has been found in subjects with long-term deficits. Volitional modulation of stable electrophysiologic structures has been maintained.

To date, EEG-based brain computer interfaces have led the field in human neuroprosthetic research. One limitation of EEG methodologies is the physical separation of the cortical source signal and the scalp based recording electrodes. Intervening meninges, bone, and scalp limits spectral and spatial resolution of the signal associated with specific cognitive processes. For an EEG electrode to record a measurable signal from the cortex, electrical potentials must be summated across an area of cortex approximately 6 cm². The spatial resolution of independent signals is thereby limited. Similarly, destructive summation of temporally overlapping signals results in cancelation of higher frequencies in EEG recordings (i.e gamma rhythms which carry substantial information on cognitive processes). These limitations may be mitigated in part by intracranial placement of recording electrodes, but at the cost of increased invasiveness (▶ Fig. 39.2).

39.4 Electrocorticography

Signals from non-penetrating electrodes on the cortical surface have features that may be optimal for clinical application. The means to obtain such signals is known as electrocorticography (ECoG). While placement of the electrodes requires surgery, such signals balance clinical risk with acceptable signal quality, durability, and reliability. They can enable a neuroprosthetic

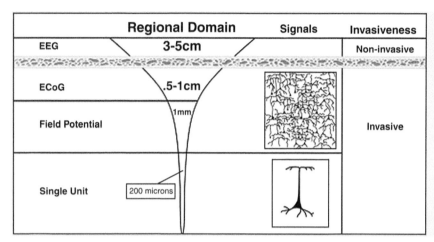

Fig. 39.2 Cortical Recording Interfaces. Cortical Recording Interfaces: Spatial scale (center) diagrammed in order of least to most invasive modality (left) with representative signal source (right). (Reproduced from Leuthardt 2006)

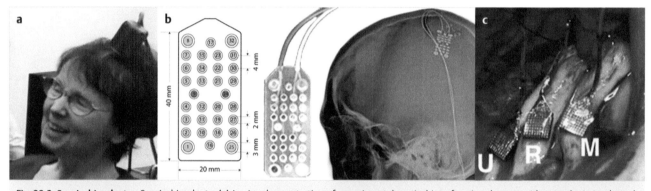

Fig. 39.3 Surgical Implants. Surgical Implants: **(a)** In vivo demonstration of experimental cortical interface in a human with tetraplegia implanted with a Utah electrode array (UEA). **(b)** Intraoperative view of an electrocorticography (ECoG) array over the convexity of a human brain. **(c)** Multiple Utah slanted electrode arrays (USEA) implanted in the ulnar, radial, and median (U, R, and M, respectively) nerves of the brachial plexus. (Adapted from Hochberg 2012, Ritaccio 2013, and Ledbetter 2013)

solution for the near future. Because ECoG electrodes record directly from the cortical surface (▶ Fig. 39.3b), the signals have excellent spatial and spectral resolution when compared to EEG. The higher signal-to-noise ratio is due in part to physical proximity, and to the reduced shielding effects of the skull (reducing ambient muscle and environmental noise). Because these electrodes do not penetrate cortex, the immunologic response to them is lessened. This improves long-term signal quality. ECoG has a long history of use in clinical neurosurgery. It was the initial application used by Penfield and Jasper in epilepsy surgery. Such a background better enables a straightforward technical transition from current methods to neuroprosthetic applications in the future.

There has been a substantial increase in the use of the ECoG approach for neuroprosthetic research since its initial demonstration of closed loop BCI control by patients undergoing invasive intracranial monitoring for epilepsy surgery. There have been numerous studies examining motor intentions to enable control of external devices. Furthermore, studies have shown that the motor physiology features that enable neuroprosthetic applications remain consistent from a pediatric age to advanced age. An additional benefit of the use of human subjects in research is that BCI research can expand beyond classic motor physiology as a signal source. While animal models have several

distinct advantages in research design, higher cognitive functions are inaccessible in non-human subjects. One example of human-specific cognitive operations used for BCI applications is the use of speech cortex and speech intentions for device control. ECoG signals over speech cortex can be modulated by imagined and overt speech production by the monitored subject. The user is then able to control the direction of a virtual cursor by saying out loud, or imagining saying covertly, various discriminating words pre-assigned to opposing direction.

ECoG also has several signal analysis advantages over non-invasive electroencephalography. Spectral resolution with EEG is limited to frequencies less than approximately 30–40 Hz (▶ Fig. 39.1b). This occurs because of the nature of the conductive properties of the skull and scalp, signal deterioration because of the increased distance between source and electrode, and the logarithmically decreasing signal power that occurs with frequency increases. These EEG limitations are overcome by intracranial electrode placement. Frequencies greater than 40 Hz, known as gamma rhythms, have been used to decode cognitive intentions associated with auditory processing, speech production, and higher cognitive functions. All of these have been used to demonstrate BCI control with ECoG in humans. Furthermore, Gaona et al., found sub-band selectivity in the high gamma range for behavior and location dependent activation during the performance of certain cognitive tasks. This is a feature not observed in the EEG frequency range.

Spatial resolution is improved by electrode placement directly onto the cortical surface. This higher anatomic fidelity translates into improved discrimination of cognitive tasks. Examples include the accurate decoding of individual finger movement (versus just hand movement) and phoneme articulation (versus just general speaking). Decreasing the size and spacing of electrode arrays increases spatial resolution. Common clinical ECoG arrays use inter electrode spacing of one centimeter. Experimental evidence suggests that less than 5 mm is plausible with microwires and continues to provide meaningful signals. Another advantage of signal source proximity is the magnitude of the voltage. While both ECoG and EEG require amplification of signals for sufficient signal analysis, scalp-based measurements are in the range of 10–100 μV. Cortical surface measurements reach up to 10–20 mV. This is several degrees of magnitude higher than with EEG. Higher voltages make it easier to filter noise and ambient signal from the environment and to reach a signal-to-noise ratio adequate for neuroprosthetic applications.

These advantages are being translated into early clinical trials for motor impaired patients. Wang et al. used a temporary ECoG implant for BCI control in a tetraplegic patient with a high cervical spinal cord injury. Their group implanted a custom designed high-density ECoG array over primary motor cortex that had been identified by fMRI. The subject had a complete C4 level spinal cord injury that occurred seven years earlier. He had no motor control of his upper extremities. Over the course of a four week implant period, the user was able to progress through a series of experiments sequentially achieving two-dimensional cursor, three-dimensional cursor, and ultimately three-dimensional robotic arm control. Vansteensel et al. implanted a chronic ECoG BCI in a patient with late-stage amyotrophic lateral sclerosis (ALS). This provided a brain–computer interface of subdural electrodes located over the motor cortex and connected to a transmitter placed subcutaneously in the left thorax. When the patient attempted to move the hand opposite to the side of the implanted electrodes, he was able to accurately and independently control a computer-typing program. The task performance required 28 weeks of training and he could type two letters per minute. The brain–computer interface offered autonomous communication that supplemented and at times supplanted the patient's eye-tracking device.

39.5 Intraparenchymal Electrodes

Recording electrodes inserted into the cortical surface, known as intra parenchymal or single unit electrodes, provide highly resolved information on neural dynamics and human intentions. Although invasive, this method yields both spatial and spectral fidelity in cortical locations less than 5 mm in size. Additionally, spike-sorting algorithms can detect action potential firing of individual neurons. These source signals are referred to as "single units." The technique is however invasive and the majority of experimental data derived from it has been in animal models.

Research in non-human primates has given insight into cortical physiology and laid the foundation for neuroprosthetic applications now in clinical trial. Macaque monkey experiments especially have contributed to current understanding of motor system electrophysiology and movement encoding. The evolution of these insights clarified that neural signals associated with intention of movement could be decoded. Beyond the ability to infer intentions from neuronal activity about endogenous limb movement, these signals can be transposed to control a robotic limb in substitution. Various research teams have shown macaque monkeys performing real-time control of robotic arms via electrode arrays implanted in the motor cortex. Several experiments have shown complex levels of control in which a monkey had sufficient dexterous robotic control to enable him to feed himself. More recently, this experience has been translated to early clinical trials in humans. (▸ Fig. 39.3a) Similar to the monkey experience, the control has been steadily increasing in complexity and capability such that humans have been able to perform simple levels of self-care.

Despite the clinical trials demonstrating exciting proof of concept in functionality, true clinical feasibility of these constructs remains a concern. Chronic recording with intra parenchymal cortical electrodes is hampered by the body's immunologic response to the presence of a foreign object in the brain. Implantation of depth electrodes initiates a process of gliosis causing scarring at the electrode interface. With time, this gliosis process insulates the electrode, limiting its recording ability, and impairs its ability to acquire neuronal signals. Research into different materials and electrode form factors is ongoing to reduce or eliminate the gliosis process from inhibiting electrode function. Despite some of the innovative novel approaches, the durability of recording remains an important hurdle to be solved before clinical grade neuroprosthetics can use intraparenchymal electrodes.

39.6 Peripheral Neuroprosthetics

Peripheral neuroprosthetic applications use remaining functional axons in peripheral nerves for device interface and restoration of function. Current techniques of peripheral nerve surgery have seen successful nerve transplant and reanimation procedures, particularly after trauma. These procedures rely on the innate ability of nerve repair and reintegration at the neuromuscular junction. Peripheral neuroprosthetics extend the concept of nerve transfer toward connection, not with a new body part, but rather a new interface with devices for functional restoration.

The peripheral nervous system offers several advantages for neural-interfacing. In general, a peripheral nerve is more easily exposed with less surgical risk, it maintains a consistent architecture, and provides direct access to both sensory and motor function. However, directly interfacing peripheral nerves to an external device also has distinct engineering and biological issues that need to be addressed for clinical application. These interfaces may be intraneural, extraneural, or may indirectly interface with the nervous system via monitoring muscle fiber activity. Nerve-based approaches are particularly advantageous for limb prosthesis control in patients who are otherwise neurologically intact.

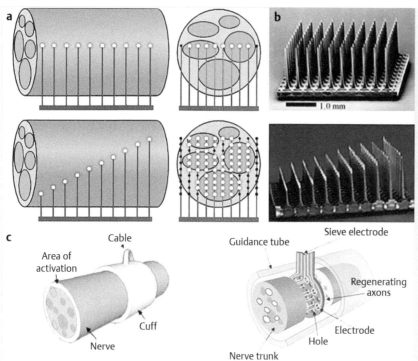

Fig. 39.4 Peripheral Electrodes. Peripheral Electrodes: **(a)** Cartoon illustrating the interface between the Utah electrode array (UEA) and Utah slanted electrode array (USEA) with a peripheral nerve in longitudinal and transverse section (left and right, respectively). **(b)** Scanning electron micrograph of the UEA and USEA (top and bottom, respectively). **(c)** Cartoon illustrating the interface between prototypical cuff and sieve peripheral nerve electrodes (left and right, respectively). The area of electrical interface is highlighted in white. (Adapted from Branner 2001 and Normann 2007)

Intra neural designs integrate a conducting electrode into the individual axons of the nerve. They have the advantage of highly selective motor activation and sensory recording. These types of electrode arrays include those developed by the University of Michigan and University of Utah. Both devices employ penetrating electrodes that interface with axons within the nerve. The Utah Slanted Electrode Array (USEA) was developed alongside the Utah Electrode Array (UEA), which is commonly used for cortical intra parenchymal recordings. The USEA uses a similar 10 X 10 electrode array configuration however, whereas the UEA electrodes have a constant length of 1.5 mm corresponding to the target depth of the cerebral cortex. The USEA is modified such that electrode lengths step along a gradient from 0.5 to 1.5 mm (▶ Fig. 39.4a, b). This design ensures uniform sampling when implanted in a peripheral nerve (▶ Fig. 39.4c). Because of the penetrating nature of the electrodes, the USEA are subject to fibrosis and signal degradation (much like their intra cerebral correlates). An alternative intra neural design is the sieve, or regenerative, electrode. The sieve electrode provides a stable, high specificity interface without the long-term signal decay seen with penetrating electrodes. Sieve electrodes rely upon nerve regeneration through small holes circumscribed by thin metal ring contacts. However, unlike penetrating electrodes arrays, the sieve electrode requires transection of the nerve for electrode positioning in the nerve's cross section so that regenerating axons grow through the device to achieve a stable interface (▶ Fig. 39.4c).

Extra neural designs do not penetrate individual nerve fascicles. They wrap the conducting material around the surface epineurium (▶ Fig. 39.4c). This class of electrodes is best known to neurosurgeons with the use of vagal nerve stimulation for epilepsy treatment. While less invasive, there is a concomitant the loss of fascicle selectivity. Prior studies have shown cuff electrodes are suboptimal for the selective sub-fascicular stimulation that is needed to achieve fine motor control. This approach is better suited for stimulation of the whole nerve. Extra neural electrodes may be extra fascicular with various means of making contact with the epineurium, or inter fascicular by penetrating the epineurium and placing contacts between the fascicles of a nerve. Examples of extra neural peripheral nerve electrodes include the button, book, helical, cuff, flat-interface nerve electrodes (FINE), and slowly penetrating inter fascicular nerve electrodes. The disadvantages of these designs include compression injury, ischemia, and poor contact.

Electromyography (EMG) is an alternate approach that is not technically a neural interface, but rather uses a signal to approximate neural intentions. This has also been used as a means for peripheral interfacing in restorative applications. Instead of directly accessing the nervous system with neural electrodes, the downstream effects of neural input to the musculoskeletal system are monitored by EMG. The EMG then becomes the source signal for device control. Examples of such control include the monitoring of volitional control of proximal muscle groups that are not neurologically impaired (e.g. the pectoralis muscle) then using signals from the monitored EMG activity to re animate distally paretic muscles groups. Thus, less functionally relevant motor activations such as a shoulder shrug may be used to restore clinically impactful actions such as elbow flexion, hand grasp, or to directly control a robotic prosthesis.

39.7 Somatosensory

The counterpart to the motor output neuroprosthesis is a somatosensory input prosthesis. Accurate control of the dynamic limb motion requires real-time visual, tactile or proprioceptive feedback. Grading of force application requires the perception of pressure. With limb amputation, peripheral nerves proximal to the injury site often are viable for direct interface. In order to achieve a peripheral interface, however, the central nervous system must be intact to process sensory input. This is often not the case in spinal cord or brain stem injury.

With higher cervical spinal cord injury, an interface with the somatic sensory cortex of the post-central gyrus is needed to provide appropriate feedback. Electrical stimulation of somatosensory cortex has been able to induce perceptions in experimental primate models. Cortical stimulation for sensory feedback has been difficult to achieve in humans because of the complex cellular architecture of the primary sensory area of the post-central gyrus and the even more difficult to access adjacent sulcus. The cause is the particular arrangement of the sensory homunculus of the post-central gyrus and the Brodmann areas along the orthogonal axis.

In the peripheral nervous system, sensation can be more readily segregated. After initial efforts showed reliable sensory perception from direct stimulation of peripheral nerves, other groups have tried to develop a bidirectional neuroprosthesis. Raspopovic et al. attached an intra fascicular electrode interface to the median and ulnar nerves to restore sensory feedback in an individual with an upper extremity traumatic amputation that had occurred ten years earlier. Motor control was achieved by translating surface EMG from more proximal muscles with which the subject had previously achieved good success. After titrating electrical stimuli through the full range of perception, from light touch to pain, these measurements were then applied to pressure recordings from the attached neuroprosthetic device. Training allowed the user in time to accurately control the motor movements of a robotic arm by modulating EMG signals and by the sensory feedback from mechanical touch sensors whose signals were transformed to electrical stimuli via intrafascicular nerve electrodes. Real-time bidirectional closed loop control was thereby possible.

39.8 Conclusion

Currently the field of neuroprosthetics is transitioning from laboratory demonstration to early clinical studies. As our insights into how neurons and neuronal populations encode human intention and perception evolve, there will be new methods to interface with the human nervous system. This evolution of technical and clinical capability will involve a convergence across the fields of neuroscience, engineering, computer science, and neurosurgery. As clinical applications develop, neurosurgeons should learn the principles that guide their creation and operation. It is a dynamic time for neural engineering; one in which neurosurgeons will need to contribute. The future holds promise from these new therapeutics options. For those patients especially who have suffered the devastating neurologic injury of degenerative central nervous system disease or limb amputation there is great hope.

Suggested Readings

[1] Vidal JJ. Toward direct brain-computer communication. Annu Rev Biophys Bioeng. 1973; 2(1):157–180

[2] Vidal JJ. Real-time detection of brain events in EEG. Proc IEEE. 1977; 65(5): 633–641

[3] Nunez PL, Srinivasan R. Electric Fields of the Brain: The Neurophysics of EEG. 2nd ed. Oxford University Press; 2005

[4] Schomer DL, Silva FLd. Niedermeyer's Electroencephalography: Basic Principles, Clinical Applications, and Related Fields. Lippincott Williams & Wilkins; 2012

[5] Crone NE, Miglioretti DL, Gordon B, et al. Functional mapping of human sensorimotor cortex with electrocorticographic spectral analysis. I. Alpha and beta event-related desynchronization. Brain. 1998; 121(Pt 12):2271–2299

[6] Buzsaki G. Rhythms of the Brain. Oxford University Press; 2011

[7] Wolpaw JR, McFarland DJ, Neat GW, Forneris CA. An EEG-based brain-computer interface for cursor control. Electroencephalogr Clin Neurophysiol. 1991; 78(3):252–259

[8] Pfurtscheller G, Brunner C, Schlögl A, Lopes da Silva FH. Mu rhythm (de)synchronization and EEG single-trial classification of different motor imagery tasks. Neuroimage. 2006; 31(1):153–159

[9] Beisteiner R, Höllinger P, Lindinger G, Lang W, Berthoz A. Mental representations of movements. Brain potentials associated with imagination of hand movements. Electroencephalogr Clin Neurophysiol/Evoked Potentials Section. 1995; 96(2):183–193

[10] Hochberg LR, Serruya MD, Friehs GM, et al. Neuronal ensemble control of prosthetic devices by a human with tetraplegia. Nature. 2006; 442(7099): 164–171

[11] Collinger JL, Wodlinger B, Downey JE, et al. High-performance neuroprosthetic control by an individual with tetraplegia. Lancet. 2013; 381(9866): 557–564

[12] Leuthardt EC, Schalk G, Moran D, Ojemann JG. The emerging world of motor neuroprosthetics: a neurosurgical perspective. Neurosurgery. 2006; 59(1):1–14, discussion 1–14

[13] Ritaccio A, Brunner P, Crone NE, et al. Proceedings of the Fourth International Workshop on Advances in Electrocorticography. Epilepsy Behav. 2013; 29(2): 259–268

[14] Penfield W. Pitfalls and success in surgical treatment of focal epilepsy. BMJ. 1958; 1(5072):669–672

[15] Leuthardt EC, Schalk G, Wolpaw JR, Ojemann JG, Moran DW. A brain-computer interface using electrocorticographic signals in humans. J Neural Eng. 2004; 1(2):63–71

[16] Leuthardt EC, Miller KJ, Schalk G, Rao RPN, Ojemann JG. Electrocorticography-based brain computer Interface-the seattle experience. IEEE Trans Neural Syst Rehabil Eng. 2006; 14(2):194–198

[17] Schalk G, Miller KJ, Anderson NR, et al. Two-dimensional movement control using electrocorticographic signals in humans. J Neural Eng. 2008; 5(1):75–84

[18] Sanchez JC, Gunduz A, Carney PR, Principe JC. Extraction and localization of mesoscopic motor control signals for human ECoG neuroprosthetics. J Neurosci Methods. 2008; 167(1):63–81

[19] Scherer R, Zanos SP, Miller KJ, Rao RPN, Ojemann JG. Classification of contralateral and ipsilateral finger movements for electrocorticographic brain-computer interfaces. Neurosurg Focus. 2009; 27(1):E12

[20] Kubánek J, Miller KJ, Ojemann JG, Wolpaw JR, Schalk G. Decoding flexion of individual fingers using electrocorticographic signals in humans. J Neural Eng. 2009; 6(6):066001

[21] Wang W, Collinger JL, Degenhart AD, et al. An electrocorticographic brain interface in an individual with tetraplegia. PLoS One. 2013; 8(2):e55344

[22] Breshears JD, Gaona CM, Roland JL, et al. Decoding motor signals from the pediatric cortex: implications for brain-computer interfaces in children. Pediatrics. 2011; 128(1):e160–e168

[23] Roland J, Miller K, Freudenburg Z, et al. The effect of age on human motor electrocorticographic signals and implications for brain-computer interface applications. J Neural Eng. 2011; 8(4):046013

[24] Leuthardt EC, Schalk G, Roland J, Rouse A, Moran DW. Evolution of brain-computer interfaces: going beyond classic motor physiology. Neurosurg Focus. 2009; 27(1):E4

[25] Leuthardt EC, Gaona C, Sharma M, et al. Using the electrocorticographic speech network to control a brain-computer interface in humans. J Neural Eng. 2011; 8(3):036004

[26] Freeman WJ, Holmes MD, Burke BC, Vanhatalo S. Spatial spectra of scalp EEG and EMG from awake humans. Clin Neurophysiol. 2003; 114(6):1053–1068

[27] Miller KJ, Sorensen LB, Ojemann JG, den Nijs M. Power-law scaling in the brain surface electric potential. PLOS Comput Biol. 2009; 5(12):e1000609

[28] Wilson JA, Felton EA, Garell PC, Schalk G, Williams JC. ECoG factors underlying multimodal control of a brain-computer interface. IEEE Trans Neural Syst Rehabil Eng. 2006; 14(2):246–250

[29] Pei X, Leuthardt EC, Gaona CM, Brunner P, Wolpaw JR, Schalk G. Spatiotemporal dynamics of electrocorticographic high gamma activity during overt and covert word repetition. Neuroimage. 2011; 54(4):2960–2972

[30] Pei X, Barbour DL, Leuthardt EC, Schalk G. Decoding vowels and consonants in spoken and imagined words using electrocorticographic signals in humans. J Neural Eng. 2011; 8(4):046028

[31] Ikeda S, Shibata T, Nakano N, et al. Neural decoding of single vowels during covert articulation using electrocorticography. Front Hum Neurosci. 2014; 8: 125

[32] Mugler EM, Patton JL, Flint RD, et al. Direct classification of all American English phonemes using signals from functional speech motor cortex. J Neural Eng. 2014; 11(3):035015

[33] Ramsey NF, van de Heuvel MP, Kho KH, Leijten FSS. Towards human BCI applications based on cognitive brain systems: an investigation of neural signals recorded from the dorsolateral prefrontal cortex. IEEE Trans Neural Syst Rehabil Eng. 2006; 14(2):214–217

[34] Gaona CM, Sharma M, Freudenburg ZV, et al. Nonuniform high-gamma (60–500 Hz) power changes dissociate cognitive task and anatomy in human cortex. J Neurosci. 2011; 31(6):2091–2100

[35] Wang W, Degenhart AD, Collinger JL, et al. Human motor cortical activity recorded with Micro-ECoG electrodes, during individual finger movements. Paper presented at: Engineering in Medicine and Biology Society, 2009. EMBC 2009. Annual International Conference of the IEEE; 3–6 Sept. 2009, 2009

[36] Leuthardt EC, Freudenberg Z, Bundy D, Roland J. Microscale recording from human motor cortex: implications for minimally invasive electrocorticographic brain-computer interfaces. Neurosurg Focus. 2009; 27(1):E10

[37] Vansteensel MJ, Pels EGM, Bleichner MG, et al. Fully Implanted Brain-Computer Interface in a Locked-In Patient with ALS. N Engl J Med. 2016; 375(21): 2060–2066

[38] Schalk G, Kubánek J, Miller KJ, et al. Decoding two-dimensional movement trajectories using electrocorticographic signals in humans. J Neural Eng. 2007; 4(3):264–275

[39] Anderson NR, Blakely T, Schalk G, Leuthardt EC, Moran DW. Electrocorticographic (ECoG) correlates of human arm movements. Exp Brain Res. 2012; 223(1):1–10

[40] Moran DW, Schwartz AB. Motor cortical representation of speed and direction during reaching. J Neurophysiol. 1999; 82(5):2676–2692

[41] Georgopoulos AP, Schwartz AB, Kettner RE. Neuronal population coding of movement direction. Science. 1986; 233(4771):1416–1419

[42] Schwartz AB. Direct cortical representation of drawing. Science. 1994; 265 (5171):540–542

[43] Heldman DA, Wang W, Chan SS, Moran DW. Local field potential spectral tuning in motor cortex during reaching. IEEE Trans Neural Syst Rehabil Eng. 2006; 14(2):180–183

[44] Georgopoulos AP, Kalaska JF, Caminiti R, Massey JT. On the relations between the direction of two-dimensional arm movements and cell discharge in primate motor cortex. J Neurosci. 1982; 2(11):1527–1537

[45] Wessberg J, Stambaugh CR, Kralik JD, et al. Real-time prediction of hand trajectory by ensembles of cortical neurons in primates. Nature. 2000; 408 (6810):361–365

[46] Taylor DM, Tillery SIH, Schwartz AB. Direct cortical control of 3D neuroprosthetic devices. Science. 2002; 296(5574):1829–1832

[47] Chapin JK, Moxon KA, Markowitz RS, Nicolelis MAL. Real-time control of a robot arm using simultaneously recorded neurons in the motor cortex. Nat Neurosci. 1999; 2(7):664–670

[48] Velliste M, Perel S, Spalding MC, Whitford AS, Schwartz AB. Cortical control of a prosthetic arm for self-feeding. Nature. 2008; 453(7198):1098–1101

[49] Hochberg LR, Bacher D, Jarosiewicz B, et al. Reach and grasp by people with tetraplegia using a neurally controlled robotic arm. Nature. 2012; 485(7398): 372–375

[50] Suner S, Fellows MR, Vargas-Irwin C, Nakata GK, Donoghue JP. Reliability of signals from a chronically implanted, silicon-based electrode array in non-human primate primary motor cortex. IEEE Trans Neural Syst Rehabil Eng. 2005; 13(4):524–541

[51] Ryu SI, Shenoy KV. Human cortical prostheses: lost in translation? Neurosurg Focus. 2009; 27(1):E5

[52] Polikov VS, Tresco PA, Reichert WM. Response of brain tissue to chronically implanted neural electrodes. J Neurosci Methods. 2005; 148 (1):1–18

[53] Viventi J, Kim D-H, Vigeland L, et al. Flexible, foldable, actively multiplexed, high-density electrode array for mapping brain activity in vivo. Nat Neurosci. 2011; 14(12):1599–1605

[54] Kellis SS, House PA, Thomson KE, Brown R, Greger B. Human neocortical electrical activity recorded on nonpenetrating microwire arrays: applicability for neuroprostheses. Neurosurg Focus. 2009; 27(1):E9

[55] Griffith RW, Humphrey DR. Long-term gliosis around chronically implanted platinum electrodes in the Rhesus macaque motor cortex. Neurosci Lett. 2006; 406(1–2):81–86

[56] Stieglitz T, Gross M. Flexible BIOMEMS with electrode arrangements on front and back side as key component in neural prostheses and biohybrid systems. Sens Actuators B Chem. 2002; 83(1–3):8–14

[57] Kozai TDY, Langhals NB, Patel PR, et al. Ultrasmall implantable composite microelectrodes with bioactive surfaces for chronic neural interfaces. Nat Mater. 2012; 11(12):1065–1073

[58] Lewitus DY, Smith KL, Landers J, Neimark AV, Kohn J. Bioactive agarose carbon-nanotube composites are capable of manipulating brain-implant interface. J Appl Polym Sci. 2014; 131(14):n/a–n/a

[59] Seymour JP, Kipke DR. Neural probe design for reduced tissue encapsulation in CNS. Biomaterials. 2007; 28(25):3594–3607

[60] Clark GA, Ledbetter NM, Warren DJ, Harrison RR. Recording sensory and motor information from peripheral nerves with Utah Slanted Electrode Arrays. Paper presented at: Engineering in Medicine and Biology Society, EMBC, 2011 Annual International Conference of the IEEE; Aug. 30 2011-Sept. 3 2011, 2011

[61] Branner A, Stein RB, Normann RA. Selective stimulation of cat sciatic nerve using an array of varying-length microelectrodes. J Neurophysiol. 2001; 85 (4):1585–1594

[62] Normann RA. Technology insight: future neuroprosthetic therapies for disorders of the nervous system. Nat Clin Pract Neurol. 2007; 3(8): 444–452

[63] Ledbetter NM, Ethier C, Oby ER, et al. Intrafascicular stimulation of monkey arm nerves evokes coordinated grasp and sensory responses. J Neurophysiol. 2013; 109(2):580–590

[64] Navarro X, Krueger TB, Lago N, Micera S, Stieglitz T, Dario P. A critical review of interfaces with the peripheral nervous system for the control of neuroprostheses and hybrid bionic systems. J Peripher Nerv Syst. 2005; 10(3):229–258

[65] Hincapie JG, Kirsch RF. EMG-based Control for a C5/C6 Spinal Cord Injury Upper Extremity Neuroprosthesis. Paper presented at: Engineering in Medicine and Biology Society, 2007. EMBS 2007. 29th Annual International Conference of the IEEE; 22–26 Aug. 2007, 2007

[66] Kuiken TA, Miller LA, Lipschutz RD, et al. Targeted reinnervation for enhanced prosthetic arm function in a woman with a proximal amputation: a case study. Lancet. 2007; 369(9559):371–380

[67] Romo R, Hernández A, Zainos A, Salinas E. Somatosensory discrimination based on cortical microstimulation. Nature. 1998; 392(6674):387–390

[68] Konrad P, Shanks T. Implantable brain computer interface: challenges to neurotechnology translation. Neurobiol Dis. 2010; 38(3):369–375

[69] Dhillon GS, Krüger TB, Sandhu JS, Horch KW. Effects of short-term training on sensory and motor function in severed nerves of long-term human amputees. J Neurophysiol. 2005; 93(5):2625–2633

[70] Raspopovic S, Capogrosso M, Petrini FM, et al. Restoring natural sensory feedback in real-time bidirectional hand prostheses. Sci Transl Med. 2014; 6 (222):222ra19

40 Exoskeletons

Hamid Shah, Dario Englot and Peter Konrad

Abstract

Spinal injury is a devastating event which currently has limited therapies. In the absence of restorative therapies, modalities to mimic motor function have been developed. These not only allow for independent motility, but can also provide much needed exercise. Exoskeletons are an example of this and heterogenous in their function. Broadly, they can be either active or passive. The simplest is external bracing and crutches in order to remain in an upright posture. More sophisticated units include feedback sensors and gait initiation sensors. In the future, even more sophisticated models may include the ability to climb stairs as well as have more normal stepping patterns.

Keywords: exoskeletons, passive, active, spinal injury

Spinal cord injury is a debilitating event defined as a fixed neurological deficit originating in the spinal cord. There are 23 million men and women living with a spinal cord injury, and globally there are 180,000 annual new cases.[1] In 2103 this represented 273,000 Americans living with a chronic spinal cord injury with 12,000 new cases that year alone.[2] The dream of every paraplegic or quadriplegic is the recovery of locomotion, toileting and sexual function. Secondary, but also meaningful consequences of spinal cord injury, are bone density homeostasis, cardiac and pulmonary dysfunction, metabolic instability and skin breakdown. Many different exoskeleton types are in development to deal with these issues.

One hour of exercise three days a week maintains cardiovascular conditioning and decreases mortality rate by 20%.[1] For a healthy person this means a daily one-hour walk at three mph three days weekly.[3,4] The sedentary lifestyle of a spinal cord injured patient also can cause muscle atrophy and have a deleterious effect on bone mineral density and body weight. Lower extremity bone mineral density decreases 3–4% per month in the first year after spinal cord injury and patients gain an average of two kilograms each year. Two-thirds of them will become obese in time, but modest increases in activity can improve both bone mineral density and body fat composition.[3,4] Exoskeleton use can help with this if an individual is able to exercise for long enough to get the benefit.

Exoskeletons are classified as passive or active devices. The simplest ones are unpowered passive devices such as hip/knee/ankle orthoses. In the spine-injured individual, the ankle is fixed in position or spring-loaded to maintain the foot in dorsiflexion. The hip and knee have joints with limited degrees of freedom. A common configuration is flexion/extension of both the hip and knee without abduction or adduction at the hip, but these unpowered devices are difficult to use.[5] There are several reasons for this. The effort to stand requires use of the arms to maintain balance and provide forward motion, since there is limited assistance from the trunk. The legs are locked in position and swung forward to execute a step. The many elements to such movement require energy exertion that cannot be sustained long enough to confer a metabolic advantage.[1,6,7]

With training, powered exoskeletons can meaningfully reduce the effort a chronically injured individual needs to be able to walk.[1] Exoskeletons diminish spasticity and improve well-being. Powered exoskeletons are classified as fully assistive or augmentative. Augmentative skeletons make use of functional electrical stimulation (FES). FES recruits local muscles by transdermal or percutaneous stimulation. A controller elicits muscle contractions to augment exoskeleton movement. FES based systems can also help with the metabolic benefits of locomotion, but there is a significant limitation. The muscular recruitment created is coarse, and there is a recruiting preference to fast twitch muscle fibers. These fatigue rapidly.[1,5] This can be painful for patients with incomplete injuries. While muscle activation can be achieved with FES, control of the limb can be quite limited. Delivery of current may induce spasms within the muscle as well as asynchronous muscle group engagement. The asynchrony can stress joints, causing pain, or it can induce resistance to the exoskeleton gaiting. Without feedback to the controller, the limb completing the movement could be hurt. Patients with chronic spinal cord injury have reduced recruitable muscle mass and the muscle that is present is often shortened causing contracture across joints. Because of high recruitment thresholds and inefficient energy usage, FES skeletons have limited useful function in sustained weight bearing walking in paraplegics. They do not eliminate the need for crutches, nor are they able to recruit abdominal wall or erector muscles in order to stabilize the torso when walking. However, FES systems can stimulate muscle tissue and generate trophic factors. This could increase muscle bulk and volume if they are incorporated into a static training regimen (▶ Fig. 40.1).

Unassisted powered exoskeletons are subdivided into the type of feedback system present. While all powered systems have some feedback system, an EMG sensing system is unique. It gets feedback from the wearer giving him volitional control to the gait.[5,6] Triggering of the EMG sensing system produces a preprogrammed gait response. For this to happen, some volitional control of the muscle group is needed to trigger the cycle. A potential shortcoming of this sort of system would be inappropriate generation of a gait cycle from a spontaneous EMG stimulus. This could arise from chronic muscle denervation or spasm. These EMG sensing systems could help chronically deconditioned but uninjured elderly users who are unable to walk for meaningful distances. This could improve the quality of their lives and maintain their independence. Unassisted powered exoskeletons have feedback systems that can initiate a gait cycle using simple gesturing. The most intuitive is one that actuates when the user leans to the side desired in order to start a gaiting cycle. Regardless of the type of powered system, the majority of units also require upper extremity involvement to maintain an upright posture. The REX bionics exoskeleton is a stand-alone unit in production that will do this, but it is not FDA approved in the United States. The unit uses hand control gesturing to initiate a gait cycle. There are three exoskeletons that are FDA approved. These are the ReWalk exoskeleton, Ekso GT and Parker Indego.

Of importance in any exoskeleton is its controller. This device determines the degrees of freedom (DOF) conferred on each active and passive joint. The hip is usually allowed passive rotation and the ankle is allowed passive dorsiflexion and plantar

Exoskeleton	Bionic Leg	Ekso	HAL	Indego	Kinesis	ReWalk	WalkTrainer	WPAL
Degrees of freedom	K	HKA	HKA	HK	KA	HKA	HaHKA	HKA
Weight-bearing devices	W	C	W/C/S	W/C	W/C	C	S	W/B
Sensor measurements	JA, JT, FF	AJA, ACF, FF, Acc/Ori (arm)	EMG, JA, FF, Acc	JA, Acc, Ori	JA, FF, IT, Ori	JA, FF, Ori	IT, JA	JA, JT
Device weight (kg)	3.6	20	15	12	9.2	23	?	13
User height (cm) limit	153–182	158–188	145–185	155–191	< 1.85	160–190	?	145–180
User weight (kg) limit	136	100	80	113	90	100	?	80
Gait initiation mode	Foot sensors and knee extension	1. Body tilt 2. Button push	Knee EMG activation	Body tilt	Button push	Body tilt	?	Button push
Unique features	Unilateral	—	—	—	Hybrid (FES)	—	Hybrid (FES), active bodyweight support suspension harness moves with exoskeleton	Frame fits between legs, easy to don within wheelchair
ClinicalTrials.gov registration		NCT02324322 NCT02132702 NCT02065830				NCT01943669 NCT02118194 NCT02104622 NCT01251549 NCT00627107 NCT01454570		

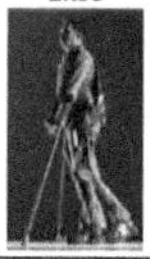

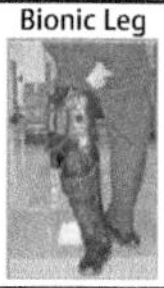

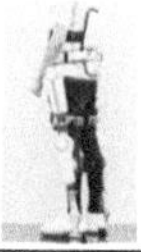

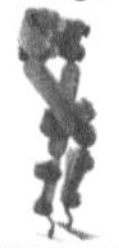

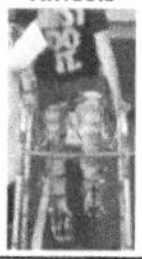

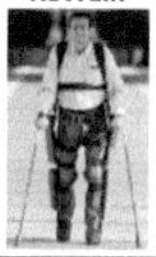

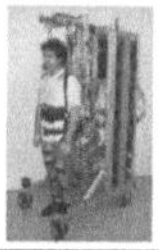

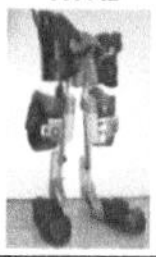

Note: Degrees of freedom: (Bilateral) Ha, hip ab/adduction; HR, hip medial/lateral rotation; H, hip (sagittal); K, knee (sagittal); A, ankle (sagittal); Av, ankle in/eversion, underline-passive.
Weight-bearing devices: C, crutches; W, walker; B, parallel safety bars; S, suspension harness.
Sensor measurements: EMG, electromyography; JA, joint angle; AJA, arm joint angle; ACF, arm crutches force; IT, interaction torque; JT, joint torque; FF, foot contacting force/pressure; Acc, acceleration; Ori, orientation.

Fig. 40.1 Summary of powered exoskeletons for individuals with SCI.
Used with permission from Contreraras-Vidal JL. Powered exoskeletons for bipedal locomotion after spinal cord injury. J Neural Eng. 2016 Jun;13 (3):031001.[8]

flexion.[7] Included in the software design is a gait cycle program that is either generated from the recorded gaits of uninjured wearers or extrapolated from a gait atlas.[7] The latter produces a more natural joint trajectory. An easier to implement and simpler gait program is a direct trajectory program based on a reference gait. Such a program can be difficult to implement since the joint trajectories tend not be natural. Also included in some controller functions are programmed positions for sitting and standing. Exoskeleton stair climbing has not yet been implemented in commercially available models. In the future, this along with slip detection and correction using a closed loop system are all desired goals.

References

[1] Miller LE, Zimmermann AK, Herbert WG. Clinical effectiveness and safety of powered exoskeleton-assisted walking in patients with spinal cord injury: systematic review with meta-analysis. Med Devices (Auckl). 2016; 9:455–466

[2] Lajeunesse V, Vincent C, Routhier F, Careau E, Michaud F. Exoskeletons' design and usefulness evidence according to a systematic review of lower limb exoskeletons used for functional mobility by people with spinal cord injury. Disabil Rehabil Assist Technol. 2016; 11(7):535–547

[3] Karelis AD, Carvalho LP, Castillo MJ, Gagnon DH, Aubertin-Leheudre M. Effect on body composition and bone mineral density of walking with a robotic exoskeleton in adults with chronic spinal cord injury. J Rehabil Med. 2017; 49 (1):84–87

[4] Miller LE, Herbert WG. Health and economic benefits of physical activity for patients with spinal cord injury. Clinicoecon Outcomes Res. 2016; 8:551–558. eCollection 2016

[5] Arazpour M, Samadian M, Bahramizadeh M, et al. The efficiency of orthotic interventions on energy consumption in paraplegic patients: a literature review. Spinal Cord. 2015

[6] Ha KH, Murray SA, Goldfarb M. An Approach for the Cooperative Control of FES With a Powered Exoskeleton During Level Walking for Persons With Paraplegia. IEEE Trans Neural Syst Rehabil Eng. 2016; 24(4):455–466

[7] Yan T, Cempini M, Oddo CM, Vitiello N. Review of assistive strategies in powered lower-limb orthoses and exoskeletons. Robot Auton Syst. 2015; 64:120–136

[8] Contreras-Vidal JL, A Bhagat N, Brantley J, et al. Powered exoskeletons for bipedal locomotion after spinal cord injury. J Neural Eng. 2016; 13(3):031001

41 Visual Prostheses

Jeffrey V. Rosenfeld and Yan Wong

Abstract

The field of electrical implants for vision restoration in the blind is rapidly advancing, though there are many blind individuals who will not be suitable for retinal electrical prostheses. The lateral geniculate nucleus and visual cortex are alternate implantation sites which bypass the retina and optic nerves. Neurosurgeons are involved in the development and implantation of bionic vision prostheses to these sites. This chapter describes how these prostheses are being designed and applied with a focus on cortical vision prostheses.

Keywords: bionic vision devices, brain computer interface, blindness, cortical implants, neuromodulation

41.1 Introduction

Electrical stimulation of the visual pathways partially restores visual function by generating phosphenes (spots of light). The aim of a bionic vision device is to create reproducible and rapidly changing patterns of phosphenes in the visual field to enable the blind person to regain sufficient vision to improve their daily activities. These activities include object recognition and safe, reliable navigation. Facial recognition is the ultimate goal. Blind individuals use their remaining senses very effectively to undertake daily activities. Visual prostheses complement these skills. Potential targets in the central nervous system for electrical stimulation to restore vision are the retina, optic nerve, lateral geniculate nucleus (LGN), and the visual cortex.

In blind individuals with retinal or optic-nerve degeneration, an approach bypassing the proximal visual pathways is required. For these patients, neurosurgeons are able to surgically access the LGN and the visual cortex. The last human trial of an implantable cortical vision prosthesis was in the year 2000.[1,2,3] Since then, there have been significant technological advances in micro-electronics, electrodes, wireless power, data transmission and human studies demonstrating that electrical stimulation of the visual cortex produces highly localized phosphenes.[4]

41.2 Sites in the Central Nervous System for Implantation of Visual Prostheses (See ▶ Table 41.1)

The retina: When photoreceptor cells are lost through inherited disease such as retinitis pigmentosa (RP), light no longer stimulates the retina and the individual becomes blind. Electrical stimulation of the residual neural components of the retina (amacrine and ganglion cells) produces phosphenes,[5] There are epiretinal, subretinal and suprachoroidal devices. Placing electrode arrays on or near to the retina provides access to a large visual field, avoids cranial surgery and allows unilateral device design. Use of such devices for severe macular degeneration is being investigated.

Optic nerve: Electrodes can be placed as a cuff on the surface of the optic nerve or, with penetrating electrodes, in the optic nerve head or the optic nerve. However, electrodes placed on the dural surface require higher currents and the spatial resolution is inferior compared with penetrating electrodes. Patients with RP could be trained to achieve some pattern recognition, shape orientation, object localization.[6,7] The indications for optic nerve electrode implantation are the same as for retinal implants. The surgical approaches to the optic nerve are by craniotomy or an intraorbital approach.[8]

Lateral geniculate nucleus (LGN): The LGN is a small nucleus (about 250-mm^3 volume and up to 10-mm long) located in the posterior/inferior part of the thalamus. The central 10 degrees of vision occupies the posterior half of the nucleus. The LGN has six layers of neurons in humans and is suitable for multi-electrode stimulation because it has retinotopic representation. The LGN remains intact after the retinas and optic nerves have lost function and this widens the number of possible indications (see ▶ Table 41.1).[9,10] The LGN could also potentially be used as a stimulation target if the visual cortices have been injured or lost (cortical blindness).

Pezaris and Eskander described their concept of a microelectrode bundle splaying out from the end of the electrode sheath into the LGN and with electrodes spaced 1 mm apart in 3 dimensions, 250 electrodes for each hemisphere could be placed on each side giving a total of 500 electrodes. Brush-like electrodes with 8 contacts have been inserted in the monkey LGN for stimulation experiments.[10] The stereotactic techniques required to place electrodes precisely in the LGN are similar to those used to place deep brain stimulation electrodes Parkinson's disease and other movement disorders.[9] Once placed, these electrodes would be stable in position. A subcutaneous lead connecting to a subclavicular or cranial stimulator is planned for the human device.[9]

Visual cortex: Electrical stimulation of the human visual cortex to restore vision in blind individuals has been evolving since the 1950s when electrodes were implanted on the surface of the visual cortex of a blind subject.[3,11,12] This allowed subjects to perceive phosphenes, identify shapes, navigate the environment, and to read Braille. These electrodes were

Table 41.1 Target causes of blindness for retinal and cortical implants

Cause of blindness	Retinal Implant	Cortical/LGN Implant
Glaucoma		x
Diabetic Retinopathy		x
Bilateral traumatic vision loss		x
Large pituitary/parasellar tumors		x
Eye tumors (e.g. bilateral retinoblastoma)		x
Optic atrophy/optic neuritis		x
Retinitis Pigmentosa	x	x
Aged Macular Degeneration	maybe	x

implanted on the cortical surface, and since then, much work has been done in developing implants that have microelectrodes that penetrate the cortex (▶ Fig. 41.1).[1,2,3,12,13] Penetrating cortical microelectrodes (intracortical microstimulation) produce more localized phosphenes (discriminable when stimulated by electrodes 700-µm apart) at currents in the µA range.[3,14,15] This is more than a 100-fold reduction in necessary current output compared to surface stimulation and significantly lowers seizure risk.

The visual cortex is a relatively large area to place electrodes for partial restoration of central and peripheral vision compared with other potential targets. The total surface area of the primary visual cortex (V1) varies between 1400 and 6300 mm², depending on the method of estimation, with approximately 67% of that area buried along the calcarine fissure.[16,17,18] If this cortex is not included in the stimulation, an hour-glass shaped visual field results. Head scanning which places the camera at different angles will help the individual 'fill in the gaps' and create a more complete picture of the visual scene.[19] Placing electrodes within the calcarine cortex may also require varying length electrodes and different carrier designs which would be more of a challenge to develop. Placement of electrodes in secondary visual cortex may cover some of the missing visual field.[12] Finally, insertion of electrodes into the medial surface of the hemisphere covers the peripheral vision and central vision but the orientation of these electrodes would be orthogonal to a transmitting coil on the scalp and wireless data transfer would be restricted unless there is some internal wired connection of the electrode carriers.

41.3 Cortical Vision Prosthesis Design

The development of a multi-electrode vision prosthesis is complex, time consuming and expensive. A collaborative interdisciplinary team of neurosurgeons, vision physiologists, electrical and computer engineers, and materials engineers is required to develop a system that is biocompatible, reliable and safe to implant. The device architecture includes a camera, a vision processing computer, the electrode interface with the brain, the interconnecting links and a power system (▶ Fig. 41.2). A vision processor is needed to run software algorithms that convert images from a small digital camera into pixelated patterns which represent relevant shapes and contours in the environment. These patterns are then sent to the implants via a wireless link.

There are many engineering challenges for the development of cortical bionic vision devices. These include: ensuring biocompatibility of the materials, electrode coverage of an anatomically variable visual cortex, wireless transmission to the arrays on the medial cortex, preventing damage to the device due to exposure to body fluids and the immune system, maintenance of hermeticity of the device, peri-electrode gliosis with gradual

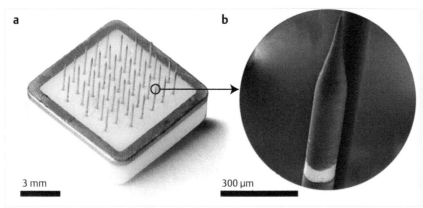

Fig. 41.1 (a) Monash Vision Group cortical vision prosthesis with the penetrating microelectrodes facing up. Electronics are hermetically encapsulated in a ceramic case (white box) with the platinum return ring return electrode surrounding the microelectrodes. The microelectrodes can be seen at a higher resolution in panel **(b)**.

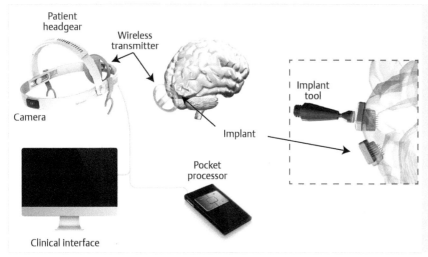

Fig. 41.2 General architecture of stimulating cortical vision prostheses. Patient's wear headgear that consists of a camera, and a wireless link that can transmit power and data to the implants. A microprocessor that patients can carry in their pocket, processes the images into the appropriate stimulation commands that are sent across the wireless link. In addition to this, most systems allow control for testing and calibration via a larger clinical interface system. Power to the implants is supplied by wireless induction. Multiple devices can be implanted into a single patient and is often achieved using a pneumatic insertor (inset).

electrode failure, electrode corrosion, and ensuring that heat generation of the electrode arrays is within safe limits.

41.4 Cortical Vision Prosthesis Operative Procedure

The patient is placed in the prone position under general anaesthesia. A unilateral occipital craniotomy passing along the edge of the sagittal and the transverse venous sinuses exposes the occipital pole and extends to the midline. The calcarine fissure and adjacent primary visual cortex are identified using frameless stereotaxy. Multi-electrode cortical arrays require an insertion tool. The Utah array insertion tool is a pneumatically controlled piston which impacts the tile pushing the electrodes through the pia (▶ Fig. 41.2, **inset**). This insertion cannot be achieved with digital pressure.

41.5 Risks of Intracranial Surgery

There is a small risk of intracranial infection and hemorrhage. There is a small risk of injury to the sagittal or transverse venous sinuses. The bone flap or synthetic material (eg.acrylic) will require contouring to avoid direct pressure on the electrodes. Pressure would result in the arrays sinking into the brain. If the active tip of the electrodes passes beyond the neurons of the grey matter and enters the white matter the electrodes will be non-functional.

Chronic focal stimulation of cerebral cortex may cause epilepsy to develop through kindling.[20,21] This will depend on the magnitude of electric currents passing through the cortex, the duration of the stimulation and the individual's threshold for seizure activation. The risk of seizures will be reduced by using very low stimulation currents, limiting temperature rise, and using intermittent stimulation of the electrodes in differing patterns and the use of prophylactic anti-epileptic drugs (AEDs).[12,22] These drugs, however, may also render the neurons less responsive (refractory) to the stimulation by the electrodes so a careful balance will have to be achieved.

41.6 Post-operative Phase

The patients will require psychophysics testing. This involves visuotopic mapping of the phosphenes and the assessments of object and shape recognition, navigational tasks, and various activities of daily living.[23,24] Individual and patterned electrode stimulation will be required. The patients will need training to use the device and then engage in daily practice sessions to optimize their performance. Psychological support should be provided throughout the rehabilitation phase and beyond.

41.7 Conclusion

Rapid advances have occurred in the development of implantable visual prostheses due to advances in computer systems, electronic micro-circuitry and wireless interfaces. The LGN and visual cortex are alternate CNS targets when the retinas and optic nerves are unavailable. Various bionic vision implants are being developed for human trial. Partial restoration of vison in blind individuals will assist them in navigation and obstacle avoidance, object recognition, and reading.

References

[1] Dobelle WH. Artificial vision for the blind by connecting a television camera to the visual cortex. ASAIO J. 2000; 46(1):3–9

[2] Schmidt EM, Bak MJ, Hambrecht FT, Kufta CV, O'Rourke DK, Vallabhanath P. Feasibility of a visual prosthesis for the blind based on intracortical microstimulation of the visual cortex. Brain. 1996; 119(Pt 2):507–522

[3] Lewis PM, Rosenfeld JV. Electrical stimulation of the brain and the development of cortical visual prostheses: An historical perspective. Brain Res. 2016; 1630:208–224

[4] Bosking WH, Sun P, Ozker M, et al. Saturation in Phosphene Size with Increasing Current Levels Delivered to Human Visual Cortex. J Neurosci. 2017; 37 (30):7188–7197

[5] Humayun MS, de Juan E , Jr, Dagnelie G. The Bionic Eye: A Quarter Century of Retinal Prosthesis Research and Development. Ophthalmology. 2016; 123 (10S) Supplement:S89–S97

[6] Brelén ME, Duret F, Gérard B, Delbeke J, Veraart C. Creating a meaningful visual perception in blind volunteers by optic nerve stimulation. J Neural Eng. 2005; 2(1):S22–S28

[7] Duret F, Brelén ME, Lambert V, Gérard B, Delbeke J, Veraart C. Object localization, discrimination, and grasping with the optic nerve visual prosthesis. Restor Neurol Neurosci. 2006; 24(1):31–40

[8] Brelén ME, De Potter P, Gersdorff M, Cosnard G, Veraart C, Delbeke J. Intraorbital implantation of a stimulating electrode for an optic nerve visual prosthesis. Case report. J Neurosurg. 2006; 104(4):593–597

[9] Pezaris JS, Eskandar EN. Getting signals into the brain: visual prosthetics through thalamic microstimulation. Neurosurg Focus. 2009; 27(1):E6

[10] Pezaris JS, Reid RC. Demonstration of artificial visual percepts generated through thalamic microstimulation. Proc Natl Acad Sci U S A. 2007; 104(18): 7670–7675

[11] Tehovnik EJ, Slocum WM, Carvey CE, Schiller PH. Phosphene induction and the generation of saccadic eye movements by striate cortex. J Neurophysiol. 2005; 93(1):1–19

[12] Lewis PM, Ackland HM, Lowery AJ, Rosenfeld JV. Restoration of vision in blind individuals using bionic devices: a review with a focus on cortical visual prostheses. Brain Res. 2015; 1595:51–73

[13] Bak M, Girvin JP, Hambrecht FT, Kufta CV, Loeb GE, Schmidt EM. Visual sensations produced by intracortical microstimulation of the human occipital cortex. Med Biol Eng Comput. 1990; 28(3):257–259

[14] Davis TS, Parker RA, House PA, et al. Spatial and temporal characteristics of V1 microstimulation during chronic implantation of a microelectrode array in a behaving macaque. J Neural Eng. 2012; 9(6):065003

[15] Lewis PM, Ayton LN, Guymer RH, et al. Advances in implantable bionic devices for blindness: a review. ANZ J Surg. 2016; 86(9):654–659

[16] Andrews TJ, Halpern SD, Purves D. Correlated size variations in human visual cortex, lateral geniculate nucleus, and optic tract. J Neurosci. 1997; 17(8): 2859–2868

[17] Stensaas SS, Eddington DK, Dobelle WH. The topography and variability of the primary visual cortex in man. J Neurosurg. 1974; 40(6):747–755

[18] Genc E, Bergmann J, Singer W, Kohler A. Surface Area of Early Visual Cortex Predicts Individual Speed of Traveling Waves During Binocular Rivalry. Cereb Cortex. 2015; 25(6):1499–508

[19] Lowery AJ, Rosenfeld JV, Lewis PM, et al. Restoration of vision using wireless cortical implants: The Monash Vision Group project. Conf Proc IEEE Eng Med Biol Soc. 2015; 2015:1041–1044

[20] Goddard GV. Development of epileptic seizures through brain stimulation at low intensity. Nature. 1967; 214(5092):1020–1021

[21] Morimoto K, Fahnestock M, Racine RJ. Kindling and status epilepticus models of epilepsy: rewiring the brain. Prog Neurobiol. 2004; 73(1):1–60

[22] Bezard E, Boraud T, Nguyen J-P, Velasco F, Keravel Y, Gross C. Cortical stimulation and epileptic seizure: a study of the potential risk in primates. Neurosurgery. 1999; 45(2):346–350

[23] Dagnelie G. Psychophysical evaluation for visual prosthesis. Annu Rev Biomed Eng. 2008; 10:339–368

[24] Chen SC, Suaning GJ, Morley JW, Lovell NH. Simulating prosthetic vision: II. Measuring functional capacity. Vision Res. 2009; 49(19):2329–2343

Index

Note: Page numbers set **bold** or *italic* indicate headings or figures, respectively.